MW01254030

Positive Nations and Communities

Cross-Cultural Advancements in Positive Psychology

Volume 6

Series Editor:

ANTONELLA DELLE FAVE
Università degli studi di Milano, Italy

Editorial Board:

The aim of the *Cross Cultural Advancements in Positive Psychology* book series is to spread a universal and culture-fair perspective on good life promotion. The series will advance a deeper understanding of the cross-cultural differences in well-being conceptualization. A deeper understanding can affect psychological theories, interventions and social policies in various domains, from health to education, from work to leisure. Books in the series will investigate such issues as enhanced mobility of people across nations, ethnic conflicts and the challenges faced by traditional communities due to the pervasive spreading of modernization trends. New instruments and models will be proposed to identify the crucial components of well-being in the process of acculturation. This series will also explore dimensions and components of happiness that are currently overlooked because happiness research is grounded in the Western tradition, and these dimensions do not belong to the Western cultural frame of mind and values.

For further volumes:
http://www.springer.com/series/8420

Helena Águeda Marujo • Luis Miguel Neto
Editors

Positive Nations and Communities

Collective, Qualitative and Cultural-Sensitive Processes in Positive Psychology

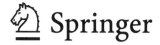 Springer

Editors
Helena Águeda Marujo
School of Social and Political
    Sciences, ISCSP
CAPP – Center for Public Policy
    and Administration
Technical University of Lisbon
Lisbon, Portugal

Luis Miguel Neto
School of Social and Political
    Sciences, ISCSP
CAPP – Center for Public Policy
    and Administration
Technical University of Lisbon
Lisbon, Portugal

ISSN 2210-5417   ISSN 2210-5425 (electronic)
ISBN 978-94-007-6868-0   ISBN 978-94-007-6869-7 (eBook)
DOI 10.1007/978-94-007-6869-7
Springer Dordrecht Heidelberg New York London

Library of Congress Control Number: 2013944062

Printed on acid-free paper

Springer is part of Springer Science+Business Media (www.springer.com)

To our loving sons, David and Thomas, who constantly expand and multiply our world views

To our dearest parents, Maria José and José Luis, Maria do Rosário e Heraldo, who birthed our daily efforts to affirm an ethical way of being

Preface

In the dark middle ages, society was seen as a God-given moral order. That view did not invite to a planned social change. In those times, earthly life was also commonly considered as a test for entrance to heaven and was not supposed to be pleasant, since God had driven man out of paradise. That view did not encourage quests for a better society either.

These views changed in the eighteenth century during the European Enlightenment. Society came to be seen as a product of human making that could be changed. Happiness came to be seen as something possible in earthly life and even desirable. These new perspectives gave rise to a widespread call for social change, which materialized in the late eighteenth century from the French revolution, in the nineteenth century through the development of political ideologies, such as liberalism and socialism, and within experiments in new societies such as the "Walden" commune. In the twentieth century, it materialized in "social engineering" by the state, which resulted in the development of "the welfare states."

This quest for a better society instigated much discussion about what a good society is like. Social philosophers, such as Karl Marx, dominated that discussion for long. As social philosophers were moral philosophers in the first place, they emphasized how a good society *should* be. For instance, they were more interested in questioning how much equality ought to be desirable in society, rather than in how livable societies actually should be. This later question was addressed by the empirical social sciences, which emerged in the second half of the twentieth century. Sociologists were the first to contribute to the discussion about the good society on the basis of fact. They started assessing actual progress on the way to a better society, in areas such as the reduction of poverty. This strand is called "Social Indicators Research" and now it is part of a wider strand of research into "quality of life." Empirical researchers have also looked for optimal combinations of desired societal characteristics and question, for instance, what degree of social inequality is functional for economic growth. This is one of the issues in the new field of "Happiness Economics."

Although psychology is, in the first place, about individual mental functioning, psychologists have not been prominent in the discussion about the good society.

So far, psychologists have mainly dealt with societal determinants of mental health, sometimes considering the context of cross-cultural psychology. Curiously, even social psychologists have remained marginal in the discussion about the good society. Nevertheless, interest in this matter is growing among psychologists. A first manifestation is the stream of "critical psychology," which emerged in the 1960s and, more recently, the development in the rise of "positive psychology" since 2000. Though the focus of positive psychology is also on individual quality of life, it also keeps an open eye for the social conditions for a good life.

Social experiments in the past have showed that realization of societal ideals might be achieved at the cost of individual happiness. Hence, one of the challenges is to find out which forms of social organization provide the best setting for human thriving. In this context, the input from psychology and in particular from positive psychology is most welcomed. This book provides such input. It is the first, of hopefully many more books, on Positive Nations.

Emeritus professor of Social Conditions for Human Happiness   *Ruut Veenhoven*
Erasmus University Rotterdam in the Netherlands
and North-West University in South Africa

Contents

Contributors

Helena Águeda Marujo School of Social and Political Sciences, ISCSP, CAPP – Center for Public Policy and Administration, Technical University of Lisbon, Lisbon, Portugal

Telmo Ferreira Alves School of Social and Political Sciences, ISCSP, CAPP – Center for Public Policy and Administration, Technical University of Lisbon, Lisbon, Portugal

George W. Burns Adjunct Professor of Psychology, Cairnmillar Institute, Melbourne, Australia

Milton H. Erickson Institute of Western Australia, Darlington, WA, Australia

Annie Chai Psychology Department and the United Nations International Council of Psychologists, Pace University, New York, NY, USA

Patrícia Jardim Da Palma School of Social and Political Sciences, ISCSP, CAPP – Center for Public Policy and Administration, Technical University of Lisbon, Lisbon, Portugal

Robert Enright Department of Educational Psychology, University of Wisconsin-Madison 859 Education Sciences, Madison, WI, USA

Antonella Delle Fave Department of Pathophysiology and Transplantation, University of Milano, Milan, Italy

Fabian Gander Department of Psychology, University of Zurich, Zurich, Switzerland

Anjali Jain Department of Humanities and Social Sciences, Indian Institute of Technology, Delhi, India

Christopher J. Kinman Executive Director, Rhizome Productions, The Rhizome Way, Vancouver, BC, Canada

Silvia Koller Department of Psychology, Federal University of Rio Grande do Sul, Institute of Psychology, Porto Alegre, Brazil

Miguel Pereira Lopes School of Social and Political Sciences, ISCSP, CAPP – Center for Public Policy and Administration, Technical University of Lisbon, Lisbon, Portugal

Mercedes A. McCormick Department of Psychology, Pace University, New York, NY, USA

Lawrence Soosai Nathan Department of Psychology, Anugraha Institute of Social Sciences (M.K University), University of Milano, Milan, Italy

Luis Miguel Neto School of Social and Political Sciences, ISCSP, CAPP – Center for Public Policy and Administration, Technical University of Lisbon, Lisbon, Portugal

Júlio Rique Neto Center for Research and Studies on Sociomoral Development (NPDSM), Universidade Federal da Paraíba – UFPB, João Pessoa, Brazil

Deborah Harris O'Brien Trinity Washington University, Washington, DC, USA

Martina Perstling Department of Psychology, Faculty of Humanities and Social Sciences, University of Namibia, Windhoek, Namibia

Clinical Psychologist Private Practice, Windhoek, Namibia

René T. Proyer Department of Psychology, University of Zurich, Zurich, Switzerland

Grant J. Rich APA Division 52 International Psychology, American Psychological Association, Juneau, AK, USA

Sebastiaan Rothmann Faculty of Humanities, North West University, Vanderbijlpark, South Africa

Willibald Ruch Department of Psychology, University of Zurich, Zurich, Switzerland

Bruna Seibel Center for Psychological Studies CEP-RUA, Universidade Federal do Rio Grande do Sul, Porto Alegre, Brazil

Dalbir Singh Geography Department, Pt. N R S Government College, Rohtak, Haryana, India

Kamlesh Singh Department of Humanities and Social Sciences, Indian Institute of Technology, Delhi, India

Q. Michael Temane School for Psychosocial Behavioural Sciences, North-West University, Potchefstroom, South Africa

Graciela Tonon Faculty of Social Sciences, Universidad de Palermo, Ciudad Autónoma de Buenos Aires, Argentina

UNI-COM, Faculty of Social Sciences, Universidad Nacional de Lomas de Zamora, Lomas de Zamora, Argentina

Ruut Veenhoven Social Conditions for Human Happiness, Erasmus University Rotterdam, Rotterdam, Netherlands

Social Conditions for Human Happiness, North-West University, Mahikeng, South Africa

Lía Rodriguez de la Vega UNI-COM, Faculty of Social Sciences, Universidad Nacional de Lomas de Zamora, Lomas de Zamora, Argentina

Sara Wellenzohn Department of Psychology, University of Zurich, Zurich, Switzerland

Marié P. Wissing School for Psychosocial Behavioural Sciences, North-West University, Potchefstroom, South Africa

Toward a Participatory and Ethical Consciousness in Positive Psychology: The Value Positioning in the Genesis of This Book

Helena Águeda Marujo and Luis Miguel Neto

> The happiest places on earth are not internal ones. They are not geographical ones. They are the places between us (…).
>
> Christopher Peterson, Pursuing the Good Life, 2013, p. 226

> The whole constitution of my spirit is one of hesitancy and of doubt. Nothing is or can be positive to me; all things oscillate around me, and all is meaning. All things are "unknown", symbolic of the Unknown.
>
> Fernando Pessoa (1888–1935), Portuguese Poet.
> Untitled excerpt

This book is the consequence of an ethical commitment and an invitation to even more participatory and polyphonic dialogues inside positive psychology.

Committed to a vision of science that honors the giant scholars of the past, and fosters a culture that appreciates its accomplishments, the editors of this book are also embedded in a scientific praxis that constantly and ethically challenges ideas and procedures while recreating and co-constructing "what is." In this sense, we encouraged a group or scholars and practitioners to look from a postmodern perspective to the field of positive psychology. While stepping upon the virtues of current models, the richness of data collected so far, and the tendencies inside the field, we were touched by Abraham Maslow's idea of "growth science" (1979, p. 113), instead of a "safety one," envisioning an approach that asks different questions, is predisposed to be mistaken, and is open to new and co-constructed versions of reality. Therefore, we invited colleagues from around the world to imagine "what if?" What if we intensely embrace the trends that are emerging (Biswas-Diener et al. 2011; Chirkov et al. 2011; Delle Fave et al. 2011a; Diener et al. 2010; Pawelski

H. Águeda Marujo • L.M. Neto
School of Social and Political Sciences, ISCSP, CAPP – Center for Public Policy and Administration, Technical University of Lisbon, Lisbon P-1349055, Portugal
e-mail: hmarujo@iscsp.utl.pt; lneto@iscsp.utl.pt

and Moores 2013), and using supplementary participatory and transformative methods (Gergen and Gergen 2003; Kotzé 2012; Mertens 2009), we actually and progressively bring a more collective, qualitative, culturally sensitive, and transformative approach to our processes of making sense and implementing the science of positive psychology? What if in particular we move beyond the individual level toward a "knowledge community" and "knowledge of the communities?"

To encourage scientific conversations around these topics, we have been bridging the postmodern relativism with a discussion about values and moral commitment (Oliver 1996), far beyond considering them as opposing grammars (Marujo and Neto 2011).

In the year 2000, Ed Diener and Eunkook M. Suh proposed a discussion about cultural issues, defending the idea that the cross-cultural comparisons of subjective well-being of societies, experienced as a value in increasingly democratic societies, is dependent of cultural relativism, addressing the need for taking into account the values of its citizens and inherent methodological challenges. In the book, they reject a complete cultural relativism, pointing out that diverse societies can be good, but that does not mean that all institutional arrangements are good (op. cit., p. 5). More than a decade has passed and we have begun responding to this complexity (Diener et al. 2010) and gradually figuring out progressively inside the positive psychology domain how to integrate in meaningful and respectful ways diversity and communality, values and science, individual and collective processes, rigor, and different and more creative forms of inquiry – with a scientific meticulousness focused not only in numbers but also in language. Nevertheless, we believe that an in-depth focus inside group, communities, and countries' dynamics can help expand the debate and convey light over some paradoxes.

The challenge of postmodernism can be traced originally to the question of *what is knowledge* – 'does it represent the world as it is?' – to the issue of *how* we congregate scientific information. It defied the dominant paradigms and discourses of the modernistic positivistic practices, where notions of objectivity, neutrality, and easy and superficial dualisms between practice and theory, researcher and subject, description and prescription, etc., where in the foreground, and brought instead to the front profound ethical concerns (Kotzé and Kotzé 1997, p. 8). These apprehensions included debating the places of context and time, disapproving a science of consensus, and questioning the angle of the "generalized other," the view from nowhere. The movement went from prescriptive ethics (knowing what is right and wrong) to participatory ethics (participation of all is a crucial obligation if we aspire to being ethical, since *to be is to participate*). The question then changed to *what are the effects of knowledge* (Kotzé 2012).

We all know how easy and inevitable it is to be caught up in the restrictions of our ways of being and reasoning, trapped in our incomplete and therefore imperfect cultural and historic perspectives, unless we are invited to new awareness through complementarities. Some of us recognize that, as a consequence, and although without intention, we marginalize and silence worldviews, particular voices and languages, and specific groups and relations. As Foucault argued (1980), we are all caught up in a web-interlacing power and knowledge and are accountable for our *moral positionings* (in White and Epston 1990). If "people exist in language" (Kotzé and Kotzé 1997, p. 31), to become aware, or from the French, "la prise de conscience," arises mainly from dialogical relations, namely from the energy and tensions uphold by the transactions with others, from that "space between us", and from the endorsing of new and diverse grammars.

That leads to the invitation to encourage new visions toward understanding human beings, groups, communities, and nations, while they are in positive relations and uplifting communion – of shared values and beliefs, routines, rituals, history, and narratives. We believe that this course of action can help positive psychology to progress through more inclusive ways of thinking and investigating and that those new processes of knowing *with* the other will permit the growth of higher forms of social accountability and a conjoint ethical consciousness, while venturing together toward more participatory processes of co-constructed knowledge.

Heshusius (1994, p. 15, cit in Kotzé 2012), while addressing the "hermeneutics of connection," describes "participatory consciousness as a freeing of ourselves from the categories imposed by the notions of objectivity and subjectivity, as a re-ordering of the understanding between the self and the other to a deep kinship of '*selfother*', between the knower and the known." A participatory consciousness then requires a "deeper level of kinship…an attitude of profound openness and receptivity." Two years later, in 1996, Heshusius goes on saying: "When the self and the other are seen as belonging to the same consciousness, all living is moral…To live morally requires, in the first instance, not moral discourse, but a relentless awareness of ourselves in the particulars of moment-to-moment living" (pp. 133–134).

What is, then, *this moment* for positive psychology? In its second decade of life, positive psychology has been "taking stock" of its field of study and is considered to be in a turning point (Sheldon et al. 2011; Wissing 2012). While designing the future, and wishing to "stay relevant to everyday human experience" (King 2011, p. 444), positive psychology is intensely debating its proposals and current paradoxes and challenges, opportunities, and obstacles, and showing four major tendencies: (a) moving from an intraindividual toward a relational, collective, and social focus (Biswas-Diener et al. 2011; Diener and Ryan 2009; Veenhoven 2011); (b) integrating objective and subjective indicators and measures and investing in the qualitative study of positive human processes due to the complexities and multifaceted proper-ties of the phenomena under study (Delle Fave et al. 2011b; Forgeard et al. 2011; Marujo and Neto 2011); (c) being less Western and middle-class centered and more sensitive to cultural and social specificities, namely, through the processes of reaching larger groups and addressing societal crucial issues and ills such as poverty and ecological sustainability (Delle Fave et al. 2011a; Marks 2009; Marks et al. 2006; Marujo and Neto 2007); and (d) dedicated to have a cultural, social, and global impact, focusing in the conditions of life and becoming an instrument for positive transformation, not only to people, but to various disciplines (Biswas-Diener 2010; Csikszentmihalyi and Nakamura 2011; Pawelski and Moores 2013; Veenhoven 2011, 2012). Therefore, these tendencies are present both when reflecting upon theoretical assumptions and the applied work of delivering empirically based interventions and also when addressing research methods (Marujo and Neto 2007, 2011). The request to align meta-theoretical and epistemological assumptions with theoretical postulates and empirical processes is hence sided with an incitement to a more sophisticated and reflective thinking inside the field and a transformative standpoint toward enhanced consciousness and different versions of the "truths."

As a consequence, at this point in time, writing one more book on positive psychology makes sense to us if we go beyond the (nevertheless important) dialectics of positive and negative, bad and good, darkness and light, and away from the pressure to create a master theory inside positive psychology. Instead, we propose to move to a clearly contextual, situated, dynamic, collaborative, and cultural transformative perspective, namely, through a social participatory and shared consciousness angle. In so doing, we believe we can diverge the tension between a value-laden or value-free, prescriptive and descriptive science, to focus more on relational and ethical issues.

In an age where governance, macroeconomics, national wealth and growth, ecology and social politics, and other vital areas such as education, work, family, the functioning of organizations, and the construction of cultures are under scrutiny and making us rethink social values and morality, the call for research on interpersonal and social connections is rising, harmonizing with the ascend of more silenced concepts such as relational goods, community, and meaning. Positive psychology is emerging, regardless of its contradictions, with a clear moral leadership toward positive relational prosperity and transformative social change (Biswas-Diener 2010; Veenhoven 2012). In order to achieve this purpose, the field needs to be increasingly more respectful of positive collective processes already in place around the world, to promote in-depth understanding of those processes, and to share its knowledge and large body of research with society at large.

This accumulative sustained engagement with society and with relevant social practices needs to honor several levels of analysis and use a community- and group-based broad-spectrum approach. It needs to consider different types of data and to give tribute to different methodologies, namely, to explore meaning around the construction of cultural and social processes. Ultimately, it should aim, not only to assess, diagnose, and amplify what is positive but also to transform the experience of participants and researchers.

Some of these purposes were present in the birth of positive psychology and can be traced to the Akumal Manifesto (Sheldon et al. 2011). There, the concept of "moral character of society" emerged, aligned with the need to address the cultural and global levels of society. Thirteen years later, the time has come.

The Dream

Accordingly, the aim of this book, affiliated with the vision of the Cross-Cultural Advancements in Positive Psychology Series, is to bring to life some data, new ideas, and deep theoretical and meta-theoretical reflections on the concepts of Positive Nations and Positive Communities. This purpose aims to complement the extraordinary and extremely relevant (Diener and Suh 2000; Diener et al. 2010; Veenhoven 2012), but also media frenzy and somehow partial, raking of happy nations and the geographical distribution of happiness and subjective well-being, namely, judged by the average self-reports of their nation's residents.

What is considered a positive nation? What qualitative processes contribute to a positive nation and to good community life? How can cross-fertilization between social sciences help promote new insights on these topics? What lies beyond and besides the added average of the happiness levels of a nation's individual citizen? What processes are we testifying and implementing inside communities and countries, and between countries, that promote a culture of positive functioning? Are diverse processes such as political revolutions, birth of countries, war and independency, youth curricular activities, or European Football Championships assets for well-being in nations? What about friendship, forgiveness, reconciliation, altruism, gift-exchange, and therapeutic indigenous practices or metrics around GNH: Can they be positive cement for citizens in a community or a nation, creating a spiral of optimal functioning? And what sustainable or episodic collective practices are signs of hope inside and among groups?

This book is tentatively trying to answer versions of these questions. It was originated in an international conference on Positive Nations that also overlapped with the 1st Portuguese Congress on Positive Psychology, held at Lisbon University on September of 2010. Some of the authors of this book were presenters at the conference, and the willingness to publish on the topic emerged as a need, after the fascinating presentations and sparkling of ideas that emerged from the speakers and audience. At the same time, what is now known as the Lisbon Group on Leadership and Culture Studies (ISCSP, Lisbon Tech University) began an international study on Positive Nations, still under process, but already with very exciting results, that connects data from countries as diverse as Portugal and Namibia.

The Creation

The book is the fruit of a group of scholars and practitioners from six continents (Asia, Australia, Africa, Europe, North America, South America) currently living and working in 12 different countries (Argentina, Australia, Canada, Brazil, India, Italy, Namibia, the Netherlands, Portugal, South Africa, Switzerland, USA), and the diversity of nations involved is even higher when we acknowledge their countries of birth, where nations like Nigeria and Austria emerge. They are authors specialized in the arenas of positive psychology, social psychology, clinical psychology, family therapy, community psychology, sociology, industrial/organizational psychology, human resources management, political science, medicine, geography, and international relations. The divergence of approaches, methods, and focus chosen by the authors and portrayed is, in our perspective, a beautiful sign of how diverse and rich this line of study is – and also how incipient – a reason that congregates us in a quest for future developments and expansions. As you will see, some of the authors answered the pledge with new points of view, more centered in the cultural sensitivity aspect, but still using methods that are closer to a more traditional discourse and line of work in positive psychology (for instance, using pure quantitative methods to analyze a collective process), while others concentrated more upon the qualitative methods, and still others risked more challenging views and analyses around collective processes and how they make communities thrive. All of them display intellectual rigor and are fascinating and prosperous, with a potential for opening up dialogical and critical perspectives, encouraging all of us to rethink our current representation and study of collective positive psychological realities.

The structure and sequence of the chapters are supported in the three-dimensional and orthogonal continuous model presented by Rom Harré (1984, pp. 45–46). In his thesis, he defends that most of our personal being may be of social origin, and that consciousness, agency, and autobiography are the three unities that compose it. He suggests that this personal being derives from the complementary powers of human beings both to display themselves socially as unique and to create novel linguistic forms. In the three-dimensional and orthogonal model he considers (1) Display, (2) Realization, and (3) Agency as way of expressing psychological attributes.

The *Display* of one's psychological attributes is represented with a pole of "private display" and "public display." *Realization* considers that those attributes can be realized as a property of one or of many, which implies that we can have "individual realization" and "collective realization." Finally, *Agency* is the third dimension that marks the degree to which, in possessing a psychological attribute or using a skill, a person is "active" or "passive," exercises power, or suffers from liability. The model helps us integrate the current movement exposed in the book from the personal being to the social being, when we are connecting and making sense of individual attributes within a global perspective.

After the Preface by the extraordinary sociologist Ruut Veenhoven, and word of value positioning by the editors regarding the story and the share vision for the book, it continues with two introductory chapters: one by Christopher J. Kinman regarding two organic visions for the community work – the rhizome and the gift-exchange – innovating beyond fixed boundaries using models of horizontal net-working, and egalitarian and open dialogue, and another by Grant J. Rich that takes a positive critical stand in what relates to methodological issues in the field, explores the richness of cross-fertilization with other disciplines, namely, anthropology, and defends the urgency of internationalizing positive psychology, to go beyond cultural universals. In the third chapter that inaugurates the session on *Display*, we have a feast of historical and cultural knowledge related to altruism as a collective vital strength, which being considered a mental attitude by the authors – Lawrence Soosai Nathan and Antonella Delle Fave – is considered to spiral in ways that have an impact upon society. The fourth chapter is written by two Argentineans, Graciela Tonon and Lía Rodriguez de la Vega, and brings interesting data from their own studies regarding friendship as relational glue for a positive nation. The fifth chapter brings a qualitative study from India, where Kamlesh Singh, Anjali Jain, and Dalbir Singh vividly analyze a cultural-specific indigenous therapeutic practice, *Satsang*, and its association with well-being of women in the rural communities. The sixth chapter addresses an issue that is very relevant but not often studied – the importance of curricular activities, in particular the belonging to an International Honor Society in Psychology, Psi Chi, to student development around the world – linking data with positive psychology and the benefits that might emerge for the construction of Positive Nations. The authors are currently linked to universities and organizations in the USA: Mercedes A. McCormick, Grant Rich, Deborah Harris O'Brien, and Annie Chai. The next chapter is already under a new heading inside the book structure, that of *Realization*. This seventh chapter presents an interesting and innovative quantitative study on the domain of sports, namely, addressing the changes encountered in character strengths of Switzerland citizens, after the European Football Championship of 2008, when Switzerland was the host country. The authors, René T. Proyer, Fabian Gander, Sara Wellenzohn, and Willibald Ruch, explore the fascinating idea of malleability of strengths at the national level. Chapter 8 brings to scientific discussion cultural data from the research on interpersonal forgiveness, using Enright's theory on the socio-moral development of forgiveness, voicing an interesting debate about the power and specificity of culture upon it. It was written by Julio R. Neto, Robert Enright, Bruna Siebel, and Silvia Koller, a team that includes Brazilians and a North American researcher. The deepness and sometimes heart-breaking narratives related to the historical process of the South Africa's Truth and Reconciliation Committee, as part of the transition process to democracy, is majestically described by Marié P. Wissing and Q. Michael Temane in the ninth chapter. The insights regarding processes to build a more just and positive society are thought provoking and extremely well supported in a profound knowledge of the positive psychology field. The final four chapters are under the umbrella of *Agency*. Chapter 10 debates Positive Nations through the lens of political philosophies and the metrics of the Gross National Happiness, exemplifying with the Himalayan Kingdom of Bhutan. The richness of its open-minded and informed analysis drives from the intense direct experience of the Australian author, George W. Burns, who has served in Bhutan as a volunteer psychologist 12 times in the last decade, studying the national processes. Chapter 11 focus extensively and interestingly on the Portuguese Revolution of the beginning of the twentieth century that allowed for the establishment of the First Portuguese Republic to explore the relationship between happiness and political revolutions and if and how political revolutions are linked to happiness in people. They also open up a rich debate regarding the ways that can be used at a macro-level by a society and a nation to increase its citizen's happiness. The case study that Miguel Pereira Lopes, Patricia Jardim da Palma, and Telmo Ferreira Alves have chosen, from their own country, brings a special light upon their conceptualization and perspectives while broadening the frontiers of the narrative to other national processes. Chapter 12 reflects upon the bridges that need to be constructed between positive psychology and community psychology, promoting what already is a new hybrid field full of potential, which dwells upon values, and rethinks research and intervention as transformative appreciative processes. The authors are the editors of the book, Luis Miguel Neto and Helena Águeda Marujo. Finally, the Chap. 13, signed by Martina Perstling (Namibia) and Ian Rothmann (South Africa), takes us to a historical and fascinating journey addressing the relationships between Namibia and South Africa and brings the studies of subjective well-being to the frontline, at the radiance of such complex experiences as war, independence, and nation building.

Grosby (2005) has defined "national identity" as a social relation of collective consciousness. In historical moments such the ones that we live, where some people believe in the sacralization of death if linked to a national project, where the fight for political freedom and the protection of peace are core values, where the comparisons and competition among nations and continents are rising, and concurrently territorial communities go far beyond that of nativity, and national boundaries are disappearing due to globalization, we, the positive psychology community, clearly need to intensify our investment in addressing societies at large and positive communal processes. We need to try to go beyond what is sometimes an oversimplification of the rich cultural and social interplay and "bring more bodies" to the conversation, as the inspirational family therapist Lynn Hoffman (2012) puts it.

This book is just a humble but yet captivating beginning for future dialogues, where discussions about values and the participatory rise of consciousness and "conscientization" (Freire 1970) can bring a new eloquence to the field.

We now want to show our deep gratitude to all the authors for their contribution and express our profound appreciation to Ana Rego and Thomas Neto for their work on revising several of the chapters. Concurrently, we convey our sincere appreciation to all the authors that helped review the chapters written by others: Antonella Delle Fave, George W. Burns, Janine Roberts, Michael Steger, Miguel Pereira Lopes, Patricia Jardim da Palma, and René Proyer.

> I've always rejected being understood. To be understood is to prostitute oneself. I prefer to be taken seriously for what I'm not, remain humanly unknown, with naturalness and all due respect.
>
> Fernando Pessoa, Portuguese Poet, The book of Disquiet, 2002

References

Biswas-Diener, R. (Ed.). (2010). *Positive psychology as a mechanism for social change*. New York: Springer.

Biswas-Diener, R., Linley, A. P., Govindji, R., & Woolston, L. (2011). Positive psychology as a force for social change. In K. Sheldon, T. B. Kashdan, & M. F. Steger (Eds.), *Designing positive psychology: Tacking stock and moving forward* (pp. 397–409). Oxford: Oxford University Press.

Chirkov, V., Ryan, R. M., & Sheldon, K. M. (Eds.). (2011). *Personal autonomy in cultural contexts: Global perspectives on the psychology of agency, freedom, and people's well-being*. Dordrecht: Springer.

Csikszentmihalyi, M., & Nakamura, J. (2011). Positive psychology: Where did it come from, where is it going? In K. M. Sheldon, T. B. Kashdan, & M. F. Steger (Eds.), *Designing positive psychology* (pp. 2–9). New York: Oxford University Press.

Delle Fave, A., Massimini, F., & Bassi, M. (2011a). *Psychological selection and optimal experience across cultures: Social empowerment through personal growth*. Dordrecht: Springer.

Delle Fave, A., Brdar, I., Freire, T., Vella-Brodrick, D., & Wissing, M. (2011b). The eudaimonic and hedonic components of happiness: Qualitative and quantitative findings. *Social Indicators Research, 100,* 158–207.

Diener, E., & Ryan, K. (2009). Subjective well-being: A general overview. *South African Journal of Psychology, 39,* 391–406.

Diener, E., & Suh, E. M. (2000). *Culture and subjective well-being.* Cambridge: A Bradford Book, The MIT Press.

Diener, E., Helliwell, J. F., & Kahneman, D. (Eds.). (2010). *International differences in well-being.* New York: Oxford University Press.

Forgeard, M. J. C., Jayawickreme, E., Kern, M., & Seligman, M. E. P. (2011). Doing the right thing: Measuring wellbeing for public policy. *International Journal of Wellbeing, 1*(1), 79–106. doi:10.5502/ijw.v1i1.15.

Foucault, M. (1980). *Power/knowledge: Selected interviews and other writings 1972–1977* (C. Gordon, Ed. and Trans.). New York: Pantheon Books.

Freire, P. (1970). *Pedagogy of the oppressed.* New York: Herder & Herder.

Gergen, K. J., & Gergen, M. M. (2003). *Social construction: A reader.* Thousands Oaks: SAGE.

Grosby, S. (2005). *Nationalism: A very short introduction.* Oxford: Oxford University Press.

Harré, R. (1984). *Personal being: A theory for individual psychology.* Boston: Harvard University Press.

Heshusius, L. (1994). Freeing ourselves from objectivity: Managing subjectivity or turning toward a participatory mode of consciousness? *Educational Researcher, 23*(3), 15–22.

Heshusius, L. (1996). Of life real and unreal. In L. Heshusius & K. Ballard (Eds.), *From positivism to interpretivism and beyond: Tales of transformation in educational and social research.* London: Teacher College Press.

Hoffman, L. (2012). *Bring in more bodies.* http://vimeo.com/56385578. Accessed 12 Jan 2012.

King, L. A. (2011). Are we there yet? What happened on the way to the demise of positive psychology. In K. Sheldon, T. B. Kashdan, & M. F. Steger (Eds.), *Designing positive psychology: Tacking stock and moving forward* (pp. 439–446). Oxford: Oxford University Press.

Kotzé, D. (2012). Doing participatory ethics. In D. Kotzé, J. Myburg, J. Roux, & Associates (Eds.), *Ethical ways of being (12–34).* Chagrin Falls: A Taos Institute Publication/WorldShare Books.

Kotzé, E., & Kotzé, D. J. (1997). Social construction as postmodern discourse: An epistemology for conversational therapeutic practice. *Acta Theologica, 17*(1), 27–50.

Marks, N. (2009). Creating national accounts of well-being: A parallel process to GNH. In K. Ura & D. Penjore (Eds.), *Gross national happiness: Practice and measurement* (pp. 102–123). Thimphu: Centre for Bhutan Studies.

Marks, N., Abdullah, S., Simms, A., & Thompson, S. (2006). *The happy planet index.* http://www.happyplanetindex.org/public-data/files/happy-planet-index-first-global.pdf. Accessed 23 June 2012.

Marujo, H. A., & Neto, L. M. (2007). *Álbuns de Família: De viva voz. Manual de Possibilidades para o Futuro.* Ponta Delgada, Açores: Instituto de Acção Social.

Marujo, H., & Neto, L. (2011). Investigação Transformativa e Apreciativa: Um elogio da Subjetividade na Contemporaneidade. *Ecos, Revista de Investigação Contemporânea da Subjetividade, 1*(1), 1–14. http://www.uff.br/periodicoshumanas/index.php/ecos/article/view/714/546. Accessed 10 Aug 2012.

Maslow, A. (1979). *The journals of A. H. Maslow.* Monterey: Brooks/Cole.

Mertens, D. (2009). *Transformative research and evaluation.* New York: Guilford Press.

Oliver, C. (1996). Systemic eloquence. *Human Systems: The Journal of Systemic Consultation and Management, 7*(4). Retrieved from http://www.christineoliver.net/docs/publications/Oliver96.htm

Pawelski, J. O., & Moores, D. J. (2013). *The eudaimonic turn: Well-being in literary studies.* Lanham: Fairleigh Dickinson University Press.

Pessoa, F. (2002). *The book of disquiet.* London: Penguin Books.

Peterson, C. (2013). *Pursuing the good life: 100 reflections on positive psychology*. Oxford: Oxford University Press.

Sheldon, K., Kashdan, T. B., & Steger, M. F. (Eds.). (2011) *Designing positive psychology: Taking stock and moving forward*. Oxford: Oxford University Press.

Veenhoven, R. (2011). Greater happiness for a greater number: Is that possible? If so, how? In K. Sheldon, T. B. Kashdan, & M. F. Steger (Eds.), *Designing positive psychology: Tacking stock and moving forward* (pp. 397–409). Oxford: Oxford University Press.

Veenhoven, R. (2012, July). *The world database of happiness: Tool for ordering the growing pile of research findings*. Paper presented at the 30th international congress of psychology, Cape Town (pp. 22–27).

White, M., & Epston, D. (1990). *Narrative means to therapeutic ends*. New York: Norton.

Wissing, M. (2012, July). *Positive psychology: Past, present and future*. Paper presented at the 30th international congress of psychology, Cape Town (pp. 22–27).

Part I
Introductory Perspectives

Chapter 1
Two Images: Rhizome and Gift-Exchange in Life and Service

Christopher J. Kinman

1.1 Introduction

> I was seeing there the roots of human symmetry, beauty and ugliness, aesthetics, the human being's very aliveness and little bit of wisdom. His wisdom, his bodily grace, and even his habit of making beautiful objects are just as "animal" as his cruelty. After all, the very word "animal" means "endowed with mind or spirit (animus)."
>
> Gregory Bateson (1979), p. 5

I begin by visiting Gregory Bateson – that maverick anthropologist and environmentalist whose thoughts played a role in inspiring the beginnings of the field of family therapy. As family therapy evolved, Bateson distanced himself from the profession. However, this very act of distancing, and the discourse around it, delivers much rich and beneficial wisdom. Bateson's thinking on what I call *the therapeutic* holds application for all professions within the human services realm, if not for all people, and is perhaps never more relevant that at this point in history. We present just a fragment of Bateson, yet, a fragment that carries with it much of that which moved him.

At times, Bateson, when with a group of students, would put before them a crab and he would ask this question:

> How could they know that this crab came from something that was alive? I want you to produce arguments which will convince me that this object is the remains of a living thing. You may imagine, if you will that you are Martians and that on Mars you are familiar with living things, being indeed yourselves alive. But, of course, you have never seen crabs or lobsters. A number of objects like this, many of them fragmentary, have arrived... You are to inspect them and arrive at the conclusion that they are remains of living things. How would you arrive at that conclusion?
>
> Bateson (1979), p. 7

C.J. Kinman (✉)
Executive Director, Rhizome Productions, The Rhizome Way, Vancouver, BC, Canada
e-mail: cjkinman@gmail.com

H. Águeda Marujo and L.M. Neto (eds.), *Positive Nations and Communities*, Cross-Cultural Advancements in Positive Psychology 6, DOI 10.1007/978-94-007-6869-7_1,
© Springer Science+Business Media Dordrecht 2014

I find this a truly beautiful question. It calls us to ponder, to wonder and to wander with the mind, the eye and the hand through the diverse spaces of life, through that vast plateau which Bateson called the Creatura. When we see a crab shell, a blade of grass, a fossil trilobite, the jaw bone of a moose, a fish scale, an earthworm, a feather, a microscopic freshwater cyclops, a humpback whale vertebrae or the hand of a loved one, how do we know these things came from something that was alive? The question does much more than invite musings over the how-to(s), those details of life's assemblages, it calls for a consideration of the movements of life itself, to a consideration of what I like to call the 'Alive'.

The question continues… Look at the wheel on your car, look at the moving lines of the road, look at the contours and patterns of a book, look at the lines of movement which are invited through the process of reading a book, look at a toothbrush, at a key, at a guitar pick, at a spoon, look at a dance, a hockey game, look at the movements of two lovers, look at the posturing of two fighters. Look at all these things. How do you know these things came from something that was alive? Human creations cannot be removed from the Alive. The movements of life are not escapable. The Alive is always evident – but we must look.

What about in the communal realm? What movements of the Alive are we able to see, to touch, to hear? How can we recognise the Alive within our varied communal interactions?

When in the midst of human institutions are we also able to sense the Alive at movement?

And, in a more particular way, are we able to sense the movements of the Alive within our work – particularly within the work of human services?

To explore these questions, I particularly lean upon the world-shifting work of two French philosophers: Gilles Deleuze and Jacques Derrida.

I explore two primary images: that of the rhizome and the gift-exchange. I suggest that these two images produce revolutionary effects upon the work of the human services industry.

1.2   Image #1 Rhizome

In order to explore the idea of the Alive within its communal movements, I introduce the idea of rhizome. This idea was developed by Gilles Deleuze, along with his friend and co-writer Felix Guattari. These writers present the idea of rhizome, but it is always paired with another image, that of 'the tree'.

> We are tired of the tree. We must no longer put our faith in trees, roots, or radicels; we have suffered enough from them. The whole arborescent culture is founded on them, from biology to linguistics. On the contrary, only underground stems and aerial roots, the adventitious and the rhizome are truly beautiful, loving or political.
>
> Deleuze and Guattari (1983), p. 33

1.2.1   The Image of a Tree

The tree, according to Deleuze and Guattari, is an image which bears resemblance to modern institutions. The 'tree of life', they suggest, became a dominant metaphor layering structure and hierarchy over much of human and non-human experience.

Trees and institutions are both:

- Concerned with power and centrality – Trees and institutions both operate from a central core, with arms that branch off yet are always securely fastened to the central structure.
- Concerned with hierarchy and structure – In both trees and institutions, things ideally move up only one cell at a time, and things move down also one cell at a time. This form of cellular transmission bears resemblance to the lines of a well-structured flow chart.
- Focus upon upward growth and progress – According to English legal traditions, institutions are treated as if they are persons. However, a person will be born, will live his or her life and, in the end, will die. Death is inescapable in her world. However, this is not so in the realms of institutions: successful institutions hold the promise of possibly living for many generations, if not forever. Institutions are supposed to be resolute upon upward movement, upon progress.
- Institutional structures hold a seeming overpowering influence in the current world.

They certainly must be taken into consideration within our movements within communal lives.

There are two sure ways for identifying institutional assemblages.

First of all, there are always higher institutions set aside for the purpose of recognising lower-level institutions.

This is always the case. A chain of recognition must occur within institutional spheres. If one looks carefully at the American dollar bill, the highest and final level of institutional recognition is provided – In God We Trust. God is thereby reduced to institutional contours. God is then to be understood through institutional eyes, as an institution, as an original and originating institution. A hierarchical chain of institutional structures is established, each in relation to the other through specified ties of control and authority or through lateral connections of competition or alliance. Divinity tops this chain, and at the bottom are an assortment of bodies and parts and relations, usually connected with women, children, animals and things. This very chain of institutions appears arborescent/tree-like in its form and function.

Much in our daily life has been connected to this tree-like language.

Even the body is understood as arborescent. This is reflected in medical discourse and practice – the body as institution – with the brain and the heart alternatively taking a 'head' or central position. It is also reflected in Christian theology, where Christ is considered the 'head' and the church is considered the 'body'. Bodies, both physical and metaphorical, become hierarchical institutional structures.

A second way of identifying institutional assemblages:

If you look carefully, you will always find lawyers lurking in the corners, accountants also. These are the bureaucratic priests of the institutional empires.

This also is always the case. The setting up of an institution, as well as the reporting requirements demanded of institutions, always necessitates the involvement of lawyers and accountants. Lawyers are to protect and challenge the boundary lines of institutional movements and expectations. Accountants ensure that institutional movements are always tied to numerical values.

Institutions are inescapable in modern life:

- Our work is defined by them.
- Money only legitimately flows along institutional lines – therefore, we cannot receive a pay cheque but through an institution.
- We buy our food, clothing, housing and other goods through them.
- We send our kids to get educated in them.
- We receive health care through them.
- We get religion through them.
- We play sports within the contexts of institutions.
- We get much of our entertainment through them.

The tree – an idea that cements us to the world of institutions and structures.

You set about opposing the rhizome to trees. And trees are not a metaphor at all, but an image of thought, a functioning, a whole apparatus that is planted in thought in order to make it go in a straight line and produce the famous correct ideas. There are all kinds of characteristics in the tree: there is a point of origin, seed, or centre; it is a binary machine or principle of dichotomy, with its perpetually divided and reproduced branchings, its points of arborescence; it is an axis of rotation which organizes things in a circle, and the circles round the centre; it is a structure, a system of points and positions which fix all of the possible within a grid, a hierarchical system or transmission of orders… it has a future and a past, roots and a peak, a whole history, an evolution, a development… Now there is no doubt that trees are planted in our heads: the tree of life, the tree of knowledge, etc. The whole world demands roots. Power is arborescent.

Deleuze and Parnet (1987), p. 24

1.2.2   The Image of a Rhizome

Deleuze and Guattari also present another concept – they call it the rhizome. This image connects us to realms that are tied to the communal:

- The rhizome is also a botanical image. It describes a certain kind of assemblage that connects together through networks of nodes and lines.
- Think of potatoes, grass, poplar trees – Many believe that the largest trees in the world are not sequoia or redwoods but rather poplar trees, for poplars are rhizomes. In the foothills of the Rocky Mountains, one will notice that, in the fall, a large section of a hill will turn yellow, while the other sections are still green.

These patches of poplar trees are actually one genetic organism, one large rhizome assemblage.
- Think of weeds, almost every weed in your garden – Rhizomes are productive spaces, enabling effective and flourishing movement through terrain and barriers often seen as impenetrable and impossible.
- Think of human creations such as telephone systems, the Internet and, to some extent, the power grid – Human creations, even institutional creations, are not always institutional in structure; sometimes they appear in rhizome form. This is especially true of some human creations that involve many diverse and loosely connected players.
- Rhizomes are typically found underground. They are not usually conspicuous – If one opens the paper or turns on the evening news, one is primarily given stories and information pertinent to institutional life. Rhizome life is not usually considered news-worthy. Rhizome movements are powerful, but are not as easily visible.
- Rhizomes are made of nodes and lines that connect the nodes – Nodes connected with numerous lines which in turn connect to other nodes and line. Now think of the American interstate system. Think of prairie dog towns. Imagine the 'communal' not as relations with local institutions, not as a realm of service institutions, but rather as rhizome connections, as lines connecting with people, places, animals, things. Think of our communal worlds as rhizome abundances.
- Rhizomes have no practical beginning, ending or centrality – Imagine that one wanted to get rid of the crab grass in one's lawn. The idea of going after the beginning grass, the one that started it all; or the latest frontiers of crab grass; or the crab grass, the boss – this type of thinking is insanity in the worlds of rhizomes. Rhizomes are not influenced by such linear and rank-oriented interests. Military-type might is notoriously ineffective at influencing rhizome community.
- Rhizomes are extremely difficult to destroy – Rhizome in nature or the communal rhizome– it is almost difficult to destroy. We must stop thinking of rhizome-like things as if they were vulnerable.

1.2.3   Overwhelming Rhizome Lines

The right way to begin to think about the pattern which connects is to think of it as primarily (whatever that means) a dance of interacting parts and only secondarily pegged down by various sorts of physical limits and by those limits which organisms characteristically impose.

Bateson (1979), pp. 13–14

As with Bateson's 'pattern which connects', so also with the rhizome, numerous lines extend, not to points/nodes, but through them, beyond them, thereby inventing a plethora of dances, connecting up entire worlds.

We are suggesting a view of humanity, of relationships, of community, even of mind and body that is like rhizome. We are suggesting worlds outside of bodily encasement, beyond familial identity, outside of what is typically thought of with the language of 'system', toward lives that are tied by uncountable lines to uncountable bodies, where relationships of many different types become engulfing and repeatedly formative. These rhizome connections are certainly about relationships with people, but they are also about so much more – they are about relationships with animals and plants; relationships with air and water; relationships with landscapes; relationships with buildings and rooms and spaces and lines of travel; relationships with relationships; relationships with countless other assemblages, whether created by people or by nature (as if that distinction can be maintained); relationships with cars and rivers and musical instruments; relationships with music; relation- ships with values and goods and affects such as love, humour, romance, sadness, loneliness, joy, annoyance. All these and numerous other assemblages not mentioned and not previously considered are connected to us and through us within rhizome space.

The rhizome is not a simple metaphor, as we often understand metaphor. It is not an image that represents something else. The rhizome is rather a physical space, as well as a spiritual space, wherein synapse-like connections form and numerous movements occur. It is a physical and spiritual space of abundances and multiplicities. After all, the brain, the nervous 'system' is itself created with rhizome abundance, with movements of electricity following chemical lines, jumping from synapse to synapse, node to node, tracing numerous possible routes, thereby creating numerous possible worlds. It is this rhizome nervous system that enables human living and movement and thought. It also creates worlds and bodies that can never be understood in simple ways, that can never be mapped out by straight lines and right angles.

> (Thinking) in terms of trees too much: the tree of knowledge, points of arborescence, the alpha and omega, the roots and the pinnacle. Trees are the opposite of grass. Not only does grass grow in the middle of things, but it grows itself through the middle…Grass has its line of flight, and does not take root. We have grass in the head, not a tree: what thinking signifies is what the brain is, a particular nervous system' of grass.

> Deleuze and Parnet (1987), p. 39

All reductionist and simple descriptions become repeatedly irrelevant. Rhizome abundance creates a necessary context for every description of things living, thereby overturning and challenging much that is considered scientific and particularly social scientific. This understanding revolutionises scientific and professionalised descriptions of life, implying that rhizome complexity and rhizome connectivity must never be absent from our descriptions. For those of us involved in work often described as 'therapeutic', for those of us who are involved in work where we are desiring to see some form of change in a social realm, there is particular relevance in the idea of rhizome. I propose that all meaningful change, everything powerful and productive and life-giving that occurs in the social realm, transpires in a rhizome-like space along rhizome-like lines.

1.2.4   A Rhizome Dilemma

For those of us who work with people in community, we find ourselves in a serious dilemma.

The work of human services, in its varied territories (from health to education, corrections to family therapy, child protection to the care of the elderly), is formed within the structures of institutions.

However, the success of this work, the capacity to connect to realms of change and productivity in life and community, is dependent upon a work that moves within the lines of rhizome relations.

This dilemma is one which we should play significant attention to. It is here, in the midst of this dilemma, that we are faced with one of the most significant difficulties and opportunities facing the human services industry.

Through my years of work, I regularly hear stories describing the pain of living with this dilemma. These stories have surfaced within realms of service as diverse as education, child protection, community corrections, the prison system, nursing, medicine, family therapy, elder care, etc. This pain is also felt, often intently, by those who receive such services, those people often called clients or patients.

It is interesting to note, however, that the pain felt in this dilemma is experienced by those who hold a value for a rhizome-honouring work. Those who hold little interest in acknowledging a rhizome work rarely experience this kind of discomfort from the context of the institutional expectations. Generally speaking, this pain is only felt on one side of the dilemma.

1.2.5   A Rhizome Work

The following statement may seem radical, may seem overstated, yet, it is a statement that I believe we should all consider.

Good work, effective work within the specific contexts of real people's lives is not, and can never be, an institutional requirement.

Following directives, maintaining the requisite flow of appropriate and designated paperwork, fitting into a specificity of work designated through a chosen model of therapeutic/professional action – these types of activities are certainly required and are often articulated as clear expectations within most (human service) institutional settings.

However, good work, effective work, is always connected by rhizome lines to real bodies living in responsivity to the worlds around them. And it is these relations of responsivity that lead us to the idea of gift-exchange (we will be discussing gift-exchange later in this chapter).

Everything flows down below, in a perpetual flux, with bits and pieces continually entering and exiting.

Deleuze and Parnet (1987), p. 80

1.2.6 Jacques Derrida and Rhizome Work

While the idea of rhizome as a philosophical concept is unique to Deleuze and Guattari, there is much comparable to the thinking of Jacques Derrida.

Derrida explores certain questions which fit in a most uneasy way into institutional realms. He talked of things such as the gift, forgiveness, friendship, hospitality and (though reluctantly) love (among many other topics). His line of thought on all these topics bears striking similarities. It often goes something like this (using forgiveness as an example):

- Forgiveness is necessary.
- Forgiveness is impossible.
- The impossibility of forgiveness does not remove it from the realm of the possible.
- The impossibility of forgiveness imbeds it in our desires, making it not only possible but impossible to not be possible.
- The impossibility possibility of forgiveness can never be realised through relations of sovereignty or through relations that are institutional.
- The impossible possibility of forgiveness can only be realised through encounters/events which are outside of the realm of sovereignty.
- The impossible possibility of forgiveness can best be realised through encounters/events where faces meet faces.
- The impossible possibility of forgiveness can never be truly realised. All these possible, impossible possibilities are prefaced by the idea of the 'perhaps'. Perhaps, they are impossibly possible. No guarantees whatsoever – just perhaps.

These ideas are seen as Derrida discusses the idea of forgiveness within the context of apartheid in South Africa. He suggests that sovereign powers can never forgive. They can assist in making restitution. They can create contexts where understandings can occur. But they cannot create forgiveness. Forgiveness is something that must come from near the bone, from flesh and blood. It must be connected to human hearts in relation – if it is possible at all, perhaps.

Derrida felt a strong connection with Deleuze's thought. He stated, upon Deleuze's death:

> Deleuze undoubtedly still remains, despite so many dissimilarities, the one among all those of my "generation" to whom I have always considered myself closest. I have never felt the slightest "objection" arising in me, not even potentially, against any of his work.

> Derrida (2001) p. 193

Derrida left room for institutions. However, the relations between institutions and things such as the gift or forgiveness are primarily relations clearly in some future. As in his 'democracy to come', the institutions of this day are not able to carry rhizome, are not able to openly and joyfully face such goods as forgiveness and the gift while refraining from doing injustice and violence to them. All of this possibility in the future was prefaced by the idea of 'perhaps'.

Derrida believed that the future can only be discoursed within the framework of the 'perhaps'. These thoughts, as outlined above, bear significant connections with Deleuze. The world Derrida describes is one where the circulation, the bringing to light of certain goods occurs in places that he describes as beyond sovereignty. He describes locations for goods like forgiveness, the gift, friendship that are outside of institution and within places that look strikingly like rhizome.

> This is what I call the 'democracy to come'. In the radical evil of which we are speaking, and consequently in the enigma of the forgiveness of the unforgivable, there is a sort of 'madness' which the juridico-political cannot approach, much less appropriate.
>
> Derrida (2004), p. 55

> In all the geopolitical scenes we have been talking about, the word most often abused is 'forgive'. Because it always has to do with negotiations more or less acknowledged, with calculated transactions, with conditions…
>
> Derrida (2001), p. 39

1.3 Image #2 – Gift-Exchange

The human services realm has built its edifices upon the ground of deficit and problem. For monies to flow, for work to be created, deficits must be produced and people must be reduced to prescribed descriptors of lack. This system or edifice feels fixed and prevailing.

Those who enter human services institutions, in their entering, must go through a filtering process of assessment and intake. They are to be sifted through words and phrases, previously designated and professionally determined words and phrases. However, for the filtering process to be effective, the object which is to be filtered, which is the person entering the human service institution, must first be pulverised. He/she must be disassembled into minute fragments/particles. Some of these tiny pieces are then caught in the filtering process. Most of the disassembled person simply washes through and evades the filtering process. These remaining pieces are reassembled. People are reassembled. This time the new assemblage is a mini-institution, but it is a defective mini-institution, an inadequate and weakened hierarchy, an organisation clearly broken and lacking.

How tragic is this tale? How limited and lifeless are the recreated assemblages?

However, this is not simply a story of oppression and tragedy; it is at the same time a story of impotence. These processes of negation emerging from the institutions of human services are unable to access the vitalities of life, those lines which open flows of change and hope. Change does not occur along these lines. Productive human living does not occur along these lines. These processes of lack and deficit simply open doors which enable money to flow, and usually the flows of money are most slim. These processes do nothing to encourage the production of the good life.

The world of deficit inevitably succumbs to its own language. It produces its own return of deficit, and it brings it upon itself. The administration of deficit within human institutions cannot but instigates its own demise.

1.3.1   The Gift

In turning from this realm of deficit, I am suggesting a certain returning emerges – a returning to the movements of life and community, a rhizome return. We all know this turning; it is an exchange; it is a repetition and returning of exchange. It is a realm where gifts flow. It is a realm where things and goods, where affections and passions, where compassions and kindnesses, where moments of life and hope turn in exchanges, from hand to hand, voice to voice, heart to heart. Not simple turns, no easy circles, just turbulent turns, exchanges that move along complicated rhizome lines.

The gift-exchange has often been associated with Aboriginal peoples. In the Pacific Northwest coast from Washington State to British Columbia and Alaska, the gift-exchange was often associated with the cultural activity of the potlatch. This was an activity where communities which were often in the midst of conflict came together and gave gifts. However, this was not an exchange of gifts like anything the Western world was familiar with, for these gift-exchanges were processes of utter abundance. Each community gave in outrageous plenitude. There seemed to be a certain competition of giving. Who could give the most?

These potlatch ceremonies were outlawed by the colonising powers in both Canada and the United States. Many believe these ceremonies were outlawed for religious reasons. These ceremonies were not Christian and thereby undermined the role of the church. I doubt that this was a significant reason for outlawing the potlatch ceremonies, however. The first contacts by the colonising powers, at least those contacts that the governing authorities would have been concerned about, were not the religious institutions but the traders, those with economic motives. I suggest that the potlatch ceremonies were outlawed because they were seen as undermining of the economic purposes of the colonising powers.

The gift, and its circulation in rhizome realms, is frequently seen as in conflict with the movements of institutions.

I must emphasise that the gift-exchange is not something that is limited to Aboriginal worlds; it is connected to all people and it is necessary for human survival. It may be marginalised in certain realms, but it cannot be removed from our worlds in its entirety. Historically, the world of gift-exchange was something that was belittled and marginalised by institutional powers. It was something seen as belonging to a world of women and heathens. It was something which may have been required but it was not viewed as an important activity, it was not perceived as of the movements of men – white, Western men, preoccupied with power, ambitious in institutions.

In spite of its subjugation, the gift is still turning in all our worlds. Imagine that you are walking on the street and you run into an old friend who you haven't seen in years. What do you do? What do you do instinctively, without conscious thought? Most people immediately engage in gift-exchange. They exchange words of greeting, they exchange hugs, handshakes. They invite further connection, going for coffee or meeting for lunch. Gifts immediately begin to circulate, and they circulate in abundance.

Imagine instead what would occur in the meeting if one of the parties behaved in a manner similar to that which is required within the human service industry.

Imagine in the meeting that instead of exchanging gifts, one of the parties immediately examined the other person, looked her up and down, searching for fault, searching for deficit. This activity would not simply halt connection it would in all probability force disconnection and dissention.

The gift-exchange is all about relationship. Deficit identification, problem description do the opposite, they engender disconnection and isolation.

1.3.2   Two Economies

In order to bring to light the movements of gift-exchange within communal life, I compare two forms of economy.

> An expected, moderate, measured, or measurable gift, a gift proportionate to the benefit or to the effect one expects from it, a reasonable gift… would no longer be a gift; at most it would be a repayment of credit, the restricted economy of difference, a calculable temporization or deferral. If it remains pure and without possible appropriation, the surprise names that instant of madness that tears time apart and interrupts every calculation.
>
> Derrida (1992), p. 147

> The idea of a gift economy seems to me important, the idea of an economy in which things move, continue to move, circulate in their excesses and heterogeneities, contrasted with economies in which wealth, money, and time are stored up, producing commodities for possession and exchange.
>
> Ross (1996), p. 19

One economy is named by Ross as the restricted economy. It is called restricted because value in these types of exchanges resides in restriction. Value is found in things which are restricted, things such as gold or real estate in Vancouver or New York City. In the restricted economy value is even found in professions which are the most restricted, where entry into these professions requires the highest cost, the most valued sacrifice, and where entrance is permitted only to those with what is considered the highest educational accomplishments.

The other form of exchange is the gift economy. In this economy value rises not in restriction but in abundance. Those things which are the most abundant are the most valuable.

I compare these two economies.

Economic Actions

Restricted Economy
Property ownership and protection

Gift Economy
Not about giving – that is more akin to charity
Emphasis on responding to the gift of the other not on the giving of the gift

Economic Quantification

Restricted Economy
The world is a place of scarcity so hoard and protect.

Gift Economy
The world is a place of abundance so give.

Economic Processes

Restricted Economy
Define the numerical 'value' of things (value as a mathematical term)

Gift Economy
Expand and enhance the capacity of things

Economic Purposes

Restricted Economy
Acquisition and accumulation

Gift Economy
Connection/relationship

Human Economics

Restricted Economy
Emphasis on the worth or value (or more typically, the lack of worth or value) inside human bodies

Gift Economy
Emphasis on the gifts and potential gifts circulating, within the lives and relationships of people

What if we were to think of the work of human services as gift-exchange? How would the work look different? What would happen to the work of assessment? How would the flows of money move in response to gift rather than deficit and problem? How would the 'therapeutic' work change? How would those realms of human services with certain police-like roles (such as child protection and corrections) look with an orientation around gift-exchange? How would medicine, education, psychiatry and psychology operate when taking seriously the gift-exchange? While gift-exchange and the purposes of institutions may seem quite at odds, somehow, through this mess, through all the challenges, the gift-exchange gets through, it leaks through, and repeatedly so.

Through those impossibilities that Derrida alludes to, through the arborescent restraints that Deleuze describes, through a virtual wall of tree-like hindrances, the gift, in its rhizome movements, still influences the work of human services, and it does so repeatedly and in abundance. It is these points of leakage, these break-throughs, these breaches in the code whereby the gift is able to emerge wherein we discover the how-to(s) of gift-exchange in institutional contexts. Pay attention to the leaks; it is there where the Alive springs forth.

1.4   Conclusion

We propose that the gift-exchange is an essential process in communal life.

We also suggest that effective work in the human services realm, work that is productive, that acknowledges and leads toward the living of the good life, is work that honours the rhizome movements of gift-exchange within people's lives and communities.

John McKnight has for many years been one who challenges the human service industry. He is also one who utilises a language of gift in his talk of other people, in his talk of those he works with, interacts with. According to McKnight (1994):

> To the degree that all of society is committed to and interested in fixing people, it creates huge and increasingly burdensome and increasingly tyrannical institutions intervening in the lives of people, when what we needed was a community that saw their gifts and said, those gifts need to be given.

A return to Bateson: to Bateson's crab shell. How do we know that this came from something that is Alive? Are we able to see those lines of Alive as they move in communal, rhizome ways? I am proposing that the Alive, the communal Alive, lives and moves in rhizome places, amidst lines of connection, complex and diverse lines which connect to numerous other people, places, animals, things, relationships, etc. Within these lines of connection, these rhizome tangles, Alive emerges. And the Alive emerges not just in the rhizome place but within the complexities of gifts as they traverse along these rhizome lines. Gifts – to be received, to be given, to pass through the giver and receiver, awaiting response, awaiting return and exchange.

References

Bateson, G. (1979). *Mind and nature: A necessary unity*. New York: Bantam.
Deleuze, G., & Guattari, F. (1983). *On the line*. New York: Semiotext(e).
Deleuze, G., & Parnet, C. (1987). *Dialogues*. New York: Columbia University Press.
Derrida, J. (1992). *Given time: 1. Counterfeit money*. Chicago: University of Chicago Press.
Derrida, J. (2001). *The work of mourning*. Chicago: University of Chicago Press.
Derrida, J. (2004). *On cosmopolitanism and forgiveness*. New York: Routledge.
McKnight, J. (1994). *Community and its counterfeits*. Ideas (Radio Program). Toronto: CBC Radio.
Ross, S. D. (1996). *The gift of beauty: The good as art*. New York: State University of New York.

Chapter 2
Positive Institutions, Communities, and Nations: Methods and Internationalizing Positive Psychology Concepts

Grant J. Rich

2.1 Introduction

Since its inception over a decade ago, positive psychology has offered a corrective to a psychology that has focused primarily on human weakness by aiming to better understand human strengths and virtues. As David Myers (2000) noted, until the launching of positive psychology in 1998, there were 21 articles on negative emotions for every article on positive emotions, as revealed by a PsycINFO database search of research since 1967. The past 10 years have brought exciting developments, such as the launching of a dedicated discipline publication, the *Journal of Positive Psychology*, the appearance of positive psychology encyclopedias (e.g., Lopez 2009) and handbooks (e.g., Lopez and Snyder 2009), and the establishment of national and international conferences and organizations, such as the International Positive Psychology Association. Currently, there are seven core positive psychology textbooks for use with university students which aim to survey this growing movement (Rich 2011a). However, despite these impressive achievements and rapid growth, positive psychology is not without its skeptics. From outside psychology, writers such as journalist Ehrenreich (2009) and English literature professor Wilson (2008) take aim at positive psychology, in part arguing that negative emotions and states such as melancholia are essential for a number of worthwhile human pursuits, such as creativity, and that positive psychology may lead to people and societies that focus on fleeting frivolity rather than on deep, meaningful engagement and values and goals that make life worth living. The strident tone and sometimes breezy dismissals by Ehrenreich and others of research may irk some psychology professors, who note that careful reading of psychological science by positive psychologists such as Seligman (2011) clearly shows that such psychologists differentiate their own science

G.J. Rich (✉)
APA Division 52 International Psychology, American Psychological Association,
Juneau, AK, USA
e-mail: optimalex@aol.com

H. Águeda Marujo and L.M. Neto (eds.), *Positive Nations and Communities*, Cross-Cultural
Advancements in Positive Psychology 6, DOI 10.1007/978-94-007-6869-7_2,
© Springer Science+Business Media Dordrecht 2014

from pop-psych "happiology" and momentary pleasures (such as from illicit drugs or junk food) from a sustained meaningful pursuit of the good life. Other scholars, such as Harvard's Derek Bok (2010), writing from a public policy point of view, also read the positive psychology research to indicate that the way to lasting happiness is through meaningful civic engagement and good works, not trivial pursuits and momentary pleasures (pp. 45–62). Nevertheless, critics of positive psychology also exist within the discipline of psychology. Though there have been earlier psychological critiques, such as a special issue of *Theory and Psychology* devoted to the topic of the limitations of a positive psychology built within an individualistic and ethnocentric perspective (Christopher et al. 2008), a recent book by Harvard psychologist Jerome Kagan (2012) demonstrates well continuing unresolved issues.

In *Psychology's Ghosts*, Kagan (2012) details his deep concern for the state of contemporary psychology, examining what he considers the flawed assumptions and practices of many psychologists. In particular, he notes several major problems that he feels plague the field, including a failure to acknowledge adequately the setting and context in which observations are made (such as participants' age and culture), the tendency to make broad inferences from a single measure or type of measure (such as a questionnaire item), and the overreliance and misinterpretation of self-reports. For instance, to illustrate problems with self-reports, he poses the hypothetical question: would society have discovered the concepts of vertebrate evolution "if natural scientists had asked the world's most experienced hunters and farmers to write down all they knew about animals"? (p. xv). Later he asks whether psychologists and other scholars should believe astrology, if 98 % of those surveyed self-report that it works (pp. 84–85). In other words, Kagan reminds psychologists that self-reports may not always be the best or most appropriate way to learn a truth or reality. Kagan devotes one full chapter to a critique of positive psychology, with a special focus on the problem of utilizing and interpreting verbal self-reports of well-being. Kagan's concern with the importance of sociocultural context in psychological research is of special relevance to the topic of this volume on collective, qualitative, and culturally sensitive processes in positive psychology. Kagan argues that as science moves from lower levels of analysis to higher levels of analysis, for example, from physics to biology to psychology, context matters increasingly more (p. 2). He reserves especially strong criticism for psychologists who make broad sweeping conclusions from their data without taking into account or even reporting details about the sociocultural context of the participants, such as historical time/ cohort of data collection, race/ethnicity, rural/urban location, religion and linguistic group, and social class. As he puts it, "too many papers assume that a result found with 40 white undergraduates at a Midwestern university responding to instructions appearing on a computer screen in a small, windowless room would be affirmed if the participants were 50-year-old South Africans administered the same procedure by a neighbor in a large room in a familiar church in Capetown" (p. xvi). While many anthropologists (such as Shweder 1991) have, like Kagan, asked why, in order to try to understand humans, psychologists put people in labs where they act as little as possible like humans, relatively few contemporary psychologists have responded adequately to this challenge. Nevertheless, some of the most well-known psychological research focuses upon just such issues of context. For instance, the debates between personality and social psychologists on the relative importance for behavior of individual personality traits versus social context are well known (e.g., Feist and Feist 2009). As another example, in the famous Milgram obedience "shock" experiments, participant obedience varied significantly depending upon social context (such as location and type of the "mock" lab setting, the qualities and appearance of the researcher, and presence or absence of witnesses) (e.g., Blass 2000).

Problems with conventional, quantitative self-report measures in positive psychology become apparent when one considers several examples of societies which have reported high personal and society well-being. For instance, Kagan dramatically offers the examples of most Germans under Hitler, who he argues would have reported higher well-being after he came to power than before, when inflation was high. Another example he mentions are Southern plantation owners before the US Civil War, whose wealth and high social position would have led to high levels of well-being. Of course, from the point of view of Jews in the first case, and enslaved African-Americans in the second case, well-being was extremely low indeed. Thus, while group level data may suggest a happy society, significant individual differences are routinely overlooked by careless analysis and interpretation. Happy societies may mask unjust societies if only select self-reports – such as questionnaire data or memoirs written by a society's power elite – are examined. To further complicate matters, an implicit goal of much positive psychology writing seems to be that persons and societies aim "to be happy," but social science does not appear to have adequate evidence to suggest that such a goal is equally endorsed by all nations and groups around the globe and across history. Additionally, societal values range across place and time. As Kagan notes, moving from modern Mao to the Maya of Mesoamerica, one society may favor state loyalty over family loyalty, while another finds it is morally appropriate to make human sacrifice to appease gods in order to benefit the community (pp. 290–291). With such variation in goals, morals, and meanings, why should a quantitative self-report approach by (mostly Western) positive psychologists be privileged when nations and communities are ranked on well-being?

Due to such difficulties with self-reports of well-being, some scholars are beginning to react against recent suggestions that legislators and governments should rely on average citizen subjective well-being to evaluate a society's success, rather than conventional measures such as economic inequality, unemployment rates, physical health, and life expectancy. For instance, Kagan is one of a few psychologists who have come out in print to argue that "it will prove more useful to rely on the objective features of a society to figure out the meaning of the answers its citizens give" (p. xix). In contrast, Derek Bok, past president of Harvard, in *The Politics of Happiness* (2010), describes what he believes government can learn from the new well-being research being produced by psychologists and economists and seems to find a middle way between skeptics and true believers. Noting the example of tiny Bhutan, which has made "Gross National Happiness" a central aim of its public policy, Bok explores how contemporary happiness research may apply to government policy in the USA toward improving marriage, family, education, health, and other institutions and reducing financial hardship. Bok concludes with a politically moderate interpretation of the positive psychology research and its relevance to building positive institutions through legislation and government, writing that it is important to remind policy makers that despite some existing methodological issues with the new happiness research, utilizing this research is more reliable than such alternatives as anecdotes or listening to a single friend, colleague, constituent, or lobbyist. For instance, imagine one was attempting to understand happiness in Russia by listening to two of its greatest writers. Should one listen to Pushkin, who writes that we may never be happy since "all we have is duty," or to Tolstoy, who wrote that "all happy families are alike; every unhappy family is unhappy in its own way"? Social science offers a solution to such debates. In addition, unlike most positive psychologists, who may be focused more on pure research than on its application, social scientist and policy maker Bok is careful to note that legislators should promote well-being as experienced by constituents, not impose their own values by deciding what type of happiness or other quality their constituents should be seeking.

At any rate, one may better understand the limitations of self-reports when one considers a 2010 Gallup poll that found that Alaska was one of the five happiest states of the 50 US states (Kagan 2012, p. 115). While the telephone poll did not directly ask about subjective well-being, it did ask participants to self-report on their health, freedom from stress, satisfaction with their community, perceived physical safety at night, job satisfaction, and several other issues. Such self-reports take on new meaning, however, when compared to objective data about various social problems that plague Alaska, a largely rural state. As Rich (2010) documents, Alaska's suicide rate is consistently one of the highest in the USA. In 2002, Alaska had almost twice the national average of 10.6 suicides for every 100,000. Compared against the national average for six types of crimes, Alaska ranked 43rd among all 50 states. Since 1976, Alaska has ranked in the worst five states for its rate of reported rape. Substance and alcohol abuse also plague the state. Some polls listed the state as fifth worst in the nation for its assault rate. Alaska ranks among the worst five states for its domestic violence rate, with Alaskan women being killed by a partner at 1.5 times the national average. Other health problems impact the state. For instance, from 2000 to 2007, Alaska had the first- or second-highest nationwide chlamydia infection rate. Alaska's school dropout rate (8 %) was double the national average in 2005–2006. An Alaskan commission found that Alaska ranks 50th (last), in the number of ninth graders who will likely have a bachelor's degree in 10 years. Alaskans also face severe financial challenges. A poll of the ten most expensive cities in the USA listed three Alaskan cities: Anchorage, Fairbanks, and Juneau. Alaska leads all states with the highest median credit card debt, based on 2006 information. Finally, the climate greatly impacts the state. In addition to the snow and extreme temperatures, Alaska ranks number one in the USA for earthquakes. The Alaskan case, with its disparity between self-reports of high satisfaction and well-being, on the one hand, and objective data on poor economic, social, and health levels, on the other hand, clearly illustrates a number of the potential problems in understanding and interpreting positive psychology research. When working toward an understanding of Positive Nations and communities, conventional quantitative psychological techniques, such as self-report single-item questionnaires of one group, are insufficient. Examination of collective, qualitative, and culturally sensitive processes is a necessary supplement to the quantitative self-report approach. However, historically psychology has focused on individual quantitative approaches with samples drawn from the majority culture groups in the USA or Europe. One historian of psychology, in his book *Even the Rats Were White* (Guthrie 2003), even noted that not only has psychological research tended to focus on convenience samples of majority culture middle-class college-aged sophomores but much research aimed at illuminating human psychology has instead utilized nonhuman participants, such as lab rats. Such limited sampling from such limited contexts hardly yields research results that one may comfortably view as representative of the diversity of the human experience around the globe. The relative paucity of cross-national and cross-cultural positive psychology research is readily apparent in the available positive psychology textbooks (Rich 2011a). While there are some examples of positive psychology research programs that focus on cultural differences in well-being, such as folk theories or philosophies of happiness (e.g., Pflug 2009; Tiberius 2004; Uchida et al. 2004; Veenhoven 2012), it makes sense to look toward other disciplines for possible models, methods, and approaches that may serve an international positive psychology. Indeed recently, disciplines including economics, sociology, and management have taken a positive turn and focused energies on issues related to positive psychology, such as the recent volume *Happiness Across Cultures*, which brings all such scholars together (Selin and Davey 2012). Such books begin conversations between disciplines, even if many of the contributing chapters still strongly reflect a disciplinary origin, rather than a multidisciplinary sensibility.

In the past, like psychology, sociology and anthropology too, in their examination of the human condition, have focused on the negative aspects of societies and cultures that disable communities; here the focus has been on social problems (such as oppression and discrimination) and on maladaptive, troubled, sick societies rather than on societies and cultures that enable flourishing (e.g., Edgerton 1992). With few exceptions, such as investigations of "lost Edens," only recently have anthropologists begun to focus on the pursuit of happiness (e.g., Mathews and Izquierdo 2009). This chapter serves to bridge the psychological research in positive psychology on the individual, with insights from psychology and related disciplines that focus upon societal and cultural institutions at the group level, to explore how positive institutions may impact well-being through their effects on positive emotions, engagement, meaning, relationships, and accomplishment. These positive institutions include such units of analysis as the family, the school, the workplace, and religion, as well as other societal and cultural level virtues. A particular emphasis of this chapter is an examination of how conceptions of well-being may vary cross-culturally, creating theoretical and measurement challenges for an international positive psychology. Thus, relevant collective, qualitative, and culturally sensitive processes will be considered relative to positive psychology.

2.2   Methodological Considerations

An examination of positive psychology cross-nationally and cross-culturally raises a legion of methodological issues. While one aim of positive psychology's founders was to offer a more rigorous approach to strengths and virtues than had been offered by humanistic psychologists in the middle of the twentieth century (Seligman and Csikszentmihalyi 2000), in practice the response to this call has been met with quantitative analysis, rather than with qualitative and other empirical work. Such a situation presents a number of challenges to a successful international positive psychology, a number of which are explored in this chapter section.

While positive psychologists have assessed a number of concepts, perhaps the most frequently examined one has been well-being/happiness/life satisfaction (Eid and Larsen 2008). Yet as Oishi (2010) correctly points out, though "many scales have been developed to assess different aspects of well-being, three types of single-item measures have dominated large scale international surveys on well-being" (p. 34), including a general life satisfaction item, a Cantril's Ladder item (the participant ranks self on an imaginary ladder), and a happiness item. Oishi examines three issues relevant to the international positive psychology of well-being, namely, historical and cultural differences in concepts of well-being, measurement issues, and issues regarding interpretations of national differences in well-being.

The issue of whether or not the concept of well-being varies cross-nationally is an important one, for a number of reasons, including the possibility that researchers fail to ask the right questions if they do not understand how a person or culture conceptualizes well-being. For instance, will a single-item assessment of well-being accurately assess the five happinesses described by Asianist Chavannes (1922/1973) in his examination of Chinese art-long life, wealth, tranquility, love of virtue, and death only after achieving one's destiny? While the idea that conceptions of emotions and psychological states and traits may vary widely across cultures is well documented by psychological anthropologists (e.g., Shweder 1991), positive psychologists have been slow to examine such differences. Even within a culture or society, changes in the concept of happiness may be seen over time, as historian Darrin McMahon (2006) has documented in detail, in his examination of the concept of happiness in (mostly) Western traditions, from ancient Greece (focus on virtue) to early Christians (focus on the afterlife), to the Enlightenment (focus on natural right), and beyond. Oishi (2010) has examined the evolution of the concept of well-being in English alone, documenting changes from the word's appearance in 1530, as reported in the Oxford English Dictionary. In an analysis of the term in the USA, including examinations of the word in the US presidential addresses since the 1790s, Oishi traces the change in meaning of the concept from connotations implying luck, to connotations suggesting satisfactions of desire, to modern connotations of pleasure and enjoyment.

Different conceptualizations of well-being may be linked to different expressions of it and to different display rules cross-nationally. For instance, if a culture views happiness as stemming from luck, then social convention may indicate that overt, extended displays of happiness are not warranted, whereas if a culture views happiness as stemming from hard work and initiative, it may be considered more socially appropriate to display happiness. As Oishi (2010) notes, such varied conceptualizations have a significant impact on survey results, such as a Gallup poll question asking participants whether they smiled a lot on the previous day. While smiles may be universal, their meaning, causes, and consequences may not. For instance, Colson (2012, p. 8) writes that her fieldwork in Zambia indicates that the Tonga say one "cannot know what someone feels or thinks from facial expression." Similarly, cultural differences in self-presentation and well-being may result from differences in reference group. When making judgments about well-being, some groups may compare themselves only to others in the same local community, state, or nation, while other groups may compare themselves to a broader reference group internationally. For instance, anthropologist Karen Kramer (2005) conducted longitudinal fieldwork among the Yucatec Maya of Mexico over a decade from 1992 to 2003. She notes that while by objective, national standards these Maya were poor when she began her fieldwork, she only heard Maya self-report feeling that they were poor, in her more recent years of fieldwork in 2003, and she attributes this difference to a change in reference group in the two time periods. In the early period, the Maya often simply compared themselves to other Maya in this relatively difficult to reach small rural village. By her later fieldwork, however, many Maya had begun to leave the village for seasonal wage-labor work in large cities such as Cancún, where they experienced their income disparity acutely and shared their experiences upon their return to the village. In addition, as television became available in the small village after electricity lines were built in the late 1990s, the villagers watched advertisements routinely depicting wealth, new products, and new lifestyles that had seemed much more remote to many in past generations. Such an experience is not unique to the Maya. As economist Carol Graham (2009) notes, once poor, rural Chinese migrate to urban areas, they begin to compare themselves to other urban dwellers, rather than to villagers from their old communities, and they experience less happiness with their material condition, even though they are better off materially than they were previous to the migration (p. 154). Oishi (2010) describes such reference group effects as "a serious threat to international comparisons on self-reports of well-being" (p. 51).

While psychometricians are well aware that assessment may be impacted by such factors as item order, item use, and item function, as well as temporary, current mood, positive psychologists have been slow to implement this knowledge in cross-national positive psychology research. Yet such factors may have a significant impact, as existing, within-nation research indicates. For instance, Marín and Marín (1991) find US Hispanics tend to use the higher and lower ends of questionnaire items as opposed to the middle, in comparison with non-Hispanic US Caucasians. Clearly such a response style, as well as other potential cultural variants, such as yeah versus nay sayers, has tremendous implications for well-being research and interpretation of scaled items, such as the Cantril Ladder or Likert-style subjective well-being and life satisfaction scales. Likewise, response and attrition rates vary within nation by religion, ethnicity, and race (e.g., Marín and Marín 1991; Schmidt and Rich 2000), and this reality often leads to underrepresentation or non-representation of various groups. For instance, in experience sampling method research with a national US sample by Schmidt and Rich (2000), despite efforts at correction, Latino, African-American, and Native youth were often under-sampled with this time intensive research tool. Internationally, similar effects may occur. For instance, one may predict that attrition or low participation rates may be especially likely to occur in authoritarian or so-called police states, in regions of political turmoil or violence, or among groups, such as isolated, rural peoples, with little experience with academic research or with filling out questionnaires. Thus, broad, sweeping reports of national differences, for instance, may obscure important differences between nations and groups that involve subgroups or subcultures, such as minority religious, linguistic, or ethnic groups.

Finally, it is worth noting that the desirability of happiness, life satisfaction, well-being, and other positive psychology strengths may vary cross-nationally. In their handbook, Peterson and Seligman (2004) offer an extensive classification of character strengths and virtues, including six broad strengths: wisdom/knowledge, courage, humanity, justice, temperance, and transcendence. Importantly, however, one nation or group may value some strengths and virtues more highly than others (e.g., Park et al. 2006). For instance, whereas one nation or group may rate creativity, love of learning, and curiosity as its most highly prized qualities, these same qualities may be seen as less desirable than bravery, social intelligence, and spirituality in another nation or group. Simplistic quantitative analysis and correlational matrices will be unlikely to illuminate the rich complexity and interrelationships between the countless variables in sociocultural context. The situation becomes even more challenging to the quantitative paradigm when group level rather than individual level concepts are examined, such as positive institutions, including families, schools, workplaces, and communities.

2.3   What Anthropology May Offer International Positive Psychology

Qualitative methods, such as the fieldwork, interviews, and participant observation, common in anthropology, offer an excellent supplement to the quantitative tools common in much psychology research. The rich, thick description offered through fieldwork and ethnography seems tailor-made for culturally sensitive investigation of collective processes of Positive Nations and communities.

The difficulty is that until quite recently, anthropologists have been even less involved in the scholarly examination of human strengths and virtues than psychologists. Additionally, in many nations, the two disciplines rarely communicate or collaborate with each other. While in the 1920s and 1930s, work by anthropologists engaged with the culture and personality movement, such as Margaret Mead and Ruth Benedict, attracted the attention of many anthropologists as well as social scientists and the general public, such multidisciplinary work by psychological anthropologists and cultural psychologists (intellectual heirs to Mead and Benedict) seems to have become more marginalized for a number of decades, at least until recently. (Note that in the USA, exceptions may include the Society for Psychological Anthropology and the Society for Cross-Cultural Research.) Anthropologist Anthony Paredes recently reported that a search of the AnthroSource database "produced only two hits on 'happiness' in all of AAA's 22 publications from 1930 to 2010… zero hits for 'life satisfaction,' three for 'optimism,' and three for 'job satisfaction'" (2012, p. 5). Similarly, anthropologist Scott Clark (2009) conducted a keyword search of the eHRAF (Human Relations Area Files) for the word pleasure coded as a drive or emotion and found only 135 matches, while a similar search of the Anthropology Index online found only 39 matches (p. 208). Thin (2009) adds that reference books and introductory textbooks on anthropology (including psycho-logical anthropology texts) "typically have no entries on happiness or well-being" (p. 27). Paredes adds that "happiness is seldom thought of as a researchable topic for anthropologists," and he and other anthropologists have noted the discipline has more typically focused upon human misery and suffering. As Johnston (2012) notes, "an engaged anthropology of trouble is a dominant concern in the discipline" (p. 6), as anthropology focuses on maladaptation, "trouble" such as the Fukushima nuclear meltdown, and "sick societies" such as those described by Edgerton (1992).

Why have anthropologists not studied well-being? The situation perhaps is sur-prising, given that no less an authority on fieldwork than Malinowski (1922/1978) wrote decades ago that "the goal [of ethnography] … is, briefly, to grasp the native's point of view; his relation to life, to realize his vision of his world…what concerns him most intimately… In each culture the values are slightly different; people aspire to different aims, follow different impulses, yearn after a different form of happiness. To study the institutions, customs, and codes or to study the behavior and mentality without the subjective desire of feeling by what these people live, or realizing the substance of their happiness…is… to miss the greatest reward which we can hope to obtain from the study of man." Thin (2009), however, suggests several reasons for the paucity of research in the anthropology discipline: (1) a relativist bias against evaluation and comparison, (2) a pathological/clinical bias and focus on suffering and a view that well-being was assumed as the default state, (3) a cognitivist/social constructivist bias that often viewed social construction as a replacement for biology rather than a complement to that approach, and (4) an anti-utilitarian/anti-hedonic bias. As he notes, "any discipline reluctant to study normality is going to have trouble studying well-being. It is this institutionalized incapacity that bedevils anthropology. It detracts from our relevance to the real world, and from our claims to scientific rigor" (p. 25).

Nevertheless, several recent publications in anthropology aim to offer a cor-rective. Colby (2009) argues that anthropology may be at a tipping point for the investigation of cultural well-being, and that the "zeitgeist is calling for it" and some anthropologists are responding (p. 55). The March 2012 issue of *Anthropology News*, a publication of the American Anthropological Association (AAA), features a series of articles on the theme, "health, well-being, and happiness." Likewise, a special section of the March 2012 issue of *American Anthropologist,* a major AAA journal, is devoted to a vital topics forum on happiness, with a half dozen articles on the subject guest edited by Barbara Rose Johnston. Finally, Mathews and Izquierdo's edited volume *Pursuits of Happiness* (2009) is subtitled "well-being in anthropological perspective," reflecting its focus relevant to international positive psychology.

What are some issues that anthropologists have with the examination of psychological states of well-being? One is skepticism of psychological assessments. Cross-cultural surveys of subjective well-being do not let participants speak in their own words, and by requiring closed-ended responses, much culture-specific content may be missed (Mathews and Izquierdo 2009, p. 7). Thus, for instance, anthropologist Colson (2012, pp. 7–8) writes that "over 50 years ago I wrote, 'We cannot measure or record happiness.' Over the years I have changed my mind about many things but not about this." She notes that the term happiness is ambiguous in English and that greater ambiguity "is introduced when we try to translate and create a happiness scale for those who speak different languages and have their own categories of emotional responses and then attempt to use such a scale to examine the benefits of given changes." Other anthropologists argue that happiness can be measured, though alternative scales and assessments should be developed and utilized to access conceptualizations of well-being that vary considerably cross-nationally and cross-culturally. For instance, Wali (2012, pp. 12–13) proposes several alternative measures of happiness based upon her experience. First, she notes that for forest dwellers in Amazonia, well-being "must include assessment of the balance between humans, other life forms, and supernatural beings, and a moral dimension that regulates relationships, especially across generations." Then she offers an example from urban Chicago, where for some people, well-being "entails freedom from work regimens (time flexibility)" and thus "people choose to earn less income to have more control over time." Finally, she notes creatively decorated products, such as pottery, spears, and baskets from around the globe, which are often produced by objectively poor people in poor nations. Wali argues that such products demonstrate humans' "irrepressible force of desire for dignity no matter what material circumstances" and that social scientists, such as psychologists and economists, perhaps ought to develop a "'dignity index' as an alternative to measuring well-being."

How may anthropologists add to the content of an international positive psychology? While anthropologists are often skeptical of proposing cultural universals (though see Brown 1991), documenting well-being as it is conceptualized cross-culturally has led anthropologist Thin (2009) to propose three basic assumptions about attitudes to well-being that may have universal validity. He argues that (1) "in all cultures, most people most of the time want to feel good and want to make other people with whom they empathize feel good" (p. 31); (2) all cultures distinguish "feeling well" from living a good, moral life; and (3) "all core moral codes…endorse the idea that it is better in principle… to try to help other people feel well and lead a good life than to try to make other people feel bad and live a bad life" (p. 31). Mathews and Izquierdo (2009) also see human universals in the "pursuit of well-being, that come to the fore differently in different societies and different social contexts but that are present in every society" (p. 254). For these authors (1) human beings need the support of their human world, often their family; (2) human beings also tend to seek freedom from coercive control; and (3) human beings also need a sense of life being worth living in a given society. If confirmed by further research, such documentation of human universals by anthropologists has significant implications for understanding positive institutions, communities, and nations. Of course anthropologists are well known, indeed better known, for documenting diverse variation around the globe, and Thin (2009) also offers a helpful list of several ways that individuals, communities, and cultures vary across several dimensions relevant to well-being. For instance, he argues that the anthropological record notes significant cross-cultural variation in (1) the degree of emphasis on hedonism (e.g., pleasure) versus meaning (e.g., value meaningful life), (2) the relative role of happiness as life purpose as opposed to other candidates for life purpose (e.g., knowledge, religious merit, or virtue), (3) the degree of deferment of well-being accepted (e.g., want to feel happy now vs. willing to defer happiness to later or to the afterlife), (4) the means by which happiness can and/or should be achieved, (5) the norms for display of well-being (e.g., is it appropriate to be happy at a wedding, funeral, or wake?), and (6) the degree to which personal well-being is seen as dependent upon others' well-being (e.g., individualistic cultures vs. collectivistic cultures).

2.4 Mixed Methods and Internationalizing Positive Psychology

While it is clear that anthropology and qualitative methods may add significantly to the examination of collective and culturally sensitive processes in positive psychology, the discipline and the method are not a substitute for more typical quantitative psychology. Rather such an approach offers an important supplement to the quantitative approach, and a few anthropologists and psychologists are realizing the advantages of putting aside any existing disciplinary turf wars and biases to combine the strengths of both disciplines and methods when conducting research on well-being. For instance, Colby (2009) writes "why can't statistics and network analyses be interlarded with a more humanized, contextual approach as well? We can use the numbers and interpersonal network relations as a guide for open-ended questions to ask some of the subjects themselves. Oral narrative, distributional analyses, statistical approaches and network analyses need not to be, mutually exclusive with traditional contextualized, ethnography" (p. 50). He further notes that "anthropology will require many perspectives, methods, and interdisciplinary contacts to meet the unprecedented challenges that lie in our future. Fresh new approaches will be needed. Yet within the discipline it is rare to find answers to this call" (p. 47). Colby writes that to understand well-being, anthropology must set aside such binary either-or, exclusionary contrasts as "theory versus description, questionnaires versus interviewing, testing versus think description, single cultural unit description versus cross-cultural comparison" (p. 47). Anthropologists Mathews and Izquierdo (2009) add that it is possible to make a comparison of different societies as to well-being, as long as this is done in a careful, culturally sensitive way. They note that "this can be done through what we… term *soft comparison*, comparison based not on- or at least not solely on- bald statistics placed side by side, but rather on all the nuances of sociocultural context ethnographically portrayed" (p. 6). They conclude their seminal book on anthropological approaches to well-being by writing that "most of the authors in [the] book, including we who edit it, believe that statistical measures of well-being are not inherently flawed, but they are incomplete (just as ethnographies themselves can have lacunae and interpretive idiosyncrasies). Only a detailed on-the-ground ethnography can provide the social and cultural context, without which, well-being, in a given society cannot be fully understood" (p. 250).

A few anthropologists have begun to venture into mixed-method research on well-being such as suggested above. Psychological anthropologist Thomas Weisner (2009) examined well-being in families in the USA with disabled children, utilizing both survey instruments and ethnographic interviews over the course of a decade. However, his research was the only contribution to the Mathews and Izquierdo book to do so, and he was the only author there to focus not on the individual basis, but instead on the collective basis of the social construction of well-being, by utilizing the family, not person, as the unit of analysis. Weisner's approach is a welcome complement to the cross-cultural psychological approach to quality of life in persons with disabilities around the globe adopted by a volume edited by two psychologists (Keith and Schlock 2000), which, while helpful, often relies more exclusively on quantitative surveys. Another recent project by anthropologists demonstrates a mixed methods approach to well-being. García-Quijano et al. (2012) investigated coastal resource use, quality of life, and well-being in Puerto Rico. The message of García-Quijano and his coauthors is that "quality of life, well-being, success, and other related constructs represent complex phenomena, influenced by multiple factors that interact with one another in multiple ways. Thus, ethnography and actual fieldwork is crucial to assess the actual ways these factors combine in ways that are relevant to local people" (p. 6). These authors note that they have engaged early on with the relevant literature in psychology and economics on assessment of well-being (such as the satisfaction with life scale) and that these measures are "proving useful for comparative purposes and we are using modified versions of some of these measures in the more quantitative survey components of our research. However, without good old-fashioned ethnography, we would have missed key elements, of what constitutes quality of life/well-being for people, in our study's region and of the relationships between coastal resource use and quality of life/well-being" (p. 6).

Like anthropologists, several psychologists have begun to utilize mixed methods in their examinations of positive psychology concepts. While it is still true that the majority of psychological research, especially in the USA, employs a quantitative bias, some psychologists have, of course, employed qualitative methods, including interviews, case studies, biographical materials, and historical document analysis. With some exceptions (e.g., Delle Fave et al. 2011a), this quantitative trend in psychology in general holds true for positive psychology in particular as well, as indicated by the contributions to a seminal book *Positive Psychological Assessment* (Lopez and Snyder 2003), which includes chapters on a range of assessments of human cognitive, emotional, interpersonal, and religious strengths.

However, to offer one example of a mixed methods approach by psychologists to a positive psychological concept related to well-being, one may look to the work of Csikszentmihalyi and colleagues on flow (e.g., Csikszentmihalyi 1990, 1996; Rich 2013). Flow is a concept that aims to define a "state of optimal experience that people report when they are intensely involved in doing something that is fun to do" (2000a, p. 381). The concept has been examined with fieldwork and interviews as well as with surveys and questionnaires, and unlike many positive psychological concepts, it has been studied in many nations, communities, and cultures (Delle Fave et al. 2011b). Indeed, based on research around the globe into the concept, Csikszentmihalyi (2000b) writes that the flow experience of enjoyment is described essentially the same way by Southeast Asian villagers, on farms in Somalia, by Navajo community members, and by industrial workers in Japan, Europe, and the USA (p. 389). Other researchers have examined flow in Taiwanese white water rafters, Dutch soccer players, and Canadian ice hockey players (Rich 2013). Additionally, the flow experience has been documented in a range of populations and contexts and at a range of levels from the biological (e.g., Dietrich 2004) to the psychological to the sociocultural, thus addressing some of the valid concerns about the need for contextualization and for a range of types of evidence in psychological research raised by Kagan (2012). Flow also has been examined in collective processes, both on smaller scales, such as in improvisational musical groups (Rich 2011b), and on larger scales, as in sociocultural and historical processes, such as the cultural evolution in complexity described in Csikszentmihalyi's (1993) discussions of such positive communities as the art worlds of Renaissance Florence or nineteenth-century Paris or ancient Athens. While there is considerable agreement about the core dimensions of flow, especially the cognitive aspects such as deep concentration and absorption, there is some variation with the emotional component, such as feeling happy/enjoyment, and often the enjoyment is reported after the end of the flow experience and not during activities such as school or work – the so-called flow paradox (e.g., Cskszentmihalyi and LeFevre 1989; Delle Fave and Massimini 2005; Rich 2013).

A major contribution of Csikszentmihalyi to the multimodal, mixed method approach to positive psychology has been his development of the experience sampling method (ESM), which combines semi-structured and open-ended interviews with quantitative survey and questionnaire techniques with more experience-near, context-sensitive capabilities than is typical of conventional psychological assessments (e.g., Csikszentmihalyi 1990). Research participants are provided with some type of alarm pager (such as a programmable watch or smart phone) and signaled at preprogrammed times to complete a brief questionnaire about the moment they were paged. Next they respond to questions about their moods, motivations, and cognitions, the activity they were doing, and their physical (and social) surroundings.

Typically the pager is programmed to beep up to a dozen times per day for a week, and a rich collection of experienced life results, leading toward development of a systematic phenomenology of many aspects of life as lived in the real world beyond the psychologist's laboratory. The ESM allows for everyday events and experiences to be reported in a much more naturalistic setting than a laboratory experience permits, allowing a real-world ecological validity that is often impossible in an artificial lab setting.

While the experience sampling method is still vulnerable to a number of the disadvantages present in all self-report measures, such as single-administration questionnaires, its sensitivity to cultural and collective processes renders it a valuable tool for psychologists exploring well-being. As with much anthropological work, which is known for its sensitivity to local knowledge and context, Csikszentmihalyi's work with the ESM, with its blending of quantitative and qualitative approaches, as well as other recent research aimed at contextualizing well-being (e.g., McNulty and Fincham 2012), offers a powerful response to Kagan's call for more contextualized research in positive psychology. The ESM has been utilized successfully to examine both individual well-being as well as collective processes such as couples' well-being (Graham 2008) and family well-being (Larson and Richards 1995), as group members' ESM responses can be compared across diverse contexts. Beyond basic research, the implications of such a technique to promote positive institutions are profound. Sample possible applications may include utilizing the assessment as a tool for counseling couples or families, for promoting optimal performance in athletic teams or musical groups, or for enhancing the group experience in classrooms and workplaces.

2.5 Conclusion

In the decade since its inception, positive psychology has grown at a dramatic pace. Yet like much of psychology, it has focused on the individual to the relative neglect of the group, community, culture, and nation. In addition, as with its individual focus, psychology's narrow emphasis on quantitative methods has limited the discipline's ability to fully understand Positive Nations and communities. By utilizing insights, evidence, and methods of related disciplines, such as anthropology, and by embracing the strengths of qualitative and mixed methods approaches to the examination of well-being, positive psychology can continue to mature. Broadening positive psychology to allow it to build upon insights from others seems to reflect a constructive approach in keeping with the spirit and mission of the original Akumal Manifesto written at the birth of the discipline. If positive psychology aims to be more than merely an intellectual exercise, it must ultimately move beyond measurement and description, and understanding and prediction, to application. Policy makers now are beginning to see how positive psychology may transform communities and nations around the globe.

References

Blass, T. (Ed.). (2000). *Obedience to authority: Current perspectives on the Milgram paradigm.* Mahwah: Lawrence Erlbaum Associates, Inc.

Bok, D. (2010). *The politics of happiness: What government can learn from the new research on well-being.* Princeton: Princeton University Press.

Brown, D. E. (1991). *Human universals.* Philadelphia: Temple University Press.

Chavannes, E. (1973). *The five happinesses: Symbolism in Chinese popular art.* New York: Weatherhill. (Original work published 1922)

Christopher, J. C., Richardson, F. C., & Slife, B. D. (2008). [Special issue]. *Theory and Psychology, 18*(5).

Clark, S. (2009). Pleasure experienced. In C. Mathews & C. Izquierdo (Eds.), *Pursuits of happiness* (pp. 189–210). New York: Berghahn Books.

Colby, B. N. (2009). Is a measure of cultural well-being possible or desirable? In C. Mathews & C. Izquierdo (Eds.), *Pursuits of happiness* (pp. 45–64). New York: Berghahn Books.

Colson, E. (2012). Happiness. *American Anthropologist, 114*(1), 7–9.

Csikszentmihalyi, M. (1990). *Flow: The psychology of optimal experience.* New York: Harper & Row.

Csikszentmihalyi, M. (1993). *The evolving self.* New York: Harper Collins.

Csikszentmihalyi, M. (1996). *Creativity.* New York: Harper Collins.

Csikszentmihalyi, M. (2000a). Flow. In A. E. Kazdin (Ed.), *Encyclopedia of psychology* (Vol. 3, pp. 381–382). Washington, DC: Oxford University Press.

Csikszentmihalyi, M. (2000b). The contribution of flow to positive psychology. In J. E. Gillham (Ed.), *The science of hope and optimism* (pp. 387–395). Philadelphia: Templeton Foundation Press.

Cskszentmihalyi, M., & LeFevre, J. (1989). Optimal experience in work and leisure. *Journal of Personality and Social Psychology, 56*, 815–822.

Delle Fave, A., & Massimini, F. (2005). The investigation of optimal experience and apathy: Developmental and psychosocial implications. *European Psychologist, 10*, 264–274.

Delle Fave, A., Brdar, I., Freire, T., Vella-Brodrick, D., & Wissing, M. (2011a). The eudaimonic and hedonic components of happiness: Qualitative and quantitative findings. *Social Indicators Research, 100*, 158–207.

Delle Fave, A., Massimini, F., & Bassi, M. (2011b). *Psychological selection and optimal experience across cultures: Social empowerment through personal growth.* Dordrecht: Springer.

Dietrich, A. (2004). Neurocognitive mechanisms underlying the experience of flow. *Consciousness and Cognition, 13*, 746–761.

Edgerton, R. B. (1992). *Sick societies.* New York: Free Press.

Ehrenreich, B. (2009). *Bright-sided: How the relentless promotion of positive thinking has undermined America.* New York: Metropolitan Books Henry Holt and Company.

Eid, M., & Larsen, R. J. (2008). *The science of subjective well-being.* New York: Guilford Press.

Feist, J., & Feist, G. J. (2009). *Theories of personality.* Boston: McGraw Hill.

García-Quijano, C., Poggie, J. J., Pitchon, A., & Del Pozo, M. (2012). Investigating coastal resource use, quality of life, and well-being in southeastern Puerto Rico. *Anthropology News, 53*(3), 6–7.

Graham, J. M. (2008). Self-expansion and flow in couples' momentary experiences. *Journal of Personality and Social Psychology, 95*(3), 679–694.

Graham, C. (2009). *Happiness around the world: The paradox of happy peasants and miserable millionaires.* New York: Oxford University Press.

Guthrie, R. V. (2003). *Even the rat was white* (2nd ed.). Boston: Allyn & Bacon.

Johnston, B. R. (Ed.). (2012). Vital topics forum: On happiness. *American Anthropologist, 114*, 6–18.

Kagan, J. (2012). *Psychology's ghosts.* New Haven: Yale University Press.

Keith, K. D., & Schlock, R. L. (2000). *Cross-cultural perspectives on quality of life.* Washington, DC: American Association on Mental Retardation.

Kramer, K. (2005). *Maya children: Helpers at the farm.* Cambridge, MA: Harvard University Press.

Larson, R., & Richards, M. (1995). *Divergent realities.* New York: Basic Books.

Lopez, S. J. (Ed.). (2009). *The encyclopedia of positive psychology*. Malden: Wiley-Blackwell.

Lopez, S. J., & Snyder, C. R. (Eds.). (2003). *Positive psychological assessment*. Washington, DC: American Psychological Association.

Lopez, S. J., & Snyder, C. R. (Eds.). (2009). *Oxford handbook of positive psychology* (2nd ed.). New York: Oxford University Press.

Malinowski, B. (1978). *Argonauts of the Western Pacific*. London: Routledge. (Original work published 1922)

Marín, G., & Marín, B. V. (1991). *Research with Hispanic populations*. Thousand Oaks: Sage.

Mathews, G., & Izquierdo, C. (Eds.). (2009). *Pursuits of happiness: Well-being in anthropological perspective*. New York: Berghahn Books.

McMahon, D. (2006). *Happiness: A history*. New York: Grove.

McNulty, J. K., & Fincham, F. D. (2012). Beyond positive psychology? Toward a contextual view of psychological processes and well-being. *American Psychologist, 67*, 101–110.

Myers, D. (2000). Hope and happiness. In J. E. Gillham (Ed.), *The science of optimism and hope* (pp. 323–336). Philadelphia: Templeton Foundation Press.

Oishi, S. (2010). Culture and well-being: Conceptual and methodological issues. In E. Diener, J. F. Helliwell, & D. Kahneman (Eds.), *International differences in well-being* (pp. 34–69). New York: Oxford University Press.

Paredes, J. A. (2012, March). In focus: Health, well-being, and happiness. *Anthropology News, 53*, 5–14.

Park, N., Peterson, C., & Seligman, M. E. P. (2006). Character strengths in fifty-four nations and the fifty US states. *The Journal of Positive Psychology, 1*, 118–129.

Peterson, C., & Seligman, M. E. P. (2004). *Character strengths and virtues*. Oxford: Oxford University Press.

Pflug, J. (2009). Folk theories of happiness: A cross-cultural comparison of conceptions of happiness in Germany and South Africa. *Social Indicators Research, 92*(3), 551–563.

Rich, G. (2010). *The state of psychology in Alaska*. Paper presented at the meeting of the International Congress of Applied Psychology, Melbourne.

Rich, G. (2011a). Teaching tools for positive psychology: A comparison of available textbooks. *The Journal of Positive Psychology, 6*(6), 492–498.

Rich, G. (2011b). *The flow experience in jazz pianists*. Paper presented at the meeting of the American Anthropological Association, Psychological Anthropology Section, Montreal.

Rich, G. (2013). Flow and positive psychology. In J. Sinnott (Ed.), *Positive psychology and adult motivation*. New York: Springer.

Schmidt, J., & Rich, G. (2000). Images of work and play. In M. Csikszentmihalyi & B. Schneider (Eds.), *Becoming adult: How teenagers prepare for the world of work* (pp. 67–94). New York: Basic Books.

Seligman, M. E. P. (2011). *Flourish: A visionary new understanding of happiness and well-being*. New York: Free Press.

Seligman, M. E. P., & Csikszentmihalyi, M. (2000). Positive psychology: An introduction. *American Psychologist, 55*, 5–14.

Selin, H., & Davey, G. (Eds.). (2012). *Happiness across cultures*. New York: Springer.

Shweder, R. (1991). *Thinking through cultures*. Cambridge, MA: Harvard University Press.

Thin, N. (2009). Why anthropology can ill afford to ignore well-being. In C. Mathews & C. Izquierdo (Eds.), *Pursuits of happiness* (pp. 23–44). New York: Berghahn Books.

Tiberius, V. (2004). Cultural differences and philosophical accounts of well-being. *Journal of Happiness Studies, 5*, 293–314.

Uchida, Y., Norasakkunkit, V., & Kitayama, S. (2004). Cultural constructions of happiness: Theory and empirical evidence. *Journal of Happiness Studies, 5*, 223–239.

Veenhoven, R. (2012). *World database of happiness*. Erasmus University, Rotterdam. Retrieved from: http://worlddatabaseofhappiness.eur.nl

Wali, A. (2012). A different measure of well-being. *American Anthropologist, 114*, 1.

Weisner, T. S. (2009). Well-being and sustainability of daily routines. In C. Mathews & C. Izquierdo (Eds.), *Pursuits of happiness* (pp. 228–247). New York: Berghahn Books.

Wilson, E. G. (2008). *Against happiness*. New York: Farrar, Straus, and Giroux.

Part II
Display of Psychological Attributes:
From Personal to Social

Chapter 3
The Altruism Spiral: An Integrated Model for a Harmonious Future

Lawrence Soosai Nathan and Antonella Delle Fave

3.1 Introduction

This chapter aims at providing a brief overview of the prominent conceptualisations of altruism, a construct widely debated from various theoretical perspectives, ranging from evolutionary biology to social psychology, philosophy and – more recently – positive psychology, but still controversial in its definition and role in human affairs. Moving from the current scientific debate, as well as delving into Western and Eastern philosophical and spiritual traditions, we attempt to build an integrated approach to the study of altruism based on the view of a substantial interconnectedness among individuals, rather than on the juxtaposition between altruism and selfishness. Within this model, altruism is defined as a general mind-set, characterised by a concern for others' welfare that implies a readiness to engage in other-oriented behaviours, bringing welfare to the agent as well. Altruism's behavioural outcomes, benefits and dangers, as well as the challenges people and communities face in cultivating and promoting an altruistic mind-set are briefly outlined.

3.2 Conceptualising Altruism: The State of the Art

What is altruism? This apparently simple question does not seem to have an indisputable answer. Altruism remains an elusive concept, even though it has been extensively explored within human sciences, such as philosophy, religion and ethics

L.S. Nathan (✉)
Department of Psychology, Anugraha Institute of Social Sciences (M.K University),
University of Milano, Milan, Italy
e-mail: lalacaps@yahoo.com

A. Delle Fave
Department of Pathophysiology and Transplantation, University of Milano,
via Francesco Sforza 35, 20122 Milan, Italy
e-mail: antonella.dellefave@unimi.it

H. Águeda Marujo and L.M. Neto (eds.), *Positive Nations and Communities*, Cross-Cultural   35
Advancements in Positive Psychology 6, DOI 10.1007/978-94-007-6869-7_3,
© Springer Science+Business Media Dordrecht 2014

(Wilson 1992; Uyenoyama and Feldman 1992; Simon 1993). Due to the varied and often contradictory perspectives, jargons like 'altruism debate' or 'altruism confusion' are often found in literature (Kerr et al. 2004; Piliavin and Charng 1990). We therefore consider the 'altruism debate' as an ideal point of departure for an exploration of this elusive topic.

3.2.1 Evolutionary Biology and the Altruism Debate

Evolutionary biology is credited to have initiated the scientific exploration of altruism, otherwise a topic of religion and ethics. However, its assumptions have become the primary source of a heated debate around altruism. Does altruism exist? Is it natural to living organisms? Within evolutionary biology, two contending positions have been developed: the egotism-altruism hypothesis and the empathy-altruism hypothesis (Piliavin and Charng 1990). Based on the Darwinian concepts of fitness and self-preservation instinct, the egotism-altruism hypothesis denies the existence of altruism in living organism. Since genes are essentially replicators and are transmitted by means of individuals' selective survival strategies, they can only be 'selfish' and not otherwise (Dawkins 1989). Altruism defined as a behaviour that simultaneously entails fitness costs to the agent and fitness benefits to the receiver is not possible (Kerr et al. 2004). Evolutionary behaviours that apparently benefit others are primarily adaptive strategies to satisfy one's needs, for example, the reduction of aversive arousal caused by seeing the suffering of others. The selfish nature of genes makes altruism not just counterintuitive but even detrimental to the actor (Simon 1993). Altruism is therefore, nothing but a myth (Dawkins 1989).

The empathy-altruism hypothesis (Batson 1991), on the contrary, acknowledges the existence of altruism in evolution based on the 'alarm-calling behaviour' (Colman 1982; Sherman 1985; Batson et al. 2008). Supported by research on mirror neurons (Rizzolatti and Craighero 2004), altruistic genes (Nedelcu and Michod 2006), sterile workers (Okasha 2005) and toddlers' social interaction patterns (Zahn-Waxler et al. 1991), altruism is proved to be natural to living organisms. Within this framework, empathy, defined as other-oriented emotional reaction to a needy neighbour, is considered a possible indicator of altruism (Batson et al. 2008; Piliavin and Charng 1990). Notwithstanding the scientific efforts of evolutionary biologists, the unresolved debate between these contending hypotheses leaves altruism still clouded with confusion. Is altruism natural to living organism or is it a myth? The debate itself seems self-contradictory, since selfish genes actually end up in serving the body, leading to the claim that genes must be altruistic rather than selfish. However, when biologists speak of selfish or altruistic behaviour, they refer to gene fitness and not to human motivations. In fact, the alleged dichotomy between selfish and altruistic genes is based on the ambiguous use of anthropomorphic terms to describe evolving genes, thus leading into a blind alley (Barash 2007).

3.2.2 The Perspective of Social Psychology

From a different perspective, social psychology contributed to the altruism debate, arguing that human beings are not just passive vehicles of fitness seeking genes but have a unique capacity to actively choose and direct their lives according to intentional motives (Jablonka and Lamb 2005). These motives – rather than fitness effects – represent the core criterion to evaluate altruism (Wilson 1992). A behaviour undertaken voluntarily and intentionally, with the sole goal of benefiting another person without expecting any external reward, is defined as altruistic (Piliavin and Charng 1990). An act becomes egoistic or altruistic on the basis of the motive – sole goal of benefiting other or not. Various studies were conducted to investigate the altruistic personality (Aronoff and Wilson 1984; Oliner and Oliner 1988), the developmental dynamics of altruism (Chambers and Ascione 1987) and its situational determinants and benefits (Latane et al. 1981; Shotland and Stebbins 1983). Motivations – the latent variable – were inferred through the assessment of prosocial behaviour, the observable variable.

Far from being resolved, within social psychology, the altruism debate continued, though with a change in focus from the existence of altruism (is there?) to criteria of altruism (what makes it?). 'Sole goal of benefiting another person' became the point of contention. A person can engage in prosocial behaviour for purely altruistic motives or for selfish motives such as to win prestige, respect, friendship and other social and psychological objectives (Andreoni 1990). Is it really possible to draw a clear distinction between purely altruistic or selfish actions? Every helping act has some remote self-benefits such as reciprocity, appreciation and feeling good about oneself (Schwartz 1992). Can some forms of self-benefit render an altruistic act to be egotistic? Given the difficulty in identifying benefit to others as the sole goal of an action (Nisbett and Wilson 1977), the proportions of observable benefits for the receiver and the agent were used to differentiate purely selfish motives from indirectly selfish motives. Consequently, the 'sole goal of benefiting another person' changed into 'sole benefits to another person', whirlpooling the debate further at two different levels. At the conceptual level, ambiguities and problems in the attempt to define altruism and egotism emerged, as occurred in evolutionary biology (Uyenoyama and Feldman 1992). At the empirical research level, altruism was investigated as a synonym with or a component of prosocial behaviour, thus being often identified with it.

3.2.3 The Binary Perspective and the Altruism Debate

The debate on altruism continues with seemingly no end, leading many scholars to either disregard it as unimportant or to consider the definition of altruism as an unattainable goal (Weinstein 2008). Should we leave it behind? Quite a number of researchers decided positively and rather started focusing on the outcome of other-regarding emotions and prosocial behaviours. In fact, altruism literature is dominated by research and evidences on the beneficial outcome of other-oriented emotions and prosocial behaviours for individuals and societies (Lyubomirsky 2007; Post 2005; Oman 2007; Tankersley et al. 2007). While this approach may seem concrete and pragmatic, the need for a clear definition of altruism cannot be ignored. Interestingly, information abounds on effects of altruism, but not on altruism per se, leaving the term elusive and often ambiguous. Yet, a concept so intimately connected to individual conduct and so central in all the value systems developed by human cultures requires an explanation or at least an exploration (Delle Fave 2004).

Clarifying the altruism debate can become a launching pad to better disentangle the potential of altruism. In our opinion, in the altruism debate, a core specific aspect of altruism definition has been neglected or often misunderstood. This aspect consists in the 'interaction process between two entities – 'self' and 'other'. From this perspective, 'self' refers to an agentic entity and 'other' as everything else other than self.

A dichotomised approach to self and other, grounded into a binary conceptualisation of the world, is the primary source of the altruism debate. The binary system or binary opposition is an epistemological methodology by which, in language and thought, two theoretical opposites are strictly defined and set off against one another, with a value hierarchy often as 'positive' and 'negative' (Smith 1996). The binary opposition is built on 'discontinuity rather than continuity' (Goody 1997, p. 81) and on the assumption that contrasting is essential as one cannot conceive of 'good' if one does not understand 'evil' (Smith 1996). It consists in organising pairs of related terms or concepts in opposition such as presence/absence, male/female and life/death. Such a binary perspective has been dominating within Western culture, language and philosophy, where organisation and structure are fundamental (Derrida 1978; Saussure 1916). The Cartesian and Newtonian worldview, considering everything – from the human body to the universe – as a machine composed of separate interacting material particles, is a vivid example of this binary methodology (Burtt 1952; Butterfield 1997). While focusing on discontinuity is beneficial in articulating crystal-clear categories, it runs the risk of an all-out dichotomisation and hierarchical organisation of reality.

Due to its focus on discontinuity, the binary system operates primarily through a methodology of differentiation and separation. Pairs of opposites – such as male and female or self and other – make sense only in their discontinuity and clear-cut boundaries. Such a dichotomised perspective represents a core paradigm guiding Western thought. Descartes is one of the most influential scholars supporting the distinction of self and other as two entirely separate and contradictory entities (Rozemond 1998). A case in point in psychoanalysis is Freud's theory on narcissism, centred on the infants' tendency to direct libido towards their own person (primary narcissism), subsequently diverting it towards other objects. If these 'object relationships' are blocked, the libido is returned to one's own person (secondary narcissism). According to Freud, there is an almost mechanical compartmentalisation of love between ego and other objects. The more love one directs towards external objects, the less love one has for oneself and vice versa (Lowen 1997). Altruism definitions within evolutionary biology and social psychology are founded on this dichotomised perspective of self and other, considered as separated and independent entities. Within this framework, authentic altruistic acts must benefit 'only the other', without any self-benefit. The notion that self and others represent two alternatives lying at opposite poles is however debatable. Can anything be completely selfish or altruistic? Can behaviours and people be divided as purely altruistic or selfish? The jigsaw puzzle of altruism is primarily due to this dichotomised perspective.

The inherent hierarchal organisation and value judgments of the binary system further complicate the debate. Binary oppositions are value laden, often as 'positive' and 'negative' poles, with an illusory order, where one of the two terms governs the other (Goody 1997). Within the white/black binary opposition, for example, the black is often less valuable and even negative (Derrida 1978). In the binary system of self/other, often self came to be less valuable in classical Western thought. A worldview spearheaded by thinkers like Augustine, Luther and Calvin reinforced devaluation of the individual self, considered as morally inferior, evil, weak and naturally drawn to close on himself/herself (Fromm 1947). In such perspective, hating oneself is considered not only a value but also a virtue. Notwithstanding the efforts to reclaim the self during Renaissance and Enlightenment, a perspective of self as narcissistic, pleasure seeking and sinful remains still influential in the binary perspective. A crucial issue in this value hierarchy is the identification of self-love with selfishness, as opposed to love for others: this assumption has been pervading Western theology, philosophy and daily life. Selfishness and self-love however remain far from being identical. The German word *Selbstsucht* (addiction to self) very adequately expresses the connection of selfishness with other kinds of *Sucht* – greediness (Fromm 1947). In particular, greediness in its various forms is characterised by insatiability, thus implying impossibility to attain real satisfaction. Selfish persons are always anxiously concerned with themselves, driven by the fear of not getting enough. The root of selfishness is basically a dislike of oneself that leads to compensation, currently identified by psychiatry and clinical psychology with the narcissistic personality disorder (American Psychiatric Association 2000; Campbell and Foster 2007). Differently from Freud's conceptualisation, narcissistic persons love neither others nor themselves; they are thus ready to die as well as to kill.

Selfishness, in fact, is opposite of self-love. However, self-love and selfishness are interchangeably used within altruism definitions. Evolutionary biology, for example, equates the natural tendency to self-preservation with selfishness and holds it a case against the possibility of altruism among living beings. The entire debate within evolutionary biology rests on this claim that selfishness is natural to organisms. Self-preservation is however self-love rather than selfishness. Ego psychology (Mahler 1968) highlights the necessity of primary narcissism for self-identity, since sense of 'self' cannot emerge without self-love. Research studies on attachment showed that in order to develop empathic skills, children must receive a secure basis of love and attention from their caregivers in early infancy (Bowlby 1958; Schore 1994). This issue is clearly addressed in most religious traditions.

Buddhist scriptures highlight the importance of the practice of *metta* (loving kindness) meditation, grounded into the assumption that 'You, yourself, as much as anybody in the entire universe deserve your love and affection' (Salzberg and Kabat-Zinn 2008). The same concept is repeatedly stated in the Bible: 'You shall love your neighbour as yourself' (Leviticus 19, 18; Matthew 22:37–39, Bible 2007).

In conclusion, the altruism debate and confusion stem from a dichotomised worldview of self/other, based on the alleged identity between self-love and selfishness. In our opinion, this view fails not only to explain altruism but also to maximise its true potential. On the basis of research highlighting that empathic concern is natural to humans, Batson et al. (2008) call for a complex perspective that integrates altruism and egotism rather than setting them in opposition. Is such a complex perspective currently available?

3.3 Interconnectedness and the Spiral Model of Altruism

Within Western philosophy, poststructuralism presents deconstruction as an alternative to binary opposition. Deconstruction challenges the inherent value hierarchy and aims at constant straining of the poles to destabilise the power in binary systems towards a balance (Derrida 1978). It argues that speech is a form of writing, presence is a certain type of absence, sanity is a kind of neurosis and man is a form of woman (Culler 1983). However, far from being a kind of monism that perceives the universe as one single entity and the differences as appearances and illusion (Kalupaha 1975), it acknowledges differences, at the same time proposing a method of integration devoid of hierarchy and power. Based on these premises, deconstruction can in principle represent an alternative perspective to understand altruism; however, its primary focus on the issue of power limits its effectiveness in clarifying such a complex issue.

In our opinion, a more universal and thus more adequate perspective to better understand and explain altruism is interconnectedness, a worldview originally developed within Asian philosophical traditions. In the Indian vision of *Rg* Veda, the universe is conceived as an ordered whole in which each part inheres the whole and the whole is balanced by the parts (Eliot 1988; James 1969). This worldview is synthesised in the concept of *Rta*. Often mistaken for a ritual law, *Rta* in Sanskrit means 'that which is properly joined', order, rule, truth, the principle of natural order that regulates and coordinates the activities of the universe and of its components (Mahony 1998). It refers to the cosmic order that knits together everything, from galaxies to atomic subparticles, influencing their nature and course. It is the supreme and ultimate foundation of everything, so that even Gods are part of it (Brown 1992). In the same vein, the Buddhist scripture Avatamsaka Sutra states that every being in the universe depends on every other being for their existence, underscoring the nature of the entire universe as made of intrinsically intertwined parts (Morgan 2010). Interconnectedness, however, is neither a static and fatalistic view (Panikkar 2001) nor an exclusively Eastern perspective derived from religious metaphysics.

In line with *Rta*, Einstein stated 'Everything is determined, the beginning as well as the end, by forces over which we have no control. It is determined for the insect, as well as for the star. Human beings, vegetables, or cosmic dust, we all dance to a mysterious tune, intoned in the distance by an invisible piper' (Einstein 1929). Scientific evidence from quantum physics, considered the cutting edge of Western science, proved to be consistent with *Rta* concept (Capra 1999; Jones 1986; Talbot 1993). In exploring probabilities of existence and energy states, quantum physics highlighted that everything in the universe is fundamentally interconnected and interdependent (Alistair 1988; Feyman et al. 1965). One of the most popular examples is the butterfly effect, referring to the sensitive dependence on initial conditions, so that the little energy arising from a butterfly's wings can affect the weather conditions of other planets.

The perspective of interconnectedness considers the entire cosmos as a mosaic, consisting in the assemblage of many different parts in unison (King 2003). In a mosaic, all tesseras differ from each other but all are connected both horizontally and vertically, according to varying patterns of complexity. The whole picture is incomplete in the absence of even just one piece, and the single unit makes no sense without the whole picture. Each part depends on the other and the whole depends on each part. In the same manner, the entire universe is interconnected. From this perspective, the extinction of a particular type of a butterfly or a tiny bird, apparently meaningless to humans, affects the universal pattern of interconnectedness and interdependence.

3.3.1 Self and Other in the Interconnected Universe

From the perspective of interconnectedness, self and other are not 'either/or' entities in binary opposition, rather they are 'intertwined' and 'dialectical'. One of the clearest examples to clarify this relationship is the Chinese conceptualisation of Yin and Yang, described as two different but complementary entities that interact within an integrated dynamic system (Graham 1986). These seemingly contrary forces are interconnected and interdependent in the natural world, to the extent that they give rise to each other in turn. Likewise, self and other are interconnected and interdependent entities. While preserving their reciprocal differentiation, they can only exist as specific 'self' and 'other' within their relation, at both the logical/conceptual and practical levels. Moreover, this relation is based on their complementariness rather than exclusiveness or opposition. The conceptualisation of self/other as inseparable and interdependent entities is not an issue of metaphysics. Systems theory strongly emphasises the interconnected and interdependent nature of self and others (Bertalanffy 1950). In Erikson's theory of development, ego identity unfolds only in the context of others, along with integration into society and culture. A deficiency in either of these factors may increase the chance of identity crisis or confusion (Cote and Levine 2002). Attachment theories underscore the role of connections in self-development (Hazan and Shaver 1994). Self-psychology claims that a child is able to develop an 'ego identity' only by three basic and fundamentally relational needs: need to be loved, need to idealise and need to belong. An individual sense of self cannot emerge without the connection to the other (Kohut 1971).

More recently, the self/other dialectical relation emerged in self-determination theory (SDT). This theory focuses on three psychological needs – need for autonomy, relatedness and competence – considering them as organismic necessities for psychological growth, integrity and well-being (Deci and Ryan 1980, 2002; Ryan and Deci 2000a, b; Ryan and Connell 1989). Even though SDT does not specifically address the issue of self/other relation, the cultural debate arisen around the need for autonomy is relevant to our discussion on altruism. The role and importance of autonomy as a basic need was called into question in light of the different conceptualisations of self endorsed by individualistic and collectivistic cultures (Markus and Kitayama 1991; Triandis 1994; Triandis et al. 1995). Claiming against a definition of autonomy as isolation and individualism, SDT underscores the importance of autonomy in connection to relatedness, and vice versa, so that autonomy without relatedness ends up to be mere individualism, while relatedness without autonomy becomes just a passive subordination (Knee and Uysal 2011). Kagitcibasi (1996, 2005) effectively contributed to this contention, arguing that autonomy at the cost of relatedness or vice versa is not helpful and proposing to address the issue in terms of 'autonomous-relational self'. We believe that this concept can be useful far beyond its original context. The term succinctly articulates the entire debate around self and other and synthesises the nature and dynamics of their relation. More specifically, it corrects the two misconceptions of altruism debate, namely, dichotomising self/other and equating self-love with selfishness. It endorses an interconnectedness perspective in which, differently from the binary, self is always 'autonomous-relational'; its focus on the 'process between self and other' contributes to better understand and explain altruism.

3.3.2 Altruism as Mind-set

The word 'altruism' per se was coined by the French philosopher Auguste Comte in 1851 from the Italian adjective *altrui*, meaning self-sacrifice for the benefit of others in the context of moral obligations and virtuous life (Comte 1852/1891). Considering the altruism debate outlined in the previous pages, terms like 'self-sacrifice' and 'benefit of others' would require extensive and explicit clarifications, as well as caution with possible underlying cultural biases. In light of the most recent advancements in scientific knowledge, we believe that a different definition of altruism founded on the perspective of interconnectedness can be more useful. We propose therefore the following definition:

> Altruism is a mind-set characterised by a concern for others' welfare that implies a readiness to engage even to the point of sacrifice and that can bring welfare to the agent as well.

Four specific aspects of this definition require thorough clarification. First, altruism is not just behaviour. In the effort to scientifically investigate altruism, evolutionary

Fig. 3.1 The altruism spiral

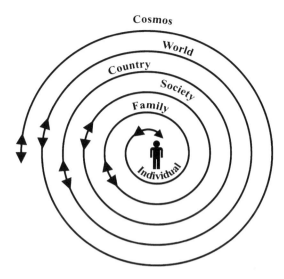

biology and social psychology reduced it to prosocial behaviour that benefits the fitness/welfare of the other at the cost of oneself. We instead propose to consider altruism as a mind-set that is a habitual or characteristic mental attitude that determines how one will interpret and respond to situations. It refers to general assumptions, methods or notations that guide an individual (Gollwitzer and Brandstaetter 1997; Gollwitzer 1999). Altruism as a mind-set refers to one's willingness to acknowledge the 'other' and to care for their well-being. The prominent motivating force in altruism, at least in the deliberative phase (Pucca and Schmalt 2001; Taylor and Gollwitzer 1995), is the benefit of the other. In the subsequent phase of implementation of intentions, outcomes can differ according to individual differences and context specificities, while mind-set serves as a general pattern that guides individuals. In this regard, altruism differs significantly from helping and prosocial behaviours that can enhance the well-being of the other with or without having it as primary focus.

The second aspect concerns the term 'other'. From the perspective of interconnectedness, it refers to a model of interaction involving a wide range of entities, characterised by different levels of structural and relational complexity. This model can be effectively depicted as a spiral that is a single continuous entity of circles with different levels (Fig. 3.1). The single individual, located at the core of the spiral, is in connection to the 'other' at different levels of the spiral. In this model, connections should not be understood in physical and quantitative terms, especially considering the variety of virtual connections existing in today's globalised and Internet-based world. Within the altruism model, connections are understood as manifestations of willingness to value others and to enhance their well-being. The inner circle is the simple level of complexity, including family and beloved ones; the outermost circle encompasses the entire cosmos and represents the most complex level of the model. In this spiral of connections, individuals can develop growing awareness of interconnectedness and cultivation of connections along a centrifugal direction, from a smaller circle to a bigger circle, from a low level of complexity to higher ones. However, such a centrifugal movement is not necessarily progressive across continuous levels of complexity. An individual can altruistically reach out to a needy person in another continent, while not doing so with neighbours living next door.

A potential danger has to be clarified in this process of connection development, related to the in-group/out-group dynamics. Establishing connections with in-group members can take place at the cost of severing connections with out-groups. In this condition, the process of moving away from the narrowly self-centred focus to connect with the other paradoxically ends up in another form of narrow-mindedness, expressed as nationalism, racism, religious hate, genocide and suicidal cults. Suicide bombing, for example, can be perceived as a higher form of altruism and self-sacrifice within a particular group, at the cost of overlooking the pain caused to the out-group. Studies on moral circles clearly highlight such danger of exclusion in the process of inclusion (Laham 2009). The perspective of interconnectedness and the model of altruism proposed here allow for a conceptual solution and mitigation of the above danger. Within a spiral model of interconnectedness, establishing connections at a particular level at the cost of severing connections at another level becomes impossible. To actualise the altruistic motivation of building a Disney world for poor children by destroying a forest inhabited by a particular human community requires to break the spiral continuity. To clarify this point, we also propose the following definition of altruistic behaviour:

> An altruistic behaviour is any other-oriented act that promotes and nourishes connections at certain level without violating connections at other levels.

The spiral analogy further underscores that altruism is neither a crystallised ideal nor a static concept. It is rather related to individual characteristics and contextual features, especially as concerns its behavioural outcomes. At the individual level, resources and potentials, skills and competences, meanings and beliefs, goals and expectations greatly influence the actualisation of the altruistic mind-set. At the contextual level, tragedies like tsunami or earthquakes strongly elicit altruistic behaviour, while a strongly competitive and consumerist environment may reduce it. In addition, the same person can fluctuate across various levels of connectedness complexity in different periods, life stages and contexts. Building on the works of Sorokin (1941, 1948, 1950), Monroe proposed an altruism continuum, classifying individuals and their behaviours in three categories: entrepreneurs, philanthropists and heroes (Monroe 1996). Entrepreneurs express the simplest level of altruism, while heroes endorse the most complex one. While the terms selected to indicate these three levels of altruism might be contentious, this perspective points to the possibility of distinguishing between different levels of complexity in the actualisation of altruism. It redeems altruism from being an ideal act of giving of one's life, as often depicted in altruism role models. Altruism need not to be identified with such extremes. Individuals can differ in the strength of their altruistic mind-set and in their willingness to act upon it.

The third aspect of the proposed definition of altruism that requires further clarification is the 'readiness to engage even to the point of sacrifice'. Although closely connected to compassion, altruism differs from it in this regard. Compassion is defined as a feeling of deep sympathy and sorrow for another who is stricken by misfortune, accompanied by a strong desire to alleviate the suffering. However, engagement to act is not an essential component of compassion. Altruism is in this respect a more active form of compassion (Weintraub 2011), which includes a strong motivation or urge to do something for the object of compassion. Altruism further differs from compassion, helping and prosocial behaviours as it is characterised by a readiness to sacrifice. Compassion, helping and prosocial behaviours may enhance the welfare of others with or without a willingness to sacrifice. The word 'sacrifice' is used here from a psychological perspective and not in relation to morality. It is rather related to a personal choice of placing others need before one's own and can derive from the human capacity for ego control and letting go. Jung proposed that ego has the power to relinquish its power to claim (Jung 1975). Therefore, though sacrifice implies placing others over oneself, it is not denial of oneself. Jung underscored that without a sense of 'me', sacrifice is not possible (Jung 1975). The act of making a sacrifice primarily consists in giving away something that belongs to an individual. Sacrifice can be thus comprised within the capacity for self-transcendence. Nevertheless, while sacrifice is a distinctive component of altruism, it is not a structural aspect of it. Altruistic engagement in its various forms does not necessarily demand a sacrifice. In addition, individuals can manifest different levels of complexity – from lower to greater ones – in sacrifice as well.

The fourth and last aspect of the proposed definition of altruism that requires clarification refers to the benefits deriving to the agent as a consequence of being altruistic. Differently from other existing definitions of altruism, a definition grounded into interconnectedness does not exclude such benefits; on the contrary, it explicitly endorses them. According to Emerson 'it is one of the most beautiful compensations of this life that no man can try to help another without helping himself' (2001, p. 65). Analogously, Victor Frankl (1988) stated that the more one helps others, the more one actually helps himself. Due to the natural condition of interconnectedness, the centrifugal movement of enhancing others' welfare actually leads to a feedback loop of one's own welfare enhancement, through a dialectical exchange process. Within the cultural evolution framework, individuals maximise their benefits in the long run by helping others than themselves (Baumeister 2005). Aristotle claimed that true human happiness, which he described as eudaimonia, was furthered more 'by loving rather than in being loved' (350 BC/1985, p. 1159). It is perhaps paradoxical that altruism often associated with going 'outside' of oneself is actually highly involving the self (Davis et al. 2004; Galinsky and Moskowitz 2000). Religious traditions often refer to this process as a 'paradoxical giving', a model of self-actualisation through self-transcendence. The Bible, for example, claims that by loosing oneself, one discovers oneself, presenting the example of a seed that dies only to germinate (John 12:24, Bible 2007). Francis of Assisi succinctly captured this idea, stating that it is in giving that one receives (Brown 1988). Buddha taught that in negating the 'self' one actually attains Nirvana (Morgan 2010).

Such an apparently paradoxical outcome seems a unique characteristic of altruism, and it can be easily reconciled only within the perspective of interconnectedness and of 'autonomous-relational self'. Perspective of interconnectedness highlights yet another important dimension of altruism: its relationship with values.

3.3.3   The Biocultural Roots of Altruism

Why do people do what they do? In the specific case of altruism, why do individuals manifest it? Exploring whether altruism is natural to living organism, evolutionary biology claimed that selfishness is natural and altruism is only due to adaptive necessity and docility to social norms (Simon 1993). Altruism is commonly perceived as an ethical doctrine and a socially imposed constraint. Comte, who coined the term, addressed the issue from the viewpoint of moral obligation to help and serve and considered altruism as a superior moral value (Comte 1852/1891). A similar perspective was also endorsed in most religious teachings and traditions that glorify altruism and advocate it as a virtue to be followed. But are people altruistic just because they believe it to be a moral value or is there something more to that?

Recent advancements in evolutionary biology consider altruism more than an external moral value and an adaptive necessity (Tankersley et al. 2007; Batson et al. 2008), assuming the existence of an altruistic impulse mediated through empathy and perspective taking (De Walls 2008). Biological foundations of altruism have been suggested by neurobiological evidence. Both pure monetary rewards and charitable donations activate the mesolimbic reward pathway, a primitive part of the brain that usually lights up in response to food and sex. In addition, when volunteers generously placed the interests of others before their own by making charitable donations, another brain circuit was selectively activated: the subgenual cortex/septal region (Moll et al. 2006). Such studies suggest that altruism is not just an acquired moral judgement imposed by the social context; it rather elicits archaic brain circuits related to pleasure and reward.

Evidences from cultural evolution theories offer further clarifications on this issue. Baumeister (2005) claims that humans are designed by nature for community, since culture alone could not sustain for long what is not natural to humans. Bounded rationality, for example, makes it impossible for humans to live alone (Simon 1993). Human newborns are more vulnerable and dependent than any other creature. It seems impossible to construct even a virtual situation where a person can manage to survive without being helped. Humans could not have achieved the current level of social development and cultural evolution without depending upon each other. Contrary to the extensive emphasis on self-preservation need, the need to belong takes precedence over in many circumstances. 'Belongingness can be almost as compelling need as food' (Baumeister and Leary 1995, p. 498). Individuals are ready to sacrifice even the self-preservation need in order to fulfil the need to belong, evolutionarily grounded together with survival and reproduction benefits (Baumeister and Leary 1995; Sedikides et al. 2006). Echoing Jean-Paul Sartre's statement 'Man is condemned to be free', we could say 'Humans are condemned to be connected'.

The need to belong is also consistently highlighted as one of the fundamental psychological needs, especially in studies conducted within the framework of self-determination theory (Deci et al. 2006; Epstein 1994; Sheldon et al. 2001; Gebauer and Maio 2012). It is plausible to claim that altruism is part of this need to belong (Moss and Barbuto 2010; Musick and Wilson 2003). As it is founded on other-orientation, altruism is inherently interpersonal and thus influences relatedness by generally promoting closeness to others, positive responses from others and intimacy. The plausibility of altruism being more than a social value is further underscored by the human need to help. Helping is identified as one of the basic human needs, being part of a more general category of 'need to belong' such as nurturance and generativity (Baumeister 2005). Caprara and Steca (2005) showed that human capacity to help is essential to the maintenance of mutually rewarding relationships and proposed that humans are evolutionarily wired to help others due to the distress response at the pain of others (Baumeister 2005). Initial support of this claim was demonstrated in a longitudinal study of volunteers (Piliavin and Siegl 2007). Based on biological evidences, and on its cultural and psychological relevance, altruism seems to be more than just a social norm and moral value. Rather than a phenomenon emerging occasionally or accidentally in extraordinary circumstances, findings suggest its relationship to both human needs and well-being.

3.3.4 Altruism and Well-Being

Research highlights a plethora of benefits of altruism at the individual level. The survival advantage of behaving altruistically is well documented in most species (Eisenberg 1986). At the biological level, altruism is associated with dopamine D4 receptors. Kindness elicits the same reward circuits activated by eating and having sex (Bachner-Melman et al. 2005; Harbaugh et al. 2007). Research indicated that people who are more altruistic have more activity in the posterior superior temporal sulcus region even while performing emotionally neutral tasks (Tankersley et al. 2007).

As concerns, the benefits of altruism on health evidence primarily emerges from studies investigating altruistic prosocial behaviours that highlighted an increase in psychophysical health after behaving prosocially (Hunter and Linn 1980; Musick and Wilson 2003). In a survey among US volunteers, participants reported better health than their peers, mediated by 'helper's high' (Luks 1988), a pleasurable and euphoric emotional sensation of energy often resulting in better health. Individuals coping with chronic pain experienced decrease of pain intensity as well as lower levels of disability and depression when they began to help their peers (Arnstein et al. 2002). Several studies showed that volunteering is consistently related to a reduction in depression levels (Hunter and Linn 1980; Musick and Wilson 2003; Thoits and Hewitt 2001). Volunteering and caring behaviours were also significantly associated with reduced or delayed mortality (Brown et al. 2003; Oman et al. 1999; Rodin and Langer 1976; Harris and Thoresen 2005). Even the thought of giving or ruminating on compassionate activities can enhance immune system. Watching a movie on Mother Teresa's compassionate work, for example, significantly increased the protective salivary immunoglobulin in comparison to watching a neutral film (McClelland et al. 1988).

Within the domain of psychology, Alice Isen conducted pioneer experimental studies showing that helping and happiness fuel each other in a circular fashion – a classic feedback loop (Isen and Levin 1972). More recently, positive psychology has provided further evidence of the role of altruism in promoting well-being. Within this framework, studies rooted in the hedonic perspective, based on the investigation of well-being as the prominence of positive affect and life satisfaction, showed that altruism elicits positive emotions (Fredrickson 2004). Prosocial spending was found to significantly increase happiness, in contrast to personal spending (Dunn et al. 2008). In a US survey, participants involved in helping professions reported higher levels of job satisfaction than those whose job did not permit altruistic gratifications (Smith 2007). Results from participants living under difficult circumstances (prostitutes, homeless people and inhabitants of Calcutta slums) suggested a link between altruism and life satisfaction (Diener et al. 2003).

From a different perspective, positive psychology research based on the eudaimonic approach – according to which well-being derives from the cultivation of personal resources and strengths through commitment to meaningful activities and pursuit of shared goals – showed that altruism promotes development (Deci and Ryan 2000) and psychological well-being (Ryff et al. 2002), fosters positive self-image (Luks 1991; Snyder and Lopez 2007) and self-esteem (Lyubomirsky 2007). As highlighted by scholars endorsing the eudaimonic perspective, to privilege others' well-being over one's own is a human capacity and a resource that can be cultivated (Keyes and Annas 2009; Sen 1987). From this perspective, altruistic behaviours can be considered eudaimonic activities par excellence. Consistently with these assumptions, research showed that, compared to hedonic activities, eudaimonic activities significantly contribute in building a meaningful and satisfying life (Steger et al. 2008). Volunteering provides meaning, a sense of self-worth, a social role, better relationships and health enhancement (Musick and Wilson 2003; Oman 2007; Schwartz et al. 2003). A simple advertisement of the American Red Cross underscores it: 'feel good about yourself – Give blood'. Prosocial behaviours based on autonomous motivation yield higher psychological need satisfaction (Weinstein and Ryan 2010). Altruism founded on an inner representation of reality as interconnectedness helps achieve the lifelong human task of building relationships and social connections (Moss and Barbuto 2010; Musick and Wilson 2003).

At the collective level, altruism enhances the communal nature of human beings as it rests on the sense of the other. Societies are, in fact, built on foundations such as mutual support, co-operation and readiness to mitigate self-focus. Altruism is essential not only for enhancing survival of societies but also for optimising their resources. The psychological processes that give rise to altruism tend to make aggression less likely (Miller and Eisenberg 1988; Spielman and Staub 2000; Staub 2003).

Altruism helps to preserve and empower the social structures that foster forgiveness and gratitude (McCullough et al. 2004). Various studies highlighted the societal benefits of empathic concern – one of the portals of altruism. It sustains the willingness to provide long-term care for those in need (Sibicky et al. 1995), reduces prejudices (Galinsky and Moskowitz 2000), increases mutual care (Gordon 2007), promotes positive consideration of stigmatised groups (Batson et al. 1997a, b) and facilitates conflict resolutions (Batson et al. 2004). Considering these societal benefits, it is no wonder then that all societies and religious traditions preach and invite their members to practice altruism.

In particular, morality, as a system of rules and prescriptions that allow people to live together (Baumeister 2005), typically invites individuals to sacrifice their own wishes and self-interests for the sake of the greater good. A study on 60 exemplary altruists detected a high sense of moral responsibility and an internalised social commitment as one of their characteristic traits (Lee et al. 2005). The process may happen because of social pressure, kin selection, empathy, perspective taking or a voluntary choice. Whatever the source may be, without such a process of keeping others' interest in mind, private morality may be not possible. In addition, if people do not practice private morality, public morality collapses. Even in free market trading, a sense of decency is expected, assuming that greed or personal gain must not dominate the transactions of the city (Wojciech and Ryan 1996). Nevertheless, formulation of the individual self as the source of value with inherently authoritative claims is one of the important cultural changes of our modern world (Baumeister and Exline 1999). One important and controversial result of this change is individualism and emphasis on personal needs and rights. Charters of rights are in the increase and often perceived as the shield to protect individuals from the others or from the societal demands. Elevation of self into a value base has generated substantial divergence on moral issues. Moral diversity, more so than demographic diversity, may pose various kinds of problems at the community level (Haidt et al. 2003), and this is a cause of concern for today's societies. The implications of this tension are numerous and far reaching, ranging from interpersonal relationships to education, economics and policy.

Given this complex picture, altruism represents a unique point of convergence in which a balanced synergy of both the traditional morality and the exaltation of self is made possible, since being altruistic seems beneficial both to the well-being of the agent and the receiver. From the perspective of interconnectedness, maintaining a balance between individual and community interests is crucial for the optimal functioning of a society. Societies cannot exist if the interests of single individuals are exalted. On the contrary, individuals will not be motivated to maintain the needs of the society if they do not receive at least a minimum guarantee for their personal needs. The concept of eudaimonia, core of Aristotle's *Nicomachean Ethics*, seems to be peculiarly consistent with this view. Resonating closely the two Greek imperatives 'know thyself' and 'become what you are', the highest good for Aristotle is to follow one's *daimon*, or true nature. This consists in engaging in meaningful living, conditioned upon self-truth and self-responsibility (Ryff and Singer 2008). The eudaimonic perspective claims that the process of fulfilling one's virtuous potentials takes place not in isolation but in the context of society, with an emphasis on belonging and benefiting others (Waterman 1993). Contribution to others is one of the essential aspects of following one's daimon, along with the pursuit of personal goals (Keyes 1998).

Could we claim that the converse is also true? In other words, could it be claimed that the absence of altruism predicts the absence of well-being in individuals and societies? Unfortunately, there are no direct and explicit works yet to prove that the absence of altruism would predict absence of well-being. However, the above hypothesis has been affirmed in humanistic psychology and in religious traditions. According to Frankl, 'when self-actualization is made an end itself and is aimed at as the objective of a primary intention, it cannot be attained' (Frankl 1967, p. 34). 'A self centred focus prevents growth, for the person can only find identity to the extent to which he commits himself to something beyond himself' (Frankl 1967, p. 63). Without a mind-set to enhance the welfare of the other, enhancing one's own welfare does not seem attainable. Religions too underscore such claim. Mahayana mediation, for example, emphasises the possibility of attaining ultimate happiness only through giving oneself completely (Neusner and Chilton 2005). Bible teaches that if anyone wants to find one's life should lose it and there seems no other alternative (Luke 17:33, Bible 2007). Bhagavad Gita proposes that liberation and happiness can be attained through selfless and desire-less action (Pande and Naidu 1992). Evolutionary theories also confirm this claim, highlighting that individuals who fail to enhance the survival of the other minimise their own survival in the long run (Simon 1993).

The debate on the nature of well-being to be individual or interpersonal offers useful insights to our discussion. A great number of studies within positive psychology remain individual focused, being grounded into the subjective well-being perspective. On the contrary, the eudaimonic perspective highlights that well-being is interpersonal and profoundly influenced by the surrounding (Ryff and Singer 2008). Eudaimonia not only affirms well-being to be interpersonal but also underscores the importance of self-gift for self-transcendence. In particular, the construct of 'flourishing' developed by Keyes (2002, 2009) corresponds to an optimal state of human functioning, characterised by goodness, generativity, growth and resilience. It refers to a life with high levels of both personal and social well-being and based on purpose, meaning and happiness (Keyes 2009). Languishing, on the contrary, is a condition devoid of illness as well as wellness, often characterised by lack of purpose, meaning and social contribution. Flourishing underscores that well-being is incomplete without social contribution. From this perspective, it is thus plausible to claim that well-being is incomplete without altruism. More research on this aspect is however needed.

3.3.5 Beyond Reductionism

As highlighted in the previous pages, the prominent challenge in altruism research consists in correcting its reduction to behaviour. By definition, reductionism refers to an approach to understand the nature of complex things by reducing them to the interactions of their parts or to simpler or more fundamental things (Cottingham et al. 1988). Existing literature on altruism primarily considers it as synonym or part of prosocial behaviour. For example, the popular self-report altruism scale comprises 18 statements referring to prosocial helping behaviours as indicators of altruism (Rushton et al. 1981).

Helping and prosocial behaviour can be considered as manifestations of altruism, but they cannot be equated to it. Altruism should also be distinguished from solidarity and philanthropy – two terms related to altruism – but characterised by an emphasis on behaviour and on collective action. Solidarity (from the Latin *solidus*: whole, compact) refers to the unity and connectedness among people belonging to a specific class, community or group. Philanthropy that originates from the ancient Greek *phil* (love) and *anthropos* (human being), has been commonly used throughout the centuries to indicate socially useful initiatives and activities mostly consisting in financial donations and material support, whose beneficiaries are usually groups and communities rather than single individuals.

Philosophy, religions and moral sciences underscore altruism as an essential value and virtue towards which humans are called forth. The definition provided by Comte in 1851 also does not tie altruism down to behaviour. Similarly, the definitions that can be found in various languages (English, Italian and Tamil dictionaries – Merriam-Webster's Online, Garzanti Online and Tamil Online Dictionary) emphasise relational and psychological features of altruism, besides the behavioural ones. Perceiving altruism as behaviour does not only reduce its richness but also discriminates between people who can perform altruistic activities, such as volunteering, and people who do not perform them (due to physical impairment or social constraints).

Proposing the mind-set model, we claim that altruism must be explored as value. Values are important and enduring beliefs or ideals of what is good and what is not. They are desirable goals that vary in importance and influence individuals' perceptions, decisions and behaviours (Rokeach 1973; Schwartz 1992). Moreover, values can be seen as a defining feature of a culture (Hofstede 2001; Schwartz 1992). Given the crucial role of values in individuals' perceptions and preferences, we assume that a deeper and broader understanding and application of altruism is possible if it is explored from the perspective of value, perceived beliefs and ideas. In fact, a glimpse of such a perspective is found in *Value in Action Inventory of Strengths* (VIA-IS, Peterson and Seligman 2004) enlisting altruism as part of the kindness strength. Similarly, Schwartz's value inventory (SVI) is grounded into a circumflex model comprising ten 'value types', grouped into four major categories: 'conservation vs. openness to change' and 'self-enhancement vs. self-transcendence' (Schwartz 1992, 1994, 2010). Although altruism is not extensively addressed, it falls into the category of self-transcendence, including universalism and benevolence. Nevertheless, in spite of its power of synthesis and clarity, Schwartz's model is built on the binary perspective of polarisation, opposing self-enhancement to self-transcendence. To the best of our knowledge, no models and investigation tools are available to explore altruism from the perspective of interconnectedness, as a human value related to both self-actualisation and social empowerment.

3.4   Promoting Altruism: Resources and Challenges

How can societies and individuals promote altruism? In other words, how can narrow self-centredness be minimised both at the level of individuals and communities?

One of the primary tasks of culture is to elicit from individuals acts that are best for the group, using mechanism like morality, laws and values (Baumeister 2005). Each culture develops specific values, expectations, rules, reward and punishment dynamics to pursue this aim. Volunteering, community services, gift-giving seasons, tax refunds for donations, curriculum adoption can be referred as few examples to it. Mandated volunteering, for example, in schools and universities, is promoted in some countries (Krehbiel and MacKay 1988; Sobus 1995). Policymakers have propounded that volunteer work be made a prerequisite for grant rewards or loan forgiveness (Newman et al. 1985; Robb and Swearer 1985). Although such methods can succeed in promoting altruistic behaviours, their efficiency is called into question in the light of studies on motivations and their role in sustaining behaviours. Programmes founded on extrinsic motivation do not have lasting influence on individuals (Frey 1997; Kunda and Schwartz 1983). Extrinsic motivation is negatively associated with volunteer satisfaction and it negatively impacts subsequent prosocial engagement (Finkelstein et al. 2005; Frey and Jegen 2001; Upton 1974). In contrast, autonomously motivated altruistic behaviours are highly correlated to well-being (Ryan and Deci 2001; Weinstein and Ryan 2010). Hence, promoting intrinsic motivation seems to have higher success rates. One of the plausible reasons for the increase in volunteering in the United States is the claim that helping promotes intrinsic rewards such as health and happiness, rather than credit hours and money (Wuthnow 1991). Role models are also beneficial to elicit autonomous motivations. The Good Samaritan story, for example, has enormous influence in shaping people's attitudes and behaviours in volunteering (Wuthnow 1991; Rushton 1980; Allison 1992). The media hike on the 'giving pledge' of some of the richest people in the United States is justified on this claim of motivating others to follow suit.

The power of values in eliciting internalisation and intrinsic motivations could be referred as another example. Some cultures enhance the sociobiological issue of reciprocity by reinforcing the value of gratitude, characterised by the belief that someone has done a favour together with a sense of guilt or obligation to reciprocate (Hardin 1982; Swidler 1986). Nurturing the value of compassion also enhances prosocial and altruistic behaviours with an internal locus of control. Studies highlighted that loving kindness (compassion) meditation promotes empathy and perspective taking, resulting in prosocial behaviours (Davis 1983; Shelton and Rogers 1981). The practice of perspective taking increases empathy and autonomously motivated altruistic tendencies (Batson et al. 1991, 1997a, b; Klen and Hodges 2001). Nurturing a sense of meaning and purpose also contributes to the development of autonomous motivation. Societies can offer various other means to elicit altruism and altruistic behaviours. The point in place is that those societies that succeed in promoting conditions for autonomous motivation (from external pressure to personal choice) stand to sustain altruistic behaviours and to optimise its benefits to individual and societal well-being.

The relevance of internal locus of control suggests that an interconnectedness mind-set is crucial to promote altruism, since mind-set serves as a basic organising principle of perceptions, motivations and behaviours, standing close to a worldview at the individual level. In our opinion, altruism can be more easily actualised if a mind-set of universal interconnectedness is promoted, consistently with in-depth studies conducted by Monroe (1996): 'To my surprise, most analysts since Hume appear to be wrong: group ties and group membership do not appear to be critical predictors of altruism' (Monroe 1996, p. 199). Myths of common ancestors and common descent extend the possibility of evoking same levels of empathy towards strangers as found towards kinship (Allison 1992; Boyd and Richerson 1985). Considering the whole world as one establishes a wider kinship of humanity. This inner representation of connectedness allows individuals to transcend a narrow self-centred focus, gaining to establish relationships not only within one's family, race and species but with the entire universe. In such a perspective, it is no more laws but a voluntary stance of morality that animates the interactions even among strangers, as happened with the Good Samaritan. In such a perspective, individuals and communities are motivated to enhance others' well-being not by occasional impulses, reciprocity or obligation, but by intentional choice. Perceived this way, altruism can mitigate if not solve many of the social problems encountered today, including controversial issues such as religious and ethnic intolerance, family crisis, health care and homelessness.

On the contrary, individuals who fail to nurture interconnectedness end up in a narrow self-focus. Given the interconnected human nature, resisting or severing connections can be compared to the dynamics of a cancer cell that gets disconnected from the other cells and multiplies itself uncontrolled, endangering the entire organism. A narrow self-focused inward movement can lead individuals towards a bottomless pit of constant need without satisfaction. 'It seems harder to care about the broader community of humanity than about one's tribe. But if we do not learn to do so, we will destroy not just the competing tribes but also all of civilization – our own selves' (Snyder and Lopez 2007, p. 494). Given the interconnected nature of the universe, there is either one human world or no world (Weinstein 2008). Therefore, promoting a sense of common humanity does not represent an extravagance but a necessity. Thanks to the technological revolution, the world is already growing in the sense of interconnectedness. A global village is becoming a reality (McLuhan and Fiore 1968) and a sense of common humanity seems part of the thought process with world institutions like UN and common concerns like environmental problem (Weinstein 2004).

However, interconnectedness is more than superficial closeness and problem-oriented bonds. Further, in spite of the opportunities for connection, there is also a sense of elusiveness of 'real' connection with growing need for individuation and separation (Snyder and Lopez 2007). Interconnectedness is awareness of a universe in relation. Such mind-set has to be further developed. The role of education remains highly important in promoting a mind-set of interconnectedness. Education at the level of family and societies must consider this urgent task.

3.4.1 Altruism and Cultural Diversity

During the last 40 years, psychologists have shown growing awareness about the role of culture in shaping human development and the importance of cultural variants in understanding individuals and their behaviours. The different dynamics of individualism/collectivism, for example, underscores this issue (Hofstede 1980). Collectivistic cultures emphasise the prominence of social norms and rules in directing individual behaviour, giving priority to social harmony; individualistic cultures focus on individual independence and autonomy, since the person is the primary unit of the society (Markus and Kitayama 1991; Triandis et al. 1995; Kitayama et al. 1997). Various studies highlighted that individualism and collectivism play a crucial role in other-oriented emotions and prosocial behaviours (Hui 1988; Iyengar and Lepper 1999; Leung and Iwawaki 1988; Miller 1994). Kemmelmeier and his colleagues (2006), for example, showed that the core values of individualistic cultures, such as self-actualisation, individual achievement and personal autonomy, contribute to the increase in prosocial behaviours. In similar line, another study highlights that certain words in a culture, for example, *simpatia* (Spanish) or *simpatico* (Portuguese), emphasising and prioritising amiability rather than achievement and productivity, increase helping behaviours towards strangers (Levin et al. 2001).

The value system of a culture and the priorities it accords play an important role in enhancing altruism. Attention to cultural specificities can not only help maximise altruism by using specific values of a culture but also minimise difficulties which are specific to a context (Kurman 2003; Guss 2004; Krishnan and Manoj 2008). In collectivistic cultures, where fulfilling needs of the society over the self is not just expected (Value) and extolled (Virtue), but to certain extent mandated (Duty), altruism may easily be elicited (Eckstein 2001; Miller et al. 1990). However, these premises run the risk of ending up with extrinsic motivations, which are counterproductive in the long run. In these contexts, it seems important to shift the focus on environmental factors that promote internalisation and integration of values, leading individuals from passive compliance to active personal commitment and engagement (Ryan and Deci 2000a, b). On the contrary, the voluntaristic stance of the individualistic societies (Kemmelmeier et al. 2006) may offer ambience for autonomous motivations to emerge, running however the risk of making altruism dependent on individual discretional power. Individual freedom without any external pressure may lead into lack of responsibility, as studies on the 'bystander effect' clearly point out (Darley and Latane 1968). In individualistic cultures, it seems important to develop explicit structures and mechanisms that enkindle intrinsic motivations for altruism rather than solely depending on individual initiative (Ryan and Deci 2000a, b; Zuckerman et al. 1978).

Overall, in order to be effective, altruism intervention programmes must consider the culture's orientation towards individualism or collectivism, as well as the independent vs. interdependent self-concepts deriving from it (Watkins et al. 2000). However, there are only a few studies on this topic, and little is known about altruism per se in the context of cultures. More explorations and research are needed.

3.4.2   The Dangers of Altruism

It may seem contradictory to discuss about dangers of altruism, after having showed the benefits it brings to individuals and societies. Nevertheless, altruism does indeed entail problems and dangers.

The first one is related to abuse. How much good is actually good? Studies indicate that the feeling of pressure and being overwhelmed is a major problem in behaving prosocially (Figley 1995; Hoffman 2008). Neglecting self-care in trying to meet the needs of others may lead to altruism burnout. In addition, overdoing negatively influences future altruism. Individuals tend to avoid and suppress empathic concern when they perceive the demands are too high leading to overall reduction in the willingness to be altruistic (Shaw et al. 1994; Bernheim and Stark 1988). A balance of self-love and love for others is important, without which altruism can become pathological.

The second danger is related to the context in which altruistic people live. At the individual level, behaving altruistically in zero-sum competitive situations will result in harm to the self (Pearson 1998; Batson et al. 2003), again prompting 'pathological altruism' (Oakley et al. 2011). At the collective level, societies may sustain practices and systems intrinsically not fair, and they can even fight to defend them. In this context, an altruistic individual may become a threat to the social system and its status quo. Further on, the average majority in this kind of society may also feel uncomfortable with altruistic people as their presence and behaviour can challenge common beliefs and attitudes or evoke a sense of guilt (Sorokin 1950). Considering altruism as a virtue renders further force to the dynamics of moral evaluation. It is not strange, therefore, that a socially desirable value like altruism is also a highly criticised one. The nature and dynamics of social evaluation and its effects on altruism need to be explored further.

Altruism entails a third risk at the societal level that consists in creating dependent individuals who shake off their responsibility. Coate (1995) showed that the certainty of altruistic helping (government security system, in his study) leads the beneficiaries to shake off their personal responsibility for insurance. Further studies in this line highlighted that individuals impoverish themselves through extravagance, hoping that an altruistic individual or the system would provide for them in future (Bernheim and Stark 1988). On the other hand, altruism could lead to dysfunctional behaviours in benefactors as well. Studies on perspective taking indicate that benefactors manifest unfair partiality towards the beneficiaries, to the extent that they may break norms and violate justice in order to help others (Batson et al. 1995a, b). Finally, altruism can be used to exploit people. Fundraisers, for example, manage to exploit the compassion of people to donate for causes, which are not often true or worthy (Shelton and Rogers 1981). The most dangerous case, in this regard, is manipulation of people's goodness for wrong ideologies. The effectiveness of Hitler's propaganda laid in the ability to tap people's best traits such as faith, hope and readiness to sacrifice towards an inherently evil ideology (Waite 1977). During the Rwandan genocide, many Hutus killed Tutsis because they believed it to be altruistically helping their society (Oakley et al. 2011). The same dynamics is used to motivate individuals in terrorist and suicidal attacks. These potential dangers have to be addressed in altruism promotion.

3.5   Conclusions

Altruism does exist. It is not just a moral virtue or a religious commandment but an integral part of human existence. It is not a mere behaviour that emerges occasionally and accidentally but an essential component of human development and well-being. Within the perspective of interconnectedness, altruism allows for both societal and individual actualisation simultaneously, without competing or contradicting dynamics. Nurturing a mind-set of interconnectedness based on the awareness of our common origin and destiny as human species is the mark of civilisation. It fosters flourishing of both individuals and communities. Martin Luther King said, 'Every man must decide whether he will walk in the light of creative altruism or in the darkness of destructive selfishness'. The dynamic force of the altruism spiral invites individuals and communities to embark a journey from mere self-preservation to self-realisation and eudaimonic well-being. Keeping alive the force of altruism spiral is a way to create flourishing individuals, communities and a positive world, which stand as a dream of humanity in the twenty-first century. Positive psychology can play an active role in this process, as a catalyst of potentials and abilities within individuals and societies. In fact, the third pillar of positive psychology is building positive communities and cultures (Seligman and Csikszentmihalyi 2000). If we do not care to keep alive the spiral of altruism, we will miss not only what we can gain – flourishing individuals and communities – but what we even have, our world itself.

References

AA. VV. Altruism. *Garzanti Italian dictionary*. Retrieved from http://garzantilinguistica.sapere.it
AA. VV. Altruism. In *Merriam-Webster's collegiate dictionary*. Retrieved from http://www.merriam-webster.com
AA. VV. Altruism. In *Tamil online dictionary*. Retrieved from http://www.tamilcube.com
Alistair, R. (1988). *Quantum physics: Illusion or reality*. London: Cambridge University Press.
Allison, P. (1992). The cultural evolution of beneficent norms. *Social Forces, 71*(2), 279–301.
American Psychiatric Association. (2000). *Diagnostic and statistical manual of mental disorders* (4th ed., text rev.). Arlington: American Psychiatric Publishing.
Andreoni, J. (1990). Impure altruism and donations to public goods: A theory of warm-glow giving. *The Economic Journal, 100*, 464–477.
Aristotle. (1985). *Nicomachean ethics* (T. Irwin, Trans.). Indianapolis: Hackett.
Arnstein, P., Vidal, M., Well-Federman, C., Morgan, B., & Caudill, M. (2002). From chronic pain patient to peer: Benefits and risks of volunteering. *Pain Management Nurses, 3*(3), 94–103.

Aronoff, J., & Wilson, J. P. (1984). *Personality in the social process*. Hillsdale: Erlbaum.

Bachner-Melman, R., Dina, C., Zohar, A. H., Constantini, N., Lerer, E., et al. (2005). *AVPR1a* and *SLC6A4* gene polymorphisms are associated with creative dance performance. *PLoS Genetics, 1*(3), e42. doi:10.1371/journal.pgen.0010042.

Barash, D. P. (2007). *Natural selection: Selfish altruists, honest liars and other realities of evolution*. New York: Bellevue Literary Press.

Batson, C. D. (1991). *The altruism question. Toward a socio-psychological answer*. Hillsdale: Erlbaum.

Batson, C. D., Batson, J. G., Slingsby, J. K., Harrell, K. L., Peekna, H. M., & Todd, R. M. (1991). Empathic joy and the empathy-altruism hypothesis. *Journal of Personality and Social Psychology, 61*, 413–426.

Batson, C. D., Batson, J. G., Todd, R. M., Brummet, B. H., Shaw, L. L., & Aldeguer, C. M. R. (1995a). Empathy and collective good: Caring for one of the others in a social dilemma. *Journal of Personality and Social Psychology, 68*, 619–631.

Batson, C. D., Klein, T. R., Highberger, L., & Shaw, L. L. (1995b). Immorality from empathy-induced altruism: When compassion and justice conflict. *Journal of Personality and Social Psychology, 68*, 1042–1054.

Batson, C. D., Polycarpou, M. P., Harmon-Jones, E., Imhoff, H. J., Mitchener, E. M., Bednar, L. L., et al. (1997a). Empathy and attitudes: Can feeling for a member of stigmatized group involve feeling toward the group. *Journal of Personality and Social Psychology, 72*, 105–118.

Batson, C. D., Sager, K., Garst, E., Kang, M., Rubchinsky, K., & Dawson, K. (1997b). Is empathy-induced helping due to self-other merging? *Journal of Personality and Social Psychology, 73*, 495–509.

Batson, C. D., Lishner, D. A., Carpenter, A., Dulin, L., Harjusola-Webb, S., Stocks, E. L., et al. (2003). "… As you would have then do unto you": Does imagining yourself in the other's place stimulate moral action? *Personality and Social Psychology Bulletin, 29*, 1190–1201.

Batson, C. D., Ahmad, N., & Stocks, E. L. (2004). Benefits and liabilities of empathy-induced altruism. In A. G. Miller (Ed.), *The social psychology of good and evil* (pp. 359–385). New York: Guilford Press.

Batson, C. D., Ahmad, N., Powell, A. A., & Stocks, E. L. (2008). Prosocial motivation. In J. Shah & W. Gardner (Eds.), *Handbook of motivational science* (pp. 135–149). New York: Guilford.

Baumeister, R. F. (2005). *The cultural animal*. New York: Oxford University Press.

Baumeister, R. F., & Exline, J. J. (1999). Virtue, personality, and social relations: Self-control as the moral muscle. *Journal of Personality, 67*, 1165–1194.

Baumeister, R. F., & Leary, M. R. (1995). The need to belong: Desire for interpersonal attachments as a fundamental human motivation. *Psychology Bulletin, 117*, 497–529.

Bernheim, B. D., & Stark, O. (1988). Altruism within the family reconsidered: Do nice guys finish last? *The American Economic Review, 78*(5), 1034–1045.

Bertalanffy, L. V. (1950). An outline of general system theory. *The British Journal for the Philosophy of Science, 1*(2), 134–165.

Bible. (2007). *NRSV international catholic edition*. Washington, DC: Harper Collins Publications.

Bowlby, J. (1958). The nature of the child's tie to his mother. *International Journal of Psycho-Analysis, XXXIX*, 1–23.

Boyd, R., & Richerson, P. J. (1985). *Culture and the evolutionary process*. Chicago: Chicago University Press.

Brown, R. (1988). *Little flowers of St. Francis*. New York: Doubleday Dell Publishing Group.

Brown, W. N. (1992). Some ethical concepts for the modern world from Hindu and Indian Buddhist tradition. In S. Radhakrishnan (Ed.), *Rabindranath Tagore: A centenary volume, 1861–1961*. Calcutta: Sahitya Akademi.

Brown, S., Nesse, R. M., Vonokur, A. D., & Smith, D. M. (2003). Providing social support may be more beneficial than receiving it: Results from a prospective study of mortality. *Psychological Science, 14*, 320–327.

Burtt, E. A. (1952). *The metaphysical foundations of modern science*. New York: Humanities Press.

Butterfield, H. (1997). *The origins of modern science*. New York: Free Press.

Campbell, W. K., & Foster, J. D. (2007). The Narcissistic self: Background and extended agency model and ongoing controversies. In C. Sedikides & S. Spencer (Eds.), *Frontiers of social psychology: The self* (pp. 115–138). Philadelphia: Psychology Press.

Capra, F. (1999). *The Tao of physics: An exploration of the parallels between modern physics and Eastern mysticism* (4th ed.). New York: Shambhala Publication.

Caprara, G. V., & Steca, P. (2005). Self-efficacy beliefs as determinants of prosocial behavior conducive to life satisfaction across ages. *Journal of Social and Clinical Psychology, 24*, 191–217.

Chambers, J. H., & Ascione, F. R. (1987). The effects of prosocial and aggressive videogames on children's donating and helping. *Journal of Genetic Psychology, 148*, 499–505.

Coate, S. (1995). Altruism, the samaritan's dilemma and government transfer policy. *The American Economic Review, 85*(1), 46–57.

Colman, A. E. (1982). *Co-operation and competition in humans and animals*. Wokingham: Van Nostrand Reinhold.

Comte, A. (1891). *Catechism of positivism* (R. Congreve, Trans.). London: Kegan Paul. (Original work published 1852)

Cote, J. E., & Levine, C. (2002). *Identity formation, agency, and culture*. Mahwah: Lawrence Erlbaum Associates.

Cottingham, J., Stoothoff, R., Kenny, A., & Murdoch, D. (1988). *The philosophical writings of Descartes in 3 vols*. Cambridge: Cambridge University Press.

Culler, J. (1983). *On deconstruction: Theory and criticism after structuralism*. Ithaca: Cornell University Press.

Darley, J. M., & Latane, B. (1968). Bystander intervention in emergencies: Diffusion of responsibility. *Journal of Personality and Social Psychology, 8*, 377–383.

Davis, M. H. (1983). Measuring individual differences in empathy: Evidences for a multidimensional approach. *Journal of Personality and Social Psychology, 44*, 113–126.

Davis, M. H., Soderlund, T., Cole, j., Gadol, E., Kute, M., Myers, M., et al. (2004). Cognitions associated with attempts to empathize: How do we imagine the perspective of another. *Personality and Social Psychology Bulletin, 30*, 1625–1635.

Dawkins, R. (1989). *The selfish gene* (2nd ed.). Oxford: Oxford University Press.

De Walls, F. B. M. (2008). Putting the altruism back into altruism: The evolution of empathy. *Annual Review of Psychology, 59*, 279–300.

Deci, E. L., & Ryan, R. M. (1980). *Intrinsic motivation and self-determination in human behavior*. New York: Springer.

Deci, E. L., & Ryan, R. M. (2000). The 'what' and 'why' of goal pursuits: Human needs and the self-determination of behavior. *Psychological Inquiry, 11*, 227–268.

Deci, E. L., & Ryan, R. M. (2002). *Handbook of self-determination research*. New York: University of Rochester Press.

Deci, E. L., La Guardia, J. G., Moller, A. C., Scheiner, M. J., & Ryan, R. M. (2006). On the benefits of giving as well as receiving autonomy support: Mutuality in close friendships. *Personality and Social Psychology Bulletin, 32*, 313–327.

Delle Fave, A. (2004). Positive psychology and the pursuit of complexity. *Ricerche di Psicologia, Special Issue on Positive Psychology, 27*, 7–12.

Derrida, J. (1978). *Writing and difference* (A. Bass, Trans.). London/New York: Routledge.

Diener, E., Oishi, S., & Lucas, R. E. (2003). Personality, culture and subjective well-being: Emotional and cognitive evaluations of life. *Annual Reviews, 54*, 403–425.

Dunn, E. W., Aknin, L. B., & Norton, M. I. (2008). Spending money on others promotes happiness. *Science, 319*(5870), 1687–1688.

Eckstein, S. (2001). Community as gift-giving: Collectivistic roots of volunteerism. *American Sociological Review, 66*, 829–851.

Einstein, A. (1929). Interview, October 26. Reprinted in G. S. Viereck. (1930). *Glimpses of the great* (p. 452). New York: The Macaulay Company.

Eisenberg, N. (1986). *Altruistic emotion, cognition and behaviour*. Hillsdale: Erlbaum.

Eliot, D. (1988). *Advaita Vedanta: A philosophical reconstruction*. Honolulu: University of Hawaii Press.

Emerson. (2001). *Essays by Ralph Waldo Emerson*. University Park: The Pennsylvania State University Publication.

Epstein, S. (1994). Integration of the cognitive and the psychodynamic unconscious. *The American Psychologist, 49*, 709–724.

Feyman, R. P., Leighton, R., & Sands, M. (1965). *The Feyman lectures on physics*. Reading: Addison- Wesley.

Figley, C. R. (1995). *Coping with secondary traumatic distress disorder in those who treat the traumatized*. New York: Brunner/Mazel.

Finkelstein, M. A., Penner, L. A., & Brannick, M. T. (2005). An examination of role identity and motives among hospice volunteers. *Social Behavior and Personality, 33*, 403–418.

Frankl, V. E. (1967). *Psychotherapy and existentialism: Selected papers on logotherapy*. New York: Washington Square Press.

Frankl, V. E. (1988). *The will to meaning: Foundations and applications of logotherapy*. New York: New American Library.

Fredrickson, B. L. (2004). Gratitude, like other positive emotions, broadens and builds. In R. A. Emmons & M. E. McCullough (Eds.), *The psychology of gratitude* (pp. 145–166). New York: Oxford University Press.

Frey, B. S. (1997). *Not just for the money: An economic theory of personal motivation*. Cheltenham: Elgar.

Frey, B. S., & Jegen, R. (2001). Motivation crowding theory. *Journal of Economic Surveys, 15*, 589–611.

Fromm, E. (1947). *Man for himself*. London: Routledge.

Galinsky, A. D., & Moskowitz, G. B. (2000). Perspective-taking: Decreasing stereotype expression, stereotype accessibility, and in-group favouritism. *Journal of Personality and Social Psychology, 78*, 708–724.

Gebauer, J. E., & Maio, G. R. (2012). The need to belong can motivate belief in God. *Journal of Personality, 80*(2), 465–501.

Gollwitzer, P. M. (1999). Implementation intentions: Strong effects of simple plans. *The American Psychologist, 54*, 493–503.

Gollwitzer, P. M., & Brandstaetter, V. (1997). Implementation intentions and effective goal pursuit. *Journal of Personality and Social Psychology, 73*, 186–199.

Goody, J. (1997). *The domestication of the savage mind*. Cambridge: Cambridge University Press.

Gordon, M. (2007). *Roots of empathy: Changing the world child by child*. Toronto: Thomas Allen.

Graham, A. C. (1986). *Yin-Yang and the nature of correlative thinking*. Singapore: The Institute of East Asian Philosophies.

Guss, C. D. (2004). Decision making in individualistic and collectivistic cultures. *Online Readings in Psychology and Culture*. Retrieved from http://scholarworks.gvsu.edu/orpc/vol4/iss1/3

Haidt, J., Rosenberg, E., & Hom, H. (2003). Differentiating diversities: Moral diversity is not like other kinds. *Journal of Applied Social Psychology, 33*, 1–36.

Harbaugh, W. T., Mayr, U., & Burghart, D. R. (2007). Neural responses to taxation and voluntary giving reveal motives for charitable donations. *Science, 316*(5831), 1622–1625.

Hardin, R. (1982). *Collective action*. Baltimore: Johns Hopkins University Press.

Harris, A. H., & Thoresen, C. E. (2005). Volunteering is associated with delayed mortality in older people: Analysis of the longitudinal study of aging. *Journal of Health Psychology, 10*(6), 739–752.

Hazan, C., & Shaver, P. R. (1994). Attachment as an organisational framework for research on close relationships. *Psychological Inquiry, 5*, 1–22.

Hoffman, M. L. (2008). Empathy and prosocial behaviour. In M. Lewis, J. Haviland-Jone, & L. F. Barrett (Eds.), *Handbook of emotions* (3rd ed., pp. 440–455). New York: Guilford Press.

Hofstede, G. (1980). *Culture's consequences: Inter-nations differences in work-related values*. Beverly Hills: Sage.

Hofstede, G. (2001). *Culture's consequences: Comparing values, behaviours, institutions and organizations across nations* (2nd ed.). Thousand Oaks: Sage.

Hui, C. H. (1988). Measurement of individualism and collectivism. *Journal of Research in Personality, 22*(1), 17–36.

Hunter, K. I., & Linn, M. W. (1980). Psychosocial differences between elderly volunteers and non-volunteers. *International Journal of Aging & Human Development, 12*(3), 205–213.

Isen, A. M., & Levin, P. F. (1972). The effect of feeling good on helping: Cookies and kindness. *Journal of Personality and Social Psychology, 21*, 384–388.

Iyengar, S. S., & Lepper, M. R. (1999). Rethinking the value of choice: A cultural perspective on intrinsic motivation. *Journal of Personality and Social Psychology, 76*(3), 349–366.

Jablonka, E., & Lamb, M. J. (2005). *Evolution in four dimensions: Genetic, epigenetic, behavioural and symbolic variations in the history of life*. Cambridge, MA: MIT Press.

James, E. O. (1969). *Creation and cosmology: A historical and comparative inquiry*. Leiden: Brill.

Jones, R. H. (1986). *Science and mysticism: A comparative study of western natural science, Theravada Buddhism and Advaita*. London: Bucknell University Press.

Jung, C. G. (1975). Psychology and religion: West and East. In H. Read, G. Adler, & R. F. C. Hull (Eds.), *The collected works of C. G. Jung* (Bollingen series, Vol. 11). Princeton: Princeton University Press.

Kagitcibasi, C. (1996). The autonomous-relational self: A new synthesis. *European Psychologist, 1*, 180–186.

Kagitcibasi, C. (2005). Autonomy and relatedness in cultural context: Implications for self and family. *Journal of Cross-Cultural Psychology, 36*, 403–422.

Kalupaha, D. (1975). *Causality: The central philosophy of Buddhism*. Honolulu: The University Press of Hawaii.

Kemmelmeier, M., Jambor, E. E., & Lenter, J. (2006). Individualism and good works: Cultural variation in giving and volunteering across the United States. *Journal of Cross-Cultural Psychology, 37*(3), 327–344.

Kerr, B., Smith, G. P., & Feldman, M. W. (2004). What is altruism? *Trends in Ecology & Evolution, 19*(3), 135–140.

Keyes, C. L. M. (1998). Social well-being. *Social Psychology Quarterly, 61*, 121–140.

Keyes, C. L. M. (2002). The mental health continuum: From languishing to flourishing in life. *Journal of Health and Social Behavior, 43*(2), 207–222.

Keyes, C. L. M. (2009). The black-white paradox in health: Flourishing in the face of social inequality and discrimination. *Journal of Personality, 77*(6), 1677–1706.

Keyes, C. L. M., & Annas, J. (2009). Feeling good and functioning well: Distinctive concepts in ancient philosophy and contemporary science. *The Journal of Positive Psychology, 4*(3), 197–201.

King, S. (2003). *Mosaic techniques and traditions*. New York: Sterling Publishing.

Kitayama, S., Markus, H. R., Matsumoto, H., & Norasakkunkit, v. (1997). Individual and collective processes in the construction of the self: Self-enhancement in the United States and self-criticism in Japan. *Journal of Personality and Social Psychology, 69*, 925–937.

Klen, K. J. K., & Hodges, S. D. (2001). Gender differences, motivation and empathic accuracy: When it pays to understand. *Personality and Social Psychology Bulletin, 27*, 720–730.

Knee, C. R., & Uysal, A. (2011). The role of autonomy in promoting healthy dyadic, familial, and parenting relationships across cultures. In V. I. Chrikov, R. M. Ryan, & K. M. Sheldon (Eds.), *Human autonomy in cross-cultural context* (pp. 95–110). London: Springer.

Kohut, H. (1971). *The analysis of the self*. New York: International Universities Press.

Krehbiel, L. E., & MacKay, K. (1988). Volunteer work by undergraduates. Retrieved from *ERIC database*. (ED308801).

Krishnan, L., & Manoj, V. R. (2008). "Giving" as a theme in the Indian psychology of values. In R. K. Rao, A. C. Paranjpe, & A. K. Dalal (Eds.), *Handbook of Indian psychology* (pp. 361–382). New Delhi: Cambridge University Press.

Kunda, Z., & Schwartz, S. H. (1983). Undermining intrinsic moral motivation: External reward and self-presentation. *Journal of Personality and Social Psychology, 45*, 763–771.

Kurman, J. (2003). Why is self-enhancement low in certain collectivist cultures? An investigation of two competing explanations. *Journal of Cross-Cultural Psychology, 34*, 496–510.

Laham, S. M. (2009). Expanding the moral circle: Inclusion and exclusion mindsets and the circle of moral regard. *Journal of Experimental Social Psychology, 45*(1), 250–253.

Latane, B., Nidas, S., & Wilson, D. (1981). The effect of group size on helping behaviour. In J. P. Rushton & R. M. Sorrentino (Eds.), *Altruism and helping behaviour* (pp. 287–317). Hillsdale: Erlbaum.

Lee, D. Y., Kang, C. H., Lee, J. Y., & Park, S. H. (2005). Characteristics of exemplary altruists. *Journal of Humanistic Psychology, 45*(2), 146–155.

Leung, K., & Iwawaki, S. (1988). Cultural collectivism and distributive behaviour. *Journal of Cross-Cultural Psychology, 19*(1), 35–49.

Levin, R. V., Norenzayan, A., & Philbrick, K. (2001). Cross-cultural differences in helping strangers. *Journal of Cross-Cultural Psychology, 32*(5), 543–560.

Lowen, A. (1997). *Narcissism: Denial of the true self.* New York: Touchstone Books.

Luks, A. (1988). Helper's high: Volunteering makes people feel good, physically and emotionally. And like "runner's calm", it's probably good for your health. *Psychology Today, 22*(10), 34–42.

Luks, A. (1991). *The healing power of doing good: The health and spiritual benefits of helping others.* New York: Columbine.

Lyubomirsky, S. (2007). *The how of happiness: A new approach to getting the life you want.* New York: Penguin.

Mahler, M. (1968). *On human symbiosis and the vicissitudes of individuation.* New York: International Universities.

Mahony, W. K. (1998). *The artful universe: An introduction to the Vedic religious imagination.* Albany: State University of New York Press.

Markus, H. R., & Kitayama, S. (1991). Culture and the self: Implications for cognition, emotion, and motivation. *Psychological Review, 98*(2), 224–253.

McClelland, D., McClelland, D. C., & Kirchnit, C. (1988). The effect of motivational arousal through films on salivary immunoglobulin A. *Psychology and Health, 2*, 31–52.

McCullough, M. E., Tsang, J., & Emmons, R. A. (2004). Gratitude in intermediate affective terrain: Links of grateful moods to individual differences and daily emotional experience. *Journal of Personality and Social Psychology, 86*, 295–309.

McLuhan, M., & Fiore, Q. (1968). *War and peace in the global village.* New York: McGraw-Hill.

Miller, J. G. (1994). Cultural diversity in the morality of caring: Individually oriented versus duty-based interpersonal moral codes. *Cross-Cultural Research, 28*(1), 3–39.

Miller, P. A., & Eisenberg, N. (1988). The relation of empathy to aggressive and externalization/antisocial behavior. *Psychological Bulletin, 103*(3), 324–344.

Miller, J. G., Bersoff, D. M., & Harwood, R. L. (1990). Perceptions of social responsibilities in India and in the United States: Moral imperatives or personal decisions? *Journal of Personality and Social Psychology, 58*, 33–47.

Moll, J., Krueger, F., Zahn, R., Pardini, M., de Oliviera-Souza, R., & Grafman, J. (2006). Human front-mesolimbic networks guide decisions about charitable donation. *Proceedings of the National Academy of Sciences, 103*, 15623–15628.

Monroe, K. R. (1996). *The heart of altruism: Perceptions of a common humanity.* Princeton: Princeton University Press.

Morgan, D. (2010). *Buddha recognizes Buddha.* Hexham: Throssel Hole Press.

Moss, J. A., & Barbuto, J. E., Jr. (2010). Testing the relationship between interpersonal political skills, altruism, leadership success and effectiveness: A multilevel model. *Journal of Behavioral and Applied Management, 11*(2), 155–174.

Musick, M. A., & Wilson, J. (2003). Volunteering and depression: The role of psychological and social resources in different age groups. *Social Sciences & Medicine, 56*(2), 259–269.

Nedelcu, A. M., & Michod, R. E. (2006). The evolutionary origin of an altruistic gene. *Molecular Biology and Evolution, 23*(8), 1460–1464.

Neusner, J., & Chilton, B. D. (2005). *Altruism in world religions.* Washington, DC: Georgetown University Press.

Newman, F., Milton, C., & Stroud, S. (1985). Community service and higher education: Obligations and opportunities. *American Association of Higher Education Bulletin, 37*, 9–13.

Nisbett, R. E., & Wilson, T. D. (1977). Telling more than we can know: Verbal reports on mental processes. *Psychological Review, 84*(3), 231–260.

Oakley, B., Knafo, A., Madhavan, G., & Wilson, D. S. (2011). *Pathological altruism*. New York: Oxford University Press.

Okasha, S. (2005). Altruism, group selection and correlated interaction. *The British Journal for the Philosophy of Science, 56*, 703–724.

Oliner, S. P., & Oliner, P. M. (1988). *The altruistic personality: Rescuers of Jews in Nazi Europe*. New York: Free Press.

Oman, D. (2007). Does volunteering foster physical health and longevity? In S. G. Post (Ed.), *Altruism and health: Perspectives from empirical research* (pp. 15–32). New York: Oxford University Press.

Oman, D., Thoresen, C. E., & McMahon, K. (1999). Volunteerism and mortality among the community-dwelling elderly. *Journal of Health Psychology, 4*, 301–316.

Pande, N., & Naidu, R. K. (1992). Anasakti and health: A study of non-attachment. *Psychology and Developing Societies, 4*, 89–104.

Panikkar, R. (2001). *The Vedic experience: Mantramañjari*. Bangalore: Motilal Banarsidass.

Pearson, C. (1998). *The hero within: Six archetypes we live by* (3rd ed.). San Francisco: Harper.

Peterson, C., & Seligman, M. E. P. (2004). *Character strengths and virtues: A handbook and classification*. New York: Oxford University Press.

Piliavin, J. A., & Charng, H. (1990). Altruism: A review of recent theory and research. *Annual Review of Sociology, 16*, 27–65.

Piliavin, J. A., & Siegl, E. (2007). Health benefits of volunteering in the Wisconsin longitudinal study. *Journal of Health and Social Behavior, 48*(4), 450–464.

Post, S. G. (2005). Altruism, happiness, and health: It is good to be good. *International Journal of Behavioural Medicine, 12*(2), 66–77.

Pucca, R. M., & Schmalt, H. D. (2001). The influence of the achievement motive on spontaneous thought in pre and post decisional action phase. *Personality and Social Psychology Bulletin, 27*, 302–308.

Rizzolatti, G., & Craighero, L. (2004). The mirror-neuron system. *Annual Review of Neuroscience, 27*, 169–192.

Robb, C., & Swearer, H. (1985). Community service and higher education: A national agenda. *American Association for Higher Education Bulletin, 37*, 3–8.

Rodin, J., & Langer, E. (1976). The effect of choice and enhanced personal responsibility for the aged: A field experiment in an institutional setting. *Journal of Personality and Social Psychology, 34*(2), 191–198.

Rokeach, M. (1973). *The nature of human values*. New York: Free Press.

Rozemond, M. (1998). *Descartes's dualism*. Cambridge: Harvard University Press.

Rushton, J. P. (1980). *Altruism, socialization, and society*. Englewood Cliffs: Prentice-Hall.

Rushton, J. P., Chrisjohn, R. D., & Fekken, G. C. (1981). The altruistic personality and the self-report altruism scale. *Personality and Individual Differences, 50*, 1192–1198.

Ryan, R. M., & Connell, J. P. (1989). Perceived locus of causality and internalization: Examining reasons for acting in two domains. *Journal of Personality and Social Psychology, 57*, 749–761.

Ryan, R. M., & Deci, E. L. (2000a). Intrinsic and extrinsic motivations: Classic definitions and new directions. *Contemporary Educational Psychology, 25*, 54–67.

Ryan, R. M., & Deci, E. L. (2000b). Self-determination theory and the facilitation of intrinsic motivation, social development, and well-being. *The American Psychologist, 55*, 68–78.

Ryan, R. M., & Deci, E. L. (2001). On happiness and human potentialities: A review of research on hedonic and eudaimonic well-being. *Annual Review of Psychology, 52*, 141–166.

Ryff, C. D., & Singer, B. H. (2008). Know thyself and become what you are: A eudaimonic approach to psychological well-being. *Journal of Happiness Studies, 9*, 13–39.

Ryff, C. D., Shmotkin, D., & Keyes, C. L. M. (2002). Optimizing well-being: The empirical encounter of two traditions. *Journal of Personality and Social Psychology, 82*(6), 1007–1022.

Salzberg, S., & Kabat-Zinn, J. (2008). *Lovingkindness: The revolutionary art of happiness*. Boston: Shambhala Publications.

Saussure, F. (1916). Nature of the linguistics sign. In C. Bally & A. Sechehaye (Eds.), *Cours de linguistique générale*. New York: McGraw-Hill Education.

Schore, A. N. (1994). *Affect regulation and the origin of the self: The neurobiology of emotional development*. Mahwah: Erlbaum.

Schwartz, S. H. (1992). Universals in the content and structure of values: Theoretical advances and empirical tests in twenty countries. In M. P. Zanna (Ed.), *Advances in experimental social psychology* (Vol. 25, pp. 1–65). San Diego: Academic.

Schwartz, S. H. (1994). Beyond individualism/collectivism: New dimensions of values. In U. Kim, H. C. Triandis, C. Kagitcibasi, S. C. Choi, & G. Yoon (Eds.), *Individualism and collectivism: Theory application and methods*. Newbury Park: Sage.

Schwartz, S. H. (2010). Are there universal aspects in the structure and contents of human values? *Journal of Social Sciences, 50*(4), 19–45.

Schwartz, C. E., Meisenhelder, J. B., Ma, Y., & Reed, G. (2003). Altruistic social interest behaviors are associated with better mental health. *Psychosomatic Medicine, 65*, 778–785.

Sedikides, C., Skowronski, J. J., & Dunbar, R. I. M. (2006). When and why did the human self evolve? In M. Schaller, J. A. Simpson, & D. T. Kenrick (Eds.), *Evolution and social psychology: Frontiers in social psychology* (pp. 55–80). New York: Psychology Press.

Seligman, M. E. P., & Csikszentmihalyi, M. (2000). Positive psychology: An introduction. *The American Psychologist, 1*, 5–14.

Sen, A. (1987). *On ethics and economics*. Oxford: Basil Blackwell.

Shaw, L. L., Batson, C. D., & Todd, R. M. (1994). Empathy avoidance: Forestalling feeling for another in order to escape the motivational consequences. *Journal of Personality and Social Psychology, 67*, 879–887.

Sheldon, K. M., Elliot, A. J., Kim, Y., & Kasser, T. (2001). What's satisfying about satisfying events? Comparing ten candidate psychological needs. *Journal of Personality and Social Psychology, 80*, 325–339.

Shelton, M. L., & Rogers, R. W. (1981). Fear-arousing and empathy-arousing appeals to help: The pathos of persuasion. *Journal of Applied Psychology, 11*, 366–378.

Sherman, P. W. (1985). Alarm calls of Belding's ground squirrels to aerial predators: Nepotism or self preservation? *Behavioral Ecology and Sociobiology, 17*, 313–323.

Shotland, R. L., & Stebbins, C. A. (1983). Emergency and cost as determinants of helping behaviour and the slow accumulation of social psychological knowledge. *Social Psychology Quarterly, 46*, 36–46.

Sibicky, M., Schroeder, D., & Dovidio, J. F. (1995). Empathy and helping: Considering the consequences of intervention. *Basic and Applied Social Psychology, 16*, 435–453.

Simon, H. A. (1993). Altruism and economics. *The American Economic Review, 83*(2), 156–161.

Smith, G. (1996). Binary opposition and sexual power in paradise lost. *Midwest Quarterly, 27*(4), 383–390.

Smith, T. (2007). *Most satisfying jobs*. Chicago: National Opinion Research Center/General Social Survey 2006.

Snyder, C. R., & Lopez, S. J. (2007). *Positive psychology: The scientific and practical explorations of human strengths*. New Delhi: Sage.

Sobus, M. S. (1995). Mandating community service: Psychological implications of requiring prosocial behavior. *Law and Psychological Review, 19*, 153–182.

Sorokin, P. A. (1941). *Crisis of our age*. New York: Dutton.

Sorokin, P. A. (1948). *The reconstruction of humanity*. Boston: Beacon.

Sorokin, P. A. (1950). *Altruistic love: A study of American "good neighbors" and Christian saints*. Boston: Beacon.

Spielman, D., & Staub, E. (2000). Reducing boys' aggression. Learning to fulfill basic needs constructively. *Journal of Applied Developmental Psychology, 21*, 165–181.

Staub, E. (2003). *The psychology of good and evil: Why children, adults and groups help and harm others*. New York: Cambridge University Press.

Steger, M. F., Kashdan, T. B., & Oishi, S. (2008). Being good by doing good: Daily eudaimonic activity and well-being. *Journal of Research in Personality, 42*, 22–42.

Swidler, A. (1986). Culture in action: Symbols and strategies. *American Sociological Review, 52*(2), 273–286.

Talbot, M. (1993). *Mysticism and the new physics* (2nd ed.). London: Arkana (Penguin Books).

Tankersley, D., Stowe, C. J., & Huettel, S. A. (2007). Altruism is associated with an increased neural response to the perception of agency. *Nature Neuroscience, 10*, 150–151.

Taylor, S. E., & Gollwitzer, P. M. (1995). Effects on mindset on positive illusions. *Journal of Personality and Social Psychology, 69*, 213–226.

Thoits, P. A., & Hewitt, L. N. (2001). Volunteer work and well-being. *Journal of Health and Social Behavior, 42*(2), 115–131.

Triandis, H. C. (1994). *Culture and social behaviour*. New York: McGraw-Hill.

Triandis, H. C., Chan, D. K. S., Bhawuk, D., Iwao, S., & Sinha, J. B. P. (1995). Multimethod probes of allocentrism and idiocentrism. *International Journal of Psychology, 30*, 461–480.

Upton, W. E., III. (1974). Altruism, attribution and intrinsic motivation in the recruitment of blood donors. In *Selected readings in donor recruitment* (Vol. 2, pp. 7–38). Washington, DC: American National Red Cross.

Uyenoyama, M. K., & Feldman, M. W. (1992). Altruism: Some theoretical ambiguities. In E. F. Keller & E. A. Lloyd (Eds.), *Keywords in evolutionary biology*. Cambridge, MA: Harvard University Press.

Waite, R. G. L. (1977). *The psychopathic God: Adolf Hitler*. New York: Basic Books.

Waterman, A. S. (1993). Two conceptions of happiness: Contrasts of personal expressiveness (eudaimonia) and hedonic enjoyment. *Journal of Personality and Social Psychology, 64*, 678–691.

Watkins, D., Mortazavi, S., & Trofimova, I. (2000). Independent and interdependent conceptions of self: An investigation of age, gender, and culture differences in importance and satisfaction ratings. *Cross-Cultural Research, 34*(2), 113–134.

Weinstein, J. (2004). Creative altruism: The prospects for a common humanity in the age of globalization. *Journal of Future Studies, 9*(1), 45–58.

Weinstein, J. (2008). Giving altruism its due: A possible world or possibly no world at all. *Journal of Applied Social Sciences, 2*(2), 39–53.

Weinstein, N., & Ryan, R. M. (2010). When helping helps: Autonomous motivation for prosocial behaviour and its influence on well-being for the helper and recipient. *Journal of Personality and Social Psychology, 98*(2), 222–244.

Weintraub, S. (2011). The absolute, the relative and the colonel. *Inquiring Mind, 28*(1). http://www.inquiringmind.com/Articles/AbsoluteRelative.html

Wilson, D. S. (1992). On the relationship between evolutionary and psychological definitions of altruism and selfishness. *Biology and Philosophy, 7*, 61–68.

Wojciech, G., & Ryan, L. V. (1996). *Human action in business: Praxiological and ethical dimensions*. New Brunswick: Transaction Publishers.

Wuthnow, R. (1991). *Acts of compassion: Caring for others and helping ourselves*. Princeton: Princeton University Press.

Zahn-waxler, C., Cummings, E. M., & Lannotti, R. (1991). *Altruism and aggression: Biological and social origin*. New York: Cambridge University Press.

Zuckerman, M., Porac, J., Lathin, D., Smith, R., & Deci, E. L. (1978). On the importance of self-determination for intrinsically motivated behaviour. *Personality and Social Psychology Bulletin, 4*, 443–446.

Chapter 4
The Importance of Friendship in the Construction of Positive Nations

Graciela Tonon and Lía Rodriguez de la Vega

Friendship is a virtue and the most necessary for life

(Aristóteles 2008,1155, a, 1–3)

4.1 Introduction

This chapter is aimed to highlight the importance of friendship in the construction of Positive Nations, considering that a nation is a soul constituted by two elements: the common possession of a legacy of memories and the desire to live together and to maintain the heritage received (Renan 1947).

Brandt and Hauser (2011) point out that the social category of "friend" became increasingly significant in the lives of human beings throughout the interconnectedness of our contemporary world. Liebler and Sandefur (2001) introduce the consideration of marital status on this subject by mentioning that exchanges of social support between friends are probably more important now than any other moment in American society, considering the high rates of divorce and extensive residential mobility away from family: married individuals can provide social support to one another, but unmarried ones may turn to friends. Zurco (2011) focuses on friendship during adolescence and sustains that friendship is one of the intimate relationships

G. Tonon (✉)
Faculty of Social Sciences, Universidad de Palermo,
Ciudad Autónoma de Buenos Aires, Argentina

UNI-COM, Faculty of Social Sciences, Universidad Nacional de Lomas de Zamora,
Lomas de Zamora, Argentina
e-mail: gracielatonon@hotmail.com

L. Rodriguez de la Vega
UNI-COM, Faculty of Social Sciences, Universidad Nacional de Lomas de Zamora,
Lomas de Zamora, Argentina
e-mail: liadelavega@yahoo.com

H. Águeda Marujo and L.M. Neto (eds.), *Positive Nations and Communities*, Cross-Cultural   65
Advancements in Positive Psychology 6, DOI 10.1007/978-94-007-6869-7_4,
© Springer Science+Business Media Dordrecht 2014

recognized as a significant source of support throughout life and that adolescence is the time when friendship is of special importance. Considering intercultural friendship, Peng (2011) mentions that among all the relationships with host and local nationals, friendship is one of the most important, while Hendrickson et al. (2010) say friendship is a very important component of individuals' lives to satisfy deep personal and emotional needs. Ying (2002) adds that it is also believed that forming friendships that are especially close with locals when overseas can reduce difficulties of adjustment for international students in a host country.

Some results of quantitative and qualitative research developed by the authors in Argentina showed that friendship was the variable that ranked as the highest value for the people interviewed. In 2003, Tonon applied the PWI (Personal Well-Being Index) to a group of 192 people (consisting of males and females aged 18–67), and "friendship" obtained an average of 8.66 of a scale of 0–10; then in 2005, Tonon applied the PWI to a group of 314 people with 16–18 years of age, and "friendship" obtained an average of 8.56 on the same scale. Toscano applied the PWI in 2006 to 276 people of 18–60 years of age, and "friendship" obtained an average of 8.61. These results mirrored what Argyle and Henderson (1984) considered about the rewards of making a friend that include emotional and social support, companionship in leisure activities, help, and satisfaction.

4.2   Friendship

We will initiate the chapter by clarifying the concepts that will guide our reflection; that is to say that we will state what theoretical conceptions we allude to when we speak about friendship and Positive Nations.

We find the first Western precedent of the concept of friendship in the work of Aristotle, *Nicomachean Ethics*, in which the author defines friendship as a virtue.

The singularity of the concept of friendship in Aristotle, if looked at with a twenty-first-century perspective, is that it is not circumscribed to relationship between friends but moreover includes the relationship between relatives and also citizens.

Aristotle acknowledges three types of friendship:

(a) *Friendship for pleasure*, defined from what is pleasing for each one and turns out to be accidental since one is not loved for what they are but for what they seek in a friendship. It is an easily resolvable relation when it is no longer pleasant.
(b) *Friendship for interest*, in which one seeks their own profit, typical of people who look for the most profitable thing for themselves.
(c) *The perfect friendship*, based on virtue and consequently superior to the former two, is that of the virtuous person who wants the best for their friend. Since virtue is stable, a confidence exists between them.

For Aristótle (2008, 1171, b, 33), friendship exists in the community and is defined as a community. Since all the communities seem to be a part of the political community, the different types of friendship correspond with the different types of community (Aristotle 2008, 1160, to, 25–30). This way, people can call friends the partners of campaign or navigation, and this is so because according to Aristotle (2008, 1159, b, 25–30), "the things of the friends are common."

Doyle and Smith (2002) mention that Stern-Gillet suggests that friendships for pleasure and for interest can be seen as processes, whereas the perfect friendships (the ones of virtue) are activities, central to living the good life. Only the last ones allow a relationship between whole persons. Osborne (2009) sustains that according to Aristotle we are oriented toward objects of attention outside ourselves and that this is the path toward fulfillment, since it is the object of attention that determines the quality of your thinking. We have different ways of seeing the world and we make value judgments and discriminate. Friends allow for other outlooks, for other perspectives.

Pahl (2003) sustains that virtuous friends enlarge each other's moral experience, whereas Kochin (2005) says that what Aristotle calls the wish to become friends with a particular person (a kind of liking – *philesis*) is what Telfer calls irrational.

Considering modern approaches to the subject, Adams and Allan (1998) mention that, by the 1990s, a new paradigm of relationships received considerable attention from different disciplines, implying the development of different researches and publications and acknowledging the importance of treating relationships (such as parenting and friendship) as emergent ties that have their own characteristics, rather than as the consequence or effect of the individual's attributes that the actors bring to the interaction.

Thus, while Kurth (1970) distinguished the differences between friendly relations and friendship, Brandt and Hauser (2011) point out that there is a problem of distinguishing friendship from other social relationships because it happens in proximity to other categories and advocate the clarification of the concept and support the need for a theory of friendship.

Authors like Allan (1989) define friendship as a voluntary relation among equals, and Beer (2001) labels it as an informal social relation, based on choice and free will, usually seen as affective although its emotional content may change. This author adds that beyond the key aspects, the notions of friendship are highly variable although, at present, an absence of information exists about friendship in different societies and even inside one given society.

Brandt and Hauser (2011), on the other hand, advocate for an inclusive understanding of this social phenomenon of multiple edges, which allows for a conceptual field for the many and even conflicting conceptions of friendship that can coexist, overlap, and even compete, depending on the context, interests, and values of the actors intervening. For that reason, they mention, as indicated by Grätz et al. (2003 quoted in Brandt and Hauser 2011), that social relations that do not qualify as friendship in the eyes of the Western–European observer can constitute "indigenous" categories of friendship, ignored or considered irrelevant in previous approaches. Krappmann (1996) summarizes saying that while there are cultural similarities in the concept of friendship in different societies, there are also cultural differences in its meaning and function. Gudykunst (1985) points out that friendship varies between cultures considering the principles entailed, its duration, its diffusion, and mutual confidence. Finally, Gareis (1995) claims that cultural elements like social structure, system of values, and sexual roles influence the formation of relations.

Then again, Keller (2004) says that there exists little knowledge about the meaning of friendship in non-Western industrialized societies and in more traditional societies. Considering that societies are not homogeneous, the definition of friendship varies within them and according to gender. She and her colleagues studied the development of expectations in parent–child and friendship relationships in a cultural context (in different Western societies and in China), and their findings show a complex interaction of development, content, and domain of reasoning and culture.

Adams and Allan (1998, p. 3) point out that "friendships do not operate in an abstract world, out of context. Like all the interpersonal relations, friendships are constructed – developed, modified, nourished and finished – by individual actors in context." These contexts impact directly in the construction of relations, shaping the conduct and the understanding of friends in several ways. By *context*, they mean the conditions external to the development and dissolution of specific friendships, the elements that surround them but that are not inherent to them, and support that what must be included as context will depend, at least partly, on the perspective of the analyst. They point out that the contexts are not one dimensional – their structural and cultural qualities, as well as the spatial and temporary organization, are important to understand friendship and all these qualities – and defend that they are dynamic and interactive. They also mention that different researchers have studied different levels of this context:

(a) The level of personal environment of individuals – economic circumstances, domestic responsibilities, labor commitments, and recreational preferences (Kaplan and Keys 1997; Rawlins 1992)
(b) The level of social network (includes the network of personal relations that every person withholds) (Allan 1989; Milardo and Allan 1997)
(c) The level of communities/subcultures (Crow and Allan 1994; Stack 1974)
(d) The level of societies (particularly the economic and social structures) (Litwak 1989; Lopata 1991)

4.3   A Positive Nation

A nation is a soul, a spiritual principle (Renan 1947, p. 11), and this is constituted by two elements: the common possession of a legacy of memories and the desire to live together and to maintain the heritage received. That's why the race, the language, the interests, the religious affinity, the geography, or the military needs do not suffice to create this spiritual principle.

Being part of a nation requires constant efforts as well as the renewal of a daily vote of allegiance, since the pleasant sensation of belonging that the nation offers is not gratuitous but it must be won and the opportunity to be safe is a certainty to be achieved, more than an accomplished fact (Bauman 2003, p. 172). According to Renan (1947, p. 11), "the existence of a nation is a plebiscite of every day."

The nation presupposes a past, but it is summed up in the present, for the assent and the clearly expressed desire to continue the common life, and consequently shapes a vast solidarity constructed by the feeling of the sacrifices already accomplished and of those that will be accomplished, in case and when it is necessary (Renan 1947, p. 11). According to Lechner (2002 p. 104), "a national society is still the habitual universe of daily life."

To be able to speak of Positive Nations, it is necessary to go back to the origins of the field of positive psychology and to follow Seligman (2002) when he identifies three paths of access to a fulfilled life: the positive emotions (pleasant life), the commitment (engagement life), and the search for sense understood in a wider global context (meaningful life). Later, in 2009, Seligman adds a fourth path of access – the positive bonds (social life).

Regarding the application of the positive qualification, referring to a nation, we will use Peterson's perspective (2006), defending that the word positive is not simply an adjective to apply in a sentence, but it is a qualification that takes us to the question: "Positive? What for?" This way the author integrates the notion of "enabling," thinking that certain institutions, more than others, make certain (positive) results possible. When referring to a positive nation, we would be defining it as the one that makes it possible for its citizens to have a better life when comparing to another nation. This way the good of a society remains defined in terms of the best thing for the majority of the people that compose it (Peterson 2006, p. 291).

4.4 Characteristics of a Modern Society

According to Bauman (2006, p. 13), the problems that affect people nowadays are uncertainty, insecurity, and lack of protection. When people feel insecure, worried about what the future holds for them, and when they are afraid for their safety, they are not truly free to face the risks that collective action involves. Being that insecure in life while in the company of other insecure people does not permit that people feel like a community (Bauman 2006, p. 32).

It becomes necessary to define three elements considered prerequisites for the achievement of self-confidence and independence: safety, certainty, and protection. Safety is what has been gained or obtained and will continue, in our power, that makes the world be considered as stable and reliable. Relational patterns of honesty also contribute to that safety; certainty implies knowing the differences between a reasonable thing and a senseless one, between reliable and deceitful, useful and useless, correct and incorrect, profitable and harmful, and all the other daily elections that help us to make decisions; and, finally, protection is based on righteousness and the belief that no danger will threaten our lives if our behavior is the correct one (Bauman 2006, p. 25).

For Castel (2004), what our recent societies constructed is what Beck (1992) names "society of risk" that is characterized by a general principle of uncertainty that governs the future of civilization. The risks are the contingencies of life that might be controlled, since the societies might develop mechanisms to be protected from those risks (in contrast to the threats from which there is no way of being protected). Being safe today turns out to be difficult, considering both the weakening of the traditional social and media coverage, and the widespread feeling of power-lessness toward possible threats (Castel 2004, pp. 76–77).

According to Lechner (2002, p. 48): "Insecurities generate pathologies in the social bond and conversely the erosion of the daily sociability accentuates the fear of one another." If it is possible to speak about a distrustful society and the erosion of the social bond, it becomes necessary either to restrict the scope of uncertainty or to increase the tolerance to it. And for Lechner (2002, p. 57), this is possible from the intersubjective link as a mechanism that facilitates the raising of the barriers of intolerance, since if the people place uncertainty as a shared problem and develop networks of confidence and cooperation among them, they might generate some frame of certainties.

Two cultural transformations have occurred: a change in the experiences that people obtain from social coexistence, settling more flexible relations that generate a thinner, more fragile social tissue, and a change in the representations of the society that people usually construe, since while earlier people imagined society as a coherent and cohesive body, now they feel that everything is possible, nothing is safe, and therefore it is difficult to feel part of a collective subject (Lechner 2002, p. 110).

In addition, another distinctive characteristic of the globalization process in which we live is the enormous facilitation of the means of contact (means of transport and communication) and the displacement of people that carry the pecu-liarities of their context of origin toward their context of residence. As a conse-quence, they will have to exchange cultural elements producing the transformation of all the participants in the contact, in different forms, and on a different scale. Accordingly, Li (2010) points out that the different cultural elements are very important for the beginning of intercultural relations of friendship that, in turn, in some cases, must face additional challenges such as the barriers of language (Chen 2002; Gareis 1995).

Some authors have paid attention to the relation of friendship and modernity. On this matter, Litwak (1989) suggests that friendship became more significant with modernity due to the increase of a need of flexibility that informal bonds provide in societies dominated by bureaucratic organizations, whereas Oliker (1989) indicates that the outcome of modernity had specific consequences of genre in friendship. Nevertheless, as Adams and Allan (1998) indicate, the arguments about the frag-mentation of social relations can seem compatible with those who support the trans-formation of the modern society in a postmodern one, in which friendship and solidity bonds will be of importance.

In view of this brief description of the characteristics of the current times in our nations, the discovery of friendship arises as a positive element, as a virtue and a value that pull people together. Let's then see how the subjects of the study in our research in Argentina have considered friendship.

4.5 The Value of Friendship in People's Quality of Life in Argentina

To study quality of life in Argentina since the beginning of the national crisis of 2001,[1] we used the Well-Being Index (The International Well-Being Group 2001). The index has two scales: the Personal Well-Being Index (PWI) and the National Well-Being Index (NWI).

The PWI is based on the Comprehensive Quality of Life Scale (ComQol) developed by Cummins and his colleagues (Cummins et al. 1994). The ComQol comprises both an objective and subjective measure of quality of life, and its domains were initially identified through a review of domain names used in the literature. This was subsequently followed by a three-phase process (Cummins et al. 1994) and empirical validation to generate the seven broad domains that comprised the scale (Cummins 1997). The PWI scale contains eight items of satisfaction, each one corresponding to a quality-of-life domain as standard of living, health, achievement in life, relationships, safety, community connectedness, future security, and spirituality/religion. These eight domains are theoretically embedded, as representing the first level of deconstruction of the global question: "How satisfied are you with your life as a whole?" (PWI-A Manual 2006). The national well-being index reflects nearly the same domains but couched in a national context (Tonon 2011, p. 548).

In 2003, we applied the index to 192 subjects of both sexes aged between 18 and 67 that were living in the Greater Buenos Aires area,[2] and in 2005, we applied it to 314 young people of ages between 16 and 18, of both sexes, that were also living in the Greater Buenos Aires area.[3] In the first study, "friendship" obtained an average of 8.66 and in the second study an average of 8.56. The variable summary of the PWI is the one that measures "the level of satisfaction with the life in general." The remarkable thing in the two research projects is that the applications of the WBI showed that the variable that scored the highest was the so-called satisfaction with friends. If we think that during this period of time Argentina had to overcome a national crisis (political, social, and economic) that began in 2001 and ensuing the presidential overturn, we might attempt a reflection that shows the importance of the

---

[1] Graciela Tonon developed the first application of the index in Argentina. She is a primary researcher of the International Well-Being Group organized by Dr. Robert Cummins in the Australian Centre on Quality of Life, Deakin University Australia. Lia Rodriguez de la Vega is project researcher.

[2] The Greater Buenos Aires area is a geographical area that surrounds the Ciudad Autónoma de Buenos Aires. It is organized in 24 departments and, in accordance with the census of 2010, possesses a population of 9,916,715 inhabitants.

[3] Research projects directed by Dr. Graciela Tonon, Quality of Life Research Program, Faculty of Social Sciences, Universidad Nacional de Lomas de Zamora, Argentina, *Quality of life of young people of the south zone of Buenos Aires Conurbano*, and *Quality of life of young people of the south zone of Buenos Aires Conurbano: public participation and access to health*. Programa Nacional de Incentivos para Docentes Investigadores, Ministerio de Educación, Argentina.

existence of friendship in terms of national and community values, as a positive element in the development of the quality of life of the nation.

From Aristotle's idea of friendship in terms of community, we can advance toward another idea of the author who differentiates concord from friendship, despite defining it as a type of civil friendship that is related to what is convenient and affects the life of the people in the community (Aristotle 2008, 1167, b, 1.3).

The idea of social bond defined by Lechner (2002 p. 49) appears here as the representation of a patrimony of knowledge and habits, of practical experiences and mental dispositions that a society accumulates, reproduces, and transforms along generations. The social bond needs active achievements of confidence and cooperation for development, as well as conversations on matters of common interest. The social bond is inserted in certain language and makes use of certain codification produced and reproduced in the public milieu (Lechner 2002, p. 57). "All action is political as long as it constructs a social bond and the above mentioned construction of the social thing by means of the struggle for the collective self-determination would be the form in which the society is constituted as a subject" (Lechner 2002, p. 118).

In a qualitative approach on civil, political, and communal participation of young people in Argentina, conducted by means of semi-structured interviews with young people of both sexes, aged between 18 and 28, and residents in the metropolitan region of Buenos Aires, the subject of friendship arose, demonstrating its continuities and flow.

As an example, C., a 28-year-old man, expresses that although he has friends of different moments of his life (school, faculty, militancy in political activism), the friends related to politics are those that he sees with greater frequency, with detriment to other friends, since politics, as he declares, is his passion.

Likewise M., a 26-year-old man, whose field of participation is mainly political, although having friends of other paths of his life, shares time especially with the friends who are part of the same political project, with whom he has common objectives.

These testimonies prove the idea supported by Bidart and Degenne (2005, p. 3):

> (friends) have a history that shows how the relations between context and behavior changes over time. Each friendship network is the result of a process of construction and re-composition that takes place along time. This process is responsible for the shaping of the friendship network as a result of the addition, disappearance, breaking or formation of friendship ties.

At the same time, Tampubolon (2005) supports that friendship is celebrated morally, partly as the expression of the skill to cope with personal relations of voluntary deed, as an expression of this individual action.

Another testimony demonstrates how socialization in sociocultural contexts and multiple life experiences not only bear multiple identifications but also contribute to the acquisition of social skills necessary for the establishment of cross-cultural friendships in life; the informal nature of friendship allows for a degree of flexibility in the construction of difference and similarity (Brandt and Hauser 2011). This is the case of M., an 18-year-old woman belonging to one of the aboriginal peoples of Argentina, who, in addition to remembering circumstances of discussion with people who did not belong to the same ethnic group for a different vision on different historical events, also remembers her years in secondary school, her meetings with other partners and friends with whom she shared, and still shares ideals, the militancy in student organizations, and the later creation of a social organization arisen from the determination of all of them. This organization has, as basic principles, horizontality, antiauthoritarianism, self-management, autonomy, independence, and decision-making, values that guide the group as result of discussion in assembly. She also points out that this process constituted a turning point in her life and that, for her friends, it was a space of collective growth. It is necessary to add to the mentioned that Brandt and Hauser (2011) have proposed the concept of trans-difference to refer to the high degree of flexibility at which the actors appraise similarity and difference in their interaction with others, accounting for multiple identifications in diverse sociocultural contexts that have multiple layers, meaning that the social actor takes cultural differences as a resource in the functioning of cross-cultural friendships. Testimonies evidence that the spaces of participation that the interviewees have at present constitute spaces which generate powerful ties of friendship, which coexist with other ties of friendship arisen in other stages of life. These spaces of participation, which concentrate the interest and the action of the interview, engage most of their time and attention, thus promoting these ties of friendship in them.

In a course of qualitative methodology,[4] we developed an exercise with our university students of psychology about the significance of the word "friendship." The analysis of the data showed us that university students expressed that friendship is a concept difficult to define, even if people think it is very clear to understand, and they recognized that it is a word with a diversity of definitions. The classification of our student's answers showed us three possibilities for the definition:

(a) Friendship as a subjective construction: based in a close social interaction
(b) Friendship as human relation: that involves feelings and respect and people affects and freedom
(c) Friendship as a group of values that need shared feelings

Different authors have indicated three reasons for the beginning of friendships: (a) the proximity or personal contact with another person (Berscheid and Walster 1991); (b) similarity in beliefs and values (Osbeck and Moghaddam 1997), to which Dod (1991 quoted in Li 2010) adds the similarity in age, gender, education, interests, etc.; and (c) the self-revelation or mutual sincerity (Berg and Archer 1980). This way, the testimonies considered allow us to indicate the presence of the reasons advocated.

---

[4]Course of *qualitative methodology* taught by Dra. Graciela Tonon in the Psychology Program. Universidad de Palermo, Argentina. April 2012.

4.6 Conclusions

As mentioned above, Seligman (2009) identifies four routes of access to a fulfilling life: the positive emotions (pleasant life), the commitment (engagement life), the search of sense understood in a wider global context (meaningful life), and the positive bonds (social life).

If, on referring to a positive nation, we understand it as the one that makes a better life possible for its citizens, more than if they were members of another nation and the good in a society remains defined in terms of what is best for the majority of its components (Peterson 2006, p. 291), then, in accordance with the quantitative approaches mentioned, besides the importance assigned by the interviewees to friendship, it is necessary to think that the Argentine nation makes the context possible for social positive bonds such as friendship.

On the other hand, the qualitative approach to which we refer shows that, as Roseneil mentions (1999, quoted in Brandt and Hauser 2011), people somehow use their friendships to construct their and others' identity in individual and group terms, and that the notions of themselves, their belongings, and personal relations are not only influenced by sociocultural processes but also updated by the actors and their interactions with others.

As we know, identity implies belonging to a social group that allows its members to distinguish among "I"/"we" and "other"/"they," being in turn carriers of different social roles that show different aspects of that identity in different situations. The otherness of the sublime is the communicative relation, which involves in itself the configuration of social and symbolic borders and a distinctive evaluation of the current axiological categories in the social and cultural group in which it is inserted. This communicative relation, inherent to identity as such, constitutes an epistemological space, while the subjects, by telling about them, tell about their group of belonging and the reality in which they are inserted, and by telling of the others, they configured social acknowledgments in which underlie, in the case of our interviewees, their intentions of change and collective social construction.

The qualitative approach shows, as we said, two of the reasons mentioned by different authors to initiate friendship: the proximity and personal contact with others and the similarity, in many cases of age, but fundamentally of interests and opinions. In view of this, we can link the first quality (proximity) to a characteristic of the participation that also becomes clear, such as the demarcation of the space or locality associated with this participation – since it alludes to the daily reality and the social practices of every interviewee – and re-signifies the collective construction. In the same way, this similarity in the construction of friendship and the solidity of friendships linked to the principal space of participation mentioned by the interviewees allows a reference to common ethics that shows a close relation between doing and personal well-being and doing and collective well-being.

That is to say, the spaces of participation and of friendship are tied to both logical perspectives and denote the existence of "founding participation" that emerges from the existential and axiological needs of subjects that interact, associated with social daily practices. On the other hand, all this seems to reveal the routes of access to a full life, enunciated by Seligman (2002).

Finally, recapturing the concept of friendship in Aristotle, which does not limit itself to friendship between friends but also includes the relation among relatives and citizens – since what every person thinks that its existence is, or what they prefer to live, is what they want to do with friends – we can link the positive emotions shown by the interviewees, their commitment, the positive bonds, and the search for meaning understood in a wider global context to the common ethics that shows a close relation between personal and group well-being and their "founding participation." This ties them to the collective construction that of the nation.

References

Adams, R. G., & Allan, G. (1998). Contextualizing friendship. In *Placing friendship in context* (pp. 1–17). Cambridge: Cambridge University Press.

Allan, G. (1989). *Friendship: Developing a sociological perspective*. Hemel Hempstead: Harvester-Wheatsheaf.

Argyle, M., & Henderson, M. (1984). The rules of friendship. *Journal of Social and Personal Relationships, 1*(2), 211–237.

Aristóteles. (2008). *Etica Nicomaquea*. Barcelona: Gredos.

Bauman, Z. (2003). *Modernidad líquida*. México: Editorial Fondo de Cultura Económica.

Bauman, Z. (2006). *En busca de la política*. Buenos Aires: Fondo de Cultura Económica.

Beck, U. (1992). *Risk society: Towards a new modernity*. London: Sage.

Beer, B. (2001). Anthropology of friendship. In *International encyclopedia of the social and behavioral sciences* (pp. 5805–5808). Kidlington: Elsevier.

Berg, J. H., & Archer, R. L. (1980). Disclosure or concern: A second look at liking for the norm breaker. *Journal of Personality, 48*, 245–257.

Berscheid, E., & Walster, E. (1991). Self-esteem and attraction. *Journal of Personality and Social Psychology, 17*, 84–91.

Bidart, C., & Degenne, A. (2005). Introduction: The dynamics of personal networks. *Social Networks, 27*(4), 283–287.

Brandt, A., & Hauser, E. A. (2011). Friendship and socio-cultural context. Experiences from New Zealand and Indonesia. In B. Descharmes et al. (Eds.), *Varieties of friendship. Interdisciplinary perspectives on social relationships* (pp. 145–174). Göttingen: V&R Unipress.

Castel, R. (2004). *La inseguridad social ¿Qué es estar protegido?* Buenos Aires: Manantial.

Chen, L. (2002). Communication in intercultural relationships. In W. Gudykunst & B. Mody (Eds.), *Handbook of international and intercultural communication* (pp. 241–258). Thousand Oaks: Sage.

Crow, G., & Allan, G. (1994). *Community life: An introduction to local social relationships*. Hemel Hempstead: Harvester-Wheatsheaf.

Cummins, R. (1997). *Comprehensive quality of life scale- Adult manual* (5th ed.). Melbourne: School of Psychology, Deakin University.

Cummins, R., McCabe, M., Romeo, Y., & Gullone, E. (1994). The comprehensive quality of life scale: Instrument development and psychometric evaluation on tertiary staff and students. *Educational and Psychological Measurement, 54*, 372–382.

Doyle, M. E., & Smith, M. K. (2002). Friendship: Theory and experience. *The encyclopaedia of informal education*, Last update: December 01, 2011. http://www.infed.org/biblio/friendship.htm

Gareis, E. (1995). *Intercultural friendship: A qualitative study*. Lanham: University Press of America.

Gudykunst, W. B. (1985). An exploratory comparison of close intracultural and intercultural friendships. *Communication Quarterly, 33*(4), 270–283.

Hendrickson, B., Rosen, D., & Aune, K. (2010). An analysis of friendship networks, social connectedness, homesickness, and satisfaction levels of international students. *International Journal of Intercultural Relations, 35*, 281–295.

Kaplan, D., & Keys, C. (1997). Sex and relationship variables as predictors of sexual attraction in cross-sex platonic friendships between young heterosexual adults. *Journal of Social and Personal Relationships, 14*, 191–206.

Keller, M. (2004). A cross-cultural perspective on friendship research. *ISBBD Newsletter, 46*(2), 10–14.

Kochin, M. S. (2005). *Friendship beyond reason.* http://www.geocities.ws/mskochin/workinprogress/friendship55.pdf

Krappmann, L. (1996). Amicitia, drujba, shin-yu, philia, Freundschaft, friendship: On the cultural diversity of human relationship. In W. M. Bukowski, A. F. Newcomb, & W. W. Hartup (Eds.), *The company they keep: Friendship in childhood and adolescence* (pp. 19–40). New York: Cambridge University Press.

Kurth, S. B. (1970). Friendships and friendly relations. In G. McCall, M. McCall, N. Denzin, G. Suttles, & S. B. Kurth (Eds.), *Social relationships* (pp. 136–170). Chicago: Aldine.

Lechner, N. (2002). *Las sombras del mañana. La dimensión subjetiva de la política.* Santiago de Chile: LOM Editorial.

Li, Z. F. (2010). *Bridging the gap: Intercultural friendship between Chinese and Americans.* Master Thesis. School of Communication, Liberty University, Lynchburg, VA.

Liebler, C. A., & Sandefur, G. D. (2001). *Gender differences in the exchange of social support with friends, neighbors, and coworkers at midlife* (CDE Working Paper No. 2001-12). Center for Demography and Ecology University of Wisconsin-Madison. http://www.ssc.wisc.edu/wlsresearch/publications/files/public/LieblerSandefur_Gender.Differences.in.the.Exchange.of.Social.Support.with.Friends.Neighbors.and.Coworkers at.Midlife_CDE_2001-12.pdf

Litwak, E. (1989). Forms of friendship among older people in industrial society. In R. G. Adams & R. Blieszner (Eds.), *Older adult friendships: Structure and process* (pp. 65–88). London: Sage.

Lopata, H. Z. (1991). Friendship: Historical and theoretical introduction. In H. Lopata & D. Maines (Eds.), *Friendship in context* (pp. 1–19). Greenwich: JAI Press.

Milardo, R. M., & Allan, G. (1997). Social networks and marital relationships. In S. Duck et al. (Eds.), *Handbook of personal relationships* (pp. 502–522). London: Wiley.

Oliker, S. (1989). *Best friends and marriage: Exchange among women.* Berkeley: University of California Press.

Osbeck, L. M., & Moghaddam, F. M. (1997). Similarity and attraction among majority and minority groups in a multicultural context. *International Journal of Intercultural Relations, 21*, 113–123.

Osborne, C. (2009). Selves and other selves in Aristotle's Eudemian ethics vii 12. *Ancient Philosophy, 29*(2), 349–371.

Pahl, R. (2003). *Sobre la Amistad.* Madrid: Siglo XXI.

Peng, F. (2011). *Intercultural friendship development between Finnish and international students.* Master Thesis. Department of Communications, Humanities Faculty, University of Jyväskylä, Jyväskylä.

Peterson, C. (2006). *A primer in positive psychology.* Oxford: Oxford University Press.

Rawlins, W. (1992). *Friendship matters: Communication, dialectics and the life course.* New York: Aldine de Gruyter.

Renan, E. (1947). *¿Qué es una nación? Cristianismo y judaísmo. Contemporáneos ilustres. Consejos del sabio.* Buenos Aires: Editorial Elevación.

Roseneil, S., & Seymour, J. (1999). *Practicing identities. Power and resistance.* Basingstoke Hampshire/London/New York: MacMillan press LTD./St. Martin's Press Inc.

Seligman, M. (2002). *La auténtica felicidad.* Barcelona: Vergara.

Seligman, M. (2009, June). *Special lecture. First world congress on positive psychology.* Philadelphia: International Positive Psychology Association.

Stack, C. (1974). *All our kin.* New York: Harper & Row.

Tampubolon, G. (2005). *Fluxes and constants in the dynamics of friendships*. ESRC Research Methods Program (Working Paper No 25). Centre for Research on Socio-Cultural Change. University of Manchester. http://www.ccsr.ac.uk/methods/publications/documents/WP25.pdf Accessed 12 Jan 2012.

The International Well-Being Group (2001) *WBI*. Manual Australian Centre on Quality of Life. Deakin University Australia. http://www.deakin.edu.au/research/acqol/bibliography/

The International Well-Being Group. *Personal well-being-adult (PWI-A)* Manual 2006.

Tonon, G. (2011). Quality of life in Argentina. In K. C. Land et al. (Eds.), *Handbook of social indicators and quality of life research* (pp. 547–554). Dordrecht: Springer Science + Business Media.

Ying, Y. W. (2002). Formation of cross-cultural relationships of Taiwanese international students in the United States. *Journal of Community Psychology, 30*(1), 45–55.

Zurco, M. (2011). Friendship during adolescence: The necessity for qualitative research of close relationships. *Polish Journal of Applied Psychology, 9*(1), 21–38.

Chapter 5
Satsang: A Culture Specific Effective Practice for Well-Being

Kamlesh Singh, Anjali Jain, and Dalbir Singh

5.1 Introduction

Considering cultural perspective, simultaneous understanding is appreciated when we consider the concepts, "happiness and well-being" in western cultures and *ananda* and *sukha* in Asian cultures. One of the aims of Positive Psychology is to improve lives. Positive interventions can either be deliberately introduced or prevailing positive practices can be evaluated and later promoted, to enhance well-being. Yoga and meditation are worldwide known practices; however, role of indigenous practice such as *satsang* is yet not explored effectively. Three consecutive studies were conducted in order to understand *satsang* as an indigenous therapeutic practice in rural India. Qualitative analysis of interviews and Focused Group Discussion indicated significant themes suggesting improvement in measures of well-being, pro-social behavior, and spiritual growth with concurrent reduction in stress and conflicts.

5.2 Culture Specificity

Cross-cultural understanding of well-being has been the focus of many researches utilizing quantitative methods (Diener et al. 2003; Park et al. 2006) and mixed methods (Delle Fave et al. 2011). Hwang (2004) talked of two microworlds: the western approach to knowledge belonging to scientific microworld and the wisdom tradition

K. Singh (✉) • A. Jain
Department of Humanities and Social Sciences, Indian Institute of Technology, Delhi, India
e-mail: singhk.iitd@gmail.com; singhk@hss.iitd.ac.in; anjalij.iitd@gmail.com

D. Singh
Geography Department, Pt. N R S Government College, Rohtak, Haryana, India
e-mail: dlbrhooda@gmail.com

H. Águeda Marujo and L.M. Neto (eds.), *Positive Nations and Communities*, Cross-Cultural
Advancements in Positive Psychology 6, DOI 10.1007/978-94-007-6869-7_5,
© Springer Science+Business Media Dordrecht 2014

as followed in Asian countries focusing on lifeworld. The present research focuses more on this aspect of lifeworld. India is historically known for its culminating diverse cultures and rich ancient ethnic traditions that set it apart from other geographical astute countries and societies. Across cultures, people aspire to lead meaningful and satisfying lives, cultivate the best in their families, and exemplify fulfilling experiences in their daily lives.

In Indian rural society, a culturally sensitive practice known as *satsang* was considered worthy of exploration. Individuals cannot be alienated from culture, and thus it is vital to appreciate the culture in order to understand the individual (Varjas et al. 2005). This suggests that an individual belonging to eastern culture may differ in indicators of well-being as compared to the characteristics influencing the western culture. For instance, in Indian rural society, cultures may promote different form of expressing gratitude, kindness, and altruistic behavior rather than performing acts of kindness or writing a letter of gratitude such as in western society where self-focused activities like as reflecting on personal strengths and weaknesses may predominate. Considering the fact that there is one psychotherapist per half million people in India, it can be contented that services of modern psychotherapy are highly inadequate to meet the massive mental health requirements of Indian community (Dalal 2007). This is compounded with unique to the culture, gender-bound health problems becoming a barrier in health care (Davar 2001). Specific to Indian tradition, the particular familial upbringing, financial constraints, socio-communal identity, and heavy dependence on social support play a categorical role in determining the health scenario (Patel et al. 1999). Also, rural areas have relatively higher prevalence of collectivism as compared to urban areas in India (Duggal Jha and Singh 2011). Together all these reasons necessitate the need to evaluate sociocultural issues in Indian subculture differently.

5.3 Happiness and Well-Being: Western Perspective

Diener (1984) defined subjective well-being as "a person's evaluative reactions to his or her life, either in terms of life satisfaction (cognitive evaluations) or affect (ongoing emotional reactions)." Ryff and Keyes (1995) proposed a multidimensional model consisting of six dimensions of well-being: self-acceptance, a sense of continued growth and development, belief that life is purposeful and meaningful, positive relations with others, and environmental mastery. Keyes (1998) similarly suggested a model of social well-being comprising of five key elements, namely, social integration, social contribution, social coherence, social actualization, and social acceptance. He later combined subjective well-being/emotional well-being and concept of psychological well-being from Ryff's (1989) model to the mental health continuum (Keyes 2002). More recently, Seligman (2011) also proposed five measurable elements of well-being: positive emotion, engagement, relationships, meaning and purpose, and accomplishment (PERMA).

5.3.1 Well-Being in Indian Context

Hindu tradition iterates that human behavior can be best understood when evaluated in the context of *desh* (place or location), *kala* (time), and *patra* (the individual) (Sinha 2002). In India, the term positive mental health is often referred to the state of mental harmony and spiritual development and not mere absence of mental affliction (Wig 1990). The Indian system is rooted in a broad ontological conceptualization where every organism is a composite entity of mind, body, and spirit. Peak personal peace and joy can be achieved by gaining knowledge of studying culturally specific indigenous approaches and learning from spiritual gurus who propagate paths involving surrendering desires and spirituality or *jnanmarg* (Bhawuk 2010).

Indian Psychology and Positive Psychology are considered birds of the same feather (Kumar 2010), both having the common aim of attaining well-being. The meaning, relevance, and pursuit of happiness is an old subject of psychological and philosophical inquiry (Halbfass 1997). Sri Aurobindo, an Indian philosopher, noted that true happiness resides at the point of harmony of spirit, mind, and body (Pande and Naidu 1992). Sanskrit equivalent of happiness is *sukham* (*su*=plenty, *kham*=space) referring to a natural state of "limitless" space. In *Bhagavad Gita*, 'happy state' denotes a larger "accommodative mental space" within the individual (Menon 1998). It is argued that humans seek for inner source of happiness called *satcitananda* (*sat* meaning being truthful, *chit* referring to being aware, and *ananda* being the bliss) (Srivastava and Misra 2011). They further reiterated in *Taittiriya Upanishad* that happiness and well-being are times when unobstructed manifestation of *ananda* or bliss is felt.

Indian philosophy proposes that every human being has his or her own unique nature or *prakriti*, and temperament or *svabhava* which is made up of three basic attributes called *Tri-gunas*, namely, *sattva, rajas,* and *tamas* (Verma and Verma 1989). *Sattva* is symbolized by purity, wisdom, bliss, serenity (peacefulness), love of knowledge, and spiritual excellence. *Rajas* is represented by egoism, activity, restlessness, and desire for wealth, power, and comforts (external locus of control), whereas *tamas* is associated with qualities such as bias, heedlessness (negligence), inertia, and perversion (distortion) in taste, thought, and action (Das 1991). Reason for obstruction or depression is *tamas,* and attitude responsible for illumination or happiness is *sattva.* More the *sattva,* greater is the experience of *ananda* (Kumar 2010). He further iterated that Positive Psychology can be redefined as the study of *sattva guna*, making use of *rajas guna* and managing *tamas guna* (Kumar 2010).

In a survey done in eight major cities of India, 75 % of respondents described their current state to be "happy", constituents being tranquility (52 %), good health (50 %), success at work (43 %), family (40 %), money (38 %), and love (33 %) (*Outlook* 2005). In East Asia, happiness often pertains to harmonious interpersonal relationships, success at work, and contentment from life (Kitayama et al. 2000; Lu et al. 2001).

Anasakti, a Sanskrit term for traits like non-attachment, equipoise, selfless duty orientation, and effort in the absence of concern for the outcome, can be regarded as a Hindu-ideal cluster of happy personality (Banth and Talwar 2012). *Anasakti,* the disengagement of consciousness from immediate outcomes and desires, is characterized by effort orientation, emotional equipoise, and limited concern for external reward (Pande and Naidu 1992). Research indicates that yogic practitioners are considerably higher in *anasakti* with large correlation between *anasakti*, meaningful life, and well-being than secular population (Banth and Talwar 2012). *Anasakti* dismisses the individual from the anxieties of success and failure. This perspective is rooted in *Bhagavad Gita* where it is purported that purpose of life is to be able to liberate oneself from suffering and realizing the true identity of self with respect to ultimate reality. Messages embedded in *bhajans* (folk songs) in *satsang* promote these human virtues thereby enhancing well-being. Indian literature also talks of five *kleshas* or mental afflictions: ignorance (*avidya*), egoism (*asmita*), attraction (*raga*), repulsion (*dvesa*), and lust for life (*abhinivesa*). As read in 18 *Puranas Vyasa*, behavior can be understood as the *dharma*. Its components are *paropkar* or helping others; *punya*, a good deed; *parapidan*, the act of hurting others which is *paap* or sin; *tyaga* the act of sacrifice; *ahinsa* referring to nonviolence, and *dana* the act of charity (Krishnan 2005). Folk songs in *satsang* contain repeated messages to abstain from five *kleshas* and to do *paropkar, punya, tyaga,* etc. Well-being can be summarized as "the subjective feeling of contentment, happiness and satisfaction with life's experiences and with one's role in the world of work, with sense of achievement, utility, belongingness and no distress, dissatisfaction or worry" (Verma and Verma 1989).

5.3.2 Well-Being Enhancing Strategies: Induced or Existing

One of the aim of Positive Psychology is that flourishing communities can be understood in two ways: by either introducing an intervention to enhance well-being or by systematically evaluating effectiveness of a existing practice in the society (Singh 2009; Singh and Dangi 2011). Efficacy of deliberately induced positive psychotherapy is well documented (Diener and Diener 1995; Gilman and Huebner 2000; Park and Huebner 2005; Seligman et al. 2005; Singh and Choubisa 2009). Urban India enjoys the luxury of existing systems such as spiritual ashrams, Yoga, and meditation which have been widely explored (Feldman et al. 2010; Jain 2007; Rauscha et al. 2006; Smith et al. 2007; Smith 2000); however, rural people yet continue only to pursue the local religious practices that may contribute to their well-being. Effectiveness of a local practice, known as *satsang* (singing local songs embedded with religious or spiritual messages in the group), in promoting well-being as any other indigenous practice suffers from dearth of scientific literature. Therefore, it was considered noteworthy to explore the existing culturally specific practice that can augment well-being of rural India. Culture specific interventions keep in consideration the beliefs, values, and language relevant to that particular culture.

Effort at bringing a "change" should not ignore culture's influence in promoting and sustaining patterns of behavior (Nastasi 1998). Moreover, results of studies may be confounded if facilitators of flow, psychological well-being, and happiness, that may be sensitive to sociocultural factors in collectivistic societies, are ignored. It is understood that direct application of western-oriented psychotherapies may not be effective in Indian regional culture (Singh and Singh 2010).

5.3.3 Well-Being Promoting Therapies

Music is a therapeutic modality that heals and progresses people mentally, physically, emotionally, and socially (Chiang 2008). Creative therapies like positive art therapy (PAT) and music therapy are non-traditional modalities that positively regulate healing in core functions of the brain which have not responded to traditional interventions (Perry 2008). PAT interplays between art therapy, positive emotions, positive character, and positive communities. It increases experiences of pleasant experiences, flow, individual and social well-being; thereby making lives more engaging and meaningful (Chilton and Wilkinson 2009). PAT also contributes in enhancement of community-based culturally sensitive models (emic). Similar is observed among Hindu village healers in northern India who use "sacred music therapy" (Cook 1997). Lyrics of music also play a key role. Listening to songs with pro-social message increases the accessibility of pro-social thoughts and result in more altruistic behavior as compared to songs with neutral lyrics (Greitemeyer 2009a). Traditional cultures have different healing practices due to prevalence of its unique religious beliefs, histories, geographies, customs, and musical traditions (Moreno 1995). "Singing religious songs" may be considered as musical and an artful act. The success of traditional healing strengthens the respective religious faith and beliefs.

Systematic practice of focused concentration, also called meditation, brings about overt and covert changes in our consciousness. Several empirical studies support that meditation in any form helps in reducing cognitive, somatic, and general state anxiety (Rauscha et al. 2006); enhances psychological well-being (Brown and Ryan 2003); and promotes social and emotional benefits for socially isolated people (Lindberg 2005). Several studies have showed efficacy of Transcendental Meditation over other therapies in enhancing mental and physical health (Alexander et al. 1989) and reducing stress and anxiety (Grosswald et al. 2008). Yoga commonly causes inhibition of instabilities of the mind. In order to attain this, *abhyasa* or constant practice and *vairagya*, i.e., detachment from worldly desires, is required. *Asanas* or physical postures are important elements in the practice of Yoga. *Dharana, Dhyana,* and *Samadhi* form the three stages of one continuous process, which may be roughly equated with meditation (Kapur 2011). All together helps in reformation of psyche (Jain 2007) and improving mental and physical health (Hadi and Hadi 2007) along with subjective well-being (Malathi et al. 2000).

5.3.4 Satsang

The enchanting and reverb hallmark of the Indian perspective of Psychology lies in its emphasis on inner-directedness and spirituality. It is said that the desire of achieving well-being for all, has been the core Indian concern that has panhuman relevance. The term *satsang* is used in various contexts. It implies "companionship of the righteous" for the "ignorant" as well as for spiritual aspirants. *Rishis* "seer or sage" used to spread the idea of *satsang* in ancient era. *Satsang* refers to company of holy people who unremittingly seek for God. It is believed that company of enlightened people radiate positive or spiritual energy to the minds, and this accelerates member's spiritual progress, as is contrary to *tamas* (Goel 2008). The member is empowered by being able to recognize his/her abilities to think, act, and feel in an integrated and complete fashion as he encounters a guru or gets guidance from some elder or other evolved member while engaging in relevant discourses. *Satsang* is a much wider term than listening to discourses (*pravachan*). Participating in the company of noble people (*satsangati*) who are enlightened or knowledge-able works like a paradigm shift for all its members. Initial group diversification automatically converges into a group cohesion where singing of discourses result in personal and spiritual growth. The life, the world, and the modes of experience get positively transformed. However, in the present research, we will be referring to *satsang* as "singing of religious songs in groups" which is common a practice in rural India. Unique to every culture, folklore has its own cultural transmission of messages through different mediums. Folk songs or *lokgeet* among women serves as catharsis for some and celebration for others, while at the same time it also reflects how they perceive, process, and communicate their experiences and feel-ings to other members of group. In rural community, women sing variety of folk songs like on the occasion of marriage, son birth in the family, and religious occa-sions. Singing folk songs or better understood as religion-driven songs, sung in groups by Indian rural women, has long been a part of Indian rural women's enter-tainment and a source that disengages them from daily stress and engages them into the thought of God. Folk songs are sung without using any musical instrument in a rhythmic manner especially as observed in the state of Haryana, India. The lyrics are straightforward and reflect variety of folk emotions, thoughts, and anec-dotes and echo the whole social system.

5.3.5 *Other Indigenous Practices Promoting Well-Being*

Almost all auspicious activities in India start with *swastika* creation. *Swastika* or universal welfare specifies happiness, safety, fertility, and prosperity (Kamat 2013). *Swastika* comes from *Swasti* meaning well-being of one and all, and *ka* refers to symbol. The four corners of the *swastika* represent four *purusharthas* (aims of life), namely, *dharma, artha, kama,* and *moksha,* and the ideal structure indicates the balance. The four stages in a man's life – *brahmacharya* (celibacy), *grihastha* (housekeeper), *vanaprashta* (seclusion), and *sanyasa* (renunciation) – represent the four corners of *swastika* and the life being the one connecting them (Kamat 2013). Indian cultures promote pro-social behavior, altruism, and oneness even by the way of celebrating several culturally profound festivals like *Holi* and *Diwali*. Festivals like *Karwa Chauth* and *Raksha Bandhan* strengthen and mobilize interpersonal relationships; religion-oriented festivity like *Kshama* day celebrated in Jainism and regionally specific harvest festival like *Makar Sankranti* (traditionally, offer gifts and honor to family elders) in Haryana and many more promote positive virtues like forgiveness, selflessness, gratitude, strong familial relationships, and well-being. However, an appreciative enquiry on these issues may considerably contribute to the literature. *Satsang*, an indigenous practice, is central theme of this chapter.

Wide-spreading religious/spiritual institutions seem to share their objectives with Applied Positive Psychology. *Radha Soami Satsang Beas* registered as *Science of the Soul Center* internationally constitutes two million members from Europe and the United States (Wolfe 2002) philosophizes that every human is entrusted with a specific purpose of life (Sachdev 2001). They propagate *Sant Mat* (teachings of the saints) and *guru pratha*, a method of attaining peace and happiness, reflecting hope, faith, and charity, as guided and mentored by gurus (Sand 1993). They foster a regime involving vegetarian diet, moralistic living, and belief in oneness of God with abstinence from tobacco and alcohol (Sachdev 2001). Meditating daily is mandatory. *Brahma Kumaris* is another such organization forming over 2.5 million members of all ethnicity. Specialized teaching programs impart lectures on positive thinking, stress management guided by principles of positive thinking, living values, and overall self-management constituting peace and humility. Unfortunately, the language of spirituality – suffering, faith, charity, forbearance, sacrifice, and transformation – have remained unfamiliar to psychologists (Pargament and Mahoney 2002). Several charitable hospitals and societal welfare centers include *satsang* and meditation centers (Larsen 2007). Other *ashrams* include *Art of Living, Shiva Yoga,* and *Sri Aurobindo Ashram*. Art of Living headed by Sri Ravi Shankar focuses on procedures such as *Sudarshankriya*, Yoga, and meditation as means to achieve relief from stress, improving relationships, enhancing health and well-being, and attaining wisdom. Guided by the motto, "all life is Yoga," *Sri Aurobindo Ashram* emphasizes development of consciousness, "becoming aware of oneself in every activity of the mind, heart, life-force and the very body" at physical, *pranic*, emotional, mental, and spiritual level by practicing *yogic kriya* ("Research Program Framework," 2012). Therefore, various spiritual and religious groups attract people for attaining wisdom and meaning in life through indigenous practices.

5.4 Relevance of the Study

In this chapter, a culture specific research question is explored: Does singing folk songs (*bhajans*) in *satsang* act as a music therapy, contributing to rural women's well-being? This research question has been absent in the documented researches, and despite the enormous issues concerning rural women they remain underprivileged. For instance, it was observed that a variety of folk songs by male singers were frequently being sung in the society and several were available on the Internet; however, there was no trace of any activity undertaken by rural women on any social media network (Singh and Singh 2010). This implied that men not only had more leisure time than women in rural culture but also were simply more at liberty to decide what they wanted to do with their time (Puchner 2003).

Sinha (2011) reported that often more than one person respond when the researcher would be talking to a person in Indian setting; they may interrupt, correct, add, and elaborate responses by adding new information, pointing out antecedent factors, and describing consequences of behavior. This was found opposing to the western concept of privacy. The shift from experimental work to culturally relevant research using qualitative method since the last decade is apparent. Moreover, blindly replicating western study's methodology may not be valid to social research conducted in India (Misra and Paranjpe 2012). Misra (1990) supported this by stating that rural and urban India constitute two independent subsystems demanding separate tools for data collection and distinct parameters for analysis since it would be misleading to understand the rural population by applying the principles and parameters derived from the urban samples. "Research methodology must follow the demand of the research questions, rather than researchers manufactured questions that fit the experimental methodology" (Bhawuk 2010). Having understood the relevance and prerequisite for culture specific therapeutic practices in enhancing well-being of rural women, certain indigenous practices or discourses have been explored in the present study to investigate their perceived influence on well-being of its participants, if any. *Bhajans* or singing prayers in *satsang* as noted has been a part of individual's entertainment since eternity. This was empirically evaluated to opine if it has been much more than a mere entertainment activity, a form of group meditation existing and unknowingly healing masses from long ago.

Series of three independent studies were conducted in this pursuit. Study 1 aimed to understand attitudes of participants toward religious activities-*satsang* – and the *guru*. Study 2 aimed to explore if folk songs (*bhajans*) acted as music therapy for Indian rural women, and finally in study 3, Focused Group Discussion (FGD) was conducted where the moderator guided the discussion to evaluate the perception and impact of *satsang* on Indian rural women.

5.4.1   Study 1

Study 1 was conducted to understand the attitudes of Indian rural women toward religious activity–*satsang* and the *guru*.

Table 5.1 Attitude toward religious activities-*satsang* – and *guru*

Question	Yes %	Neutral %	No %	Missing values %
Participation in *satsang*	37.7	6.1	52.8	3.3
Listening to religious gurus (via television or other medium)	47.6	7.5	42.5	2.4
Belief if peace of mind can be attained through *satsang*	73.1	10.8	14.2	1.9
Attending *satsang* decreases problems/anxiety	64.2	14.2	19.3	2.4
Belief in religious rituals	83.0	8.5	5.7	2.8
Belief that gurus show the right path	59.9	17.0	20.3	2.8
Gurus are impostors (*dhongi*)	18.9	14.6	63.2	3.3

Participants

One hundred and fifty Indian rural women from the rural area of Haryana (India) constituted the sample. Their mean age was 39 years (SD = 16 years), ranging from 17 to 85 years. Demographic information indicated that majority of women were married and had completed their secondary level education. Most women participants were homemakers belonging to a nuclear family and mothered three to four children. Family income varied from Rs. 1,000 to 3,000 per month for most.

Keeping in mind the aim of the study, participants were interviewed on how they felt about participating in *satsang* and about the *guru pratha*. Questions were directive in nature, and respondent's responses are tabulated in Table 5.1. Responses were collected in written and verbal modes.

Results and Discussion

Folk songs that have spiritual/religious-driven messages are known as *bhajans*, and the setting where it takes place is called *satsang*. They carry religious anecdotes of God, Rama, Krishna, and Shiva along with other spiritual messages. Table 5.1 shows that 37.7 % of women participated in satsang. This can be explained by the fact that owing to the wide variation in age (17–85 years) of participants, younger participants though interested in *satsang* found lesser time from their daily routine to invest in *satsang*. This is supported by study 2 where majority of women participants were from an older age group, as they explained that they had more free time relatively, to participate in such group activities. Participants shared that 47.6 % attended to religious guru talks as against to a close 42.5 % who did not follow any religious guru on a regular basis. These figures indicate that majority of women do continue to follow this belief and the spiritual talks of gurus, however, a section of population in dilemma do not follow their preaching. 73.1 % of participants admitted that attending *satsang* may bring peace of mind. 64.2 % of total participants believed that *satsang* may reduce various kinds of problems and/or anxiety.

When participants were questioned about the credibility of *gurus*, they showed a positive opinion. They were asked if they believed guru could show them the "right path." 59.9 % responded affirmative as against to 20.3 % who did not believe in wisdom imparted by the *gurus*. This is in confirmation with the fact that 63.2 % of people disagreed for gurus to be impostors. However, 18.9 % of people were in agreement that potential *gurus* could be imposters and 14.6 % people did not have an opinion on this. This reflects the great bewilderment that perhaps people still hold when it concerns the viability of Indian *gurus*. Where 60 % people agreed on relying on *gurus* for sense of right direction to growth and well-being 18.9 % believed that there were mere imposters to the devotees. This is perhaps because in India today, there exist an overflowing number of upsurging gurus hailing from diverse backgrounds (professional or religious) and common man yet has no stable reference to confirm the *guru's* credibility. Indian healing traditions emphasize on the supportive–suggestive processes. The role of a *guru* as healer of emotional and somatic suffering is well known in Indian tradition. It is understood that here, when a disciple forms a relationship with a *guru*, the disciple is in fact forming a relationship with his own best self. Degree of faith in religious rituals as represented in Table 5.1 indicates that 83 % of participants held faith in religious rituals. Therefore, though people held positive attitude toward religious and spiritual sects and activities like *satsang*, they still were unsure about their blind faith over gurus. Their belief in the capacity of a *guru* to show them the right path remains unflinching however, as true for the Indian tradition at large.

5.4.2 Study 2

Study 1 was followed by study 2 where it was aimed to explore if folk songs-*satsang* acted as music therapy for Indian rural women.

Participants

The group comprised of 25–30 women who participated in *satsang* on a daily basis, from more than 10 to 15 years. The average age was 55 years, ranging from 45 years (eight members) to 85 years (four members). Fifty percent of participants had high school education (tenth grade) with formal teacher's training. Twenty-five percent of participants were educated till eighth grade, and the remaining 25 % of them were uneducated. Most of them were homemakers by occupation, and a few of were retired school teachers.

Procedure

Participants were interviewed about how participating in *satsang* may be influencing their lives. Data was collected with the help of semi-structured interview schedule and Focus Group Discussion.

Main Group Activities

It was gathered that the group performed certain activities together. Their message was sensitive to their region. Some folk songs were propagating specific religious beliefs. These are characteristically known as *bhajans*. They carry the messages such as *zindagi me iutar chadhav ayenge par inmei behna nahi* which meant that there will be ups and downs (benefits and loses) in an individual's life, and so, one should not be elated during the "up" times and neither should be depressed when "downs" are faced, and hence, an attempt should be made towards maintaining a balanced life. Certain examples of extensively populated folk songs themes were prayer/*aarti* (*om jai jagdeesh*) for well-being and peace (*om shanti*), asking for God's blessings, surrendering to God (*nahi bhagat ki haar*), chanting, and inviting to join *satsang* (*sathanaao*).

They would get together every day in the ground (3:30–5:30 PM) at evening and sing spiritual/religious message-driven folk songs. They also distributed *prasada* at the end of *satsang* to all available people. It resulted in a pleasant interaction with other members of *satsang*. This made participants happy and enhanced their interpersonal relationships. It was observed that in addition, the group also collected donations/charity on different religious occasions like *Purnima, Sankranti, Holi, Diwali,* and other local festivals. They would later donate collected money to *aanathaashram, gaushala,* and *vridha-aashram* and to other charitable institutions including the disadvantaged individuals. The sum of contribution would be anywhere from Rs. 50 to Rs. 500 per head on a voluntary basis, and the entire collection would mount to be from Rs. 3,000 to Rs. 5,000 per occasion. Participants revealed that they would feel immense joy during the process of donations and *prasada* distribution. Meeting regularly for *satsang* also led the group to share their familial joys and sorrows. All of them also visited bereaved families and offered social support whenever warranted.

Results and Discussion

Analysis of Focused Group Discussions (FGD) revealed various percepts of information. It indicated the various categories of folk songs, embedded diverse messages in them, and different group activities in which they participated all year round. Specific categories emerged from thematic analysis of the data:

1. Messages in the song would comprise of spiritual/religious message. Religious songs were based on various mythological stories such as on *Gopi Chand,*

Shivji-Parvati, Raja Mordawj, Savitri-Satyavan, and *Sri Krishna's* life events. *Bhajans* sometimes took the form of a *Katha* like *Bhagwat Geeta, Mahabharat, Ramayan,* etc., and would narrate the epic stories of different representations of God. Each member would derive wisdom and apply to their everyday lives for gaining respite from hassles and learn in effect from their domestic and spiritual unrest.

2. Participants reported to be free from stressors during singing. Some of them even perceived this practice as entertainment of the day.
3. It was observed that *prasada* (sweet) distribution formed an essential part of the *bhajan or satsang.* Participants would always distribute *prasada* as a mandatory practice to all attendees at the end of *satsang.* On careful consideration, it was understood that *prasada* was not a mere sweet distribution but a religious belief that God sweetened it with his love and blessings and its *grahan* (consumption) will make people more pious; it was essentially the *God's ashirwad* (blessing) to his *bhakt* (disciple). On the other hand, from a pragmatic socialistic view, it can also be seen as a happy exchange and interface of interaction among people who can be future embodied active participants.
4. *Satsang* paved the way for healthier interpersonal relations and a resource for strong social support. In some cases, women would bring their grandchildren along, which helped in family responsibilities.
5. This purposefully formed group in the study, served functions like collecting money on religious occasions such as *Purnima, Sankranti, Holi, Diwali,* and other local festivals along with giving donations by volunteer members to orphanages *(aanathaashram), gaushala,*(cow ranch), and *vridha-aashra* (old age home) and to other people in need. This observation revealed that folk songs served a platform for sharing member's joys and sorrows, as a by-product.

It was contended that in village communities such as the one like rural Haryana, which was studied, psychological well-being was made up of constituents, namely: activities involving sharing behavior with the same age group, a felt purposeful life, active involvement in pro-social behavior patterns, women being allowed to make visits outside the village community, an activity which formed the entertainment of the day, healthier interpersonal relationships, and singing of folk songs that made them free from stressors. Folk songs can be understood as a culturally specific form of music therapy (Singh and Singh 2010). In order to confirm the drawn conclusions and for further in-depth understanding, study 3 was conducted.

5.4.3 Study 3

To evaluate the perception of Indian rural women and the impact that *satsang* may have had on their lives, study 3 was conducted for in-depth understanding.

Participants

Six groups comprising of 15–20 women participants in each were included. The study utilized Focused Group Discussions that was conducted in one town (*Mansarover Park, Rohtak*) and four villages (*Kahni, Jasiya, Chhoti Bahu,* and *Singhpura*) in Haryana. Overall, the age range of participant women was 18–80 years, comprising in six groups (two groups from Rohtak and one group from each village). All participants were married. Majority of the participants belonged to middle socioeconomic status. More than half of the participants were housewives, whereas a small percentage was working outside home. Of the entire sample, more than half were uneducated and hence, communicated their responses verbally. Even those who were educated (class 12) preferred to participate and share in verbatim as opposed to writing. Participants had been practicing *satsang* on regular basis; moreover, they were very well aware of the practice.

Procedure

Convenient sampling was followed. In towns, women who were spotted sitting in groups in parks or who had gathered for *satsang* were contacted by the principal investigator. Their consent was sought after explaining to them in detail the purpose of the research. Help of *anganwadi* workers was sought to approach the rural women and to seek their consent and cooperation for participation in the study. Focused Group Discussions were recorded. They were organized to facilitate uninhibited interaction with women participants and to know of their perception and impact of *satsang* in their lives. Recorded data in their regional dialect was later translated for coding purposes. All obtained themes in first two studies were probed and explored, centered on issues that encompassed the objectives. The moderator focused on themes such as the following: what did *satsang* mean to them, what motivated them to join the group, and if there was any other concurrent or separate activity in which they had divulged themselves for the same purpose. They were asked about the duration of their participation in *satsang*; what was their opinion of gains/losses, if any, from the participation; and if they had derived similar benefits from any other similar mode. Additionally, they were also asked for their agreement/disagreement on the findings from the previous two studies conducted, i.e., if they felt subjectively free from daily hassles at the time of doing satsang, if they indulged in sharing with same age group participants, and if the activity was perceived purposeful, or if holding religious/spiritual beliefs helped them gain peace of mind and enhanced their well-being.

Results and Discussion

Group discussions were recorded with prior permission. The Focused Group Discussions transformed into sharing occasions. The Focused Group "sharing sessions" helped most women to give up their inhibitions and share their perceptions, feelings, and views more openly. In the rapport formation stage itself, the self-consciousness and discomfort level of participants was reduced and they actively participated. The transcribed data was analyzed with reference with the focus of each objective and theme.

1. All participants accepted that *satsang* was not just a mere activity that distracted them from their daily tussles of life but unquestionably a medium by which they are able to connect to their own "higher self" and God.

2. They mentioned that it reduced *virodhbhav* (jealousy) in them. That is, *satsang* reduced the negative attitude in them to retaliate or that of destruction. It makes made them more positive and accepting and increased their tolerance for differences. They were better able to understand diverse perspectives of beings and were able to integrate it in themselves.

3. They felt a deep sense of inner peace which was soulful in experience. They expressed it as *aatmik shanti*.

4. They disclosed that in addition to being a part of a pious group, attending to the teachings, and learning of spiritual members, *satsang* helped them to cultivate good habits and refrain from gossiping, backbiting, and from becoming a party to needless quarrels of other village members.

5. Few participants reported that at times they needed to sneak from their house to participate in *satsang* since they are not openly allowed to spend time purely for themselves, given the existence of a patriarchal society. Whereas at the same time, some women shared that with time they felt empowered and were no more scared of their "unpermitting" husbands or mother-in-laws.

6. *Aatmicshuddhi* (cleansing of soul) was another common benefit voiced by participants. They revealed that satsang evoked a sense of purity of soul in them. *Sat ka sang* taught them forgiveness, helped them to let go, and brought the realization in them about their own strengths and individuality. They learned to assert against oppression if required, to be more tolerant of differences, believe in self, as the soul was the most powerful entity which was pure and audacious. This have also been true for an upwardly mobile society where high level of material comfort may yet be not able to provide mental and spiritual support.

7. Additionally, members shared that participation in *satsang* was not only helping them in their self-growth, but their families were benefited as well. As all *vichar* (thoughts), *prakriti* (nature), and *bhav* (emotion) get transmitted from mother to children and from one generation to another, the sanctity and wisdom obtained by them on being the participant of *satsang* got inevitably transferred to their children and families. Moreover, they shared that most of them have been successfully able to encourage many other participants from neighborhood to join *satsang*.

8. *Satsang* also became a ground for self-healing through sharing and consequent strengthening of emotions between members.

9. Every new member brought their own values, *bhajans* (folk songs), and beliefs to the group. Diversification of the group gets transcended into cohesion with individual bolstering.

10. All members would assemble at a predetermined time; however, on occasions and on special requests, *satsang* was also performed by members in individual's houses. Free and open membership and the flexibility of attendance and exit hours made *satsang* as a pure benevolent and an altruistic intervention.
11. Singing religious songs brought happiness to members. They experienced flow, unity, and satisfaction within themselves and in their lives. People got united for a selfless cause and consciously or unconsciously forgot their sorrows and problems. They were able to concentrate and gain strength and wisdom to deal with disturbances and find solutions to their problems.
12. Majority voiced that it was an attractive medium that helped them promote their well-being. They were able to unburden themselves, shed their shortcomings and "evil" ideas, and learned to maintain confidentiality when they returned to their subjective homes.
13. *Seva-bhav and sadh-bhav* as taught through satsang was propagated by all. *Bhajan* preached them about wellness and torched the practical path for them on which they learn about love and forgiveness. They learn that they should *tyaga-hem bhav*. That is, they should always think of "other's" welfare before their own. They should try to wish well for other fellow beings and give up "I" (ego).
14. *Satsang* instilled in them the motivation to prosper and propelled them to conduct themselves in behaviors that will enhance their families and their own physical and mental well-being.
15. *Satsang* not only prepared them for tomorrow but also helped them in an improved functioning with regard to daily tasks. For example, a participant, who was attending *satsang* for 10–12 years, reported that regular *satsang* has improved her quality of sleep. Now whenever she wakes up in middle of night, her attention naturally goes back to *satsang*, and it inhibits any intruding or disturbing thought to her mind.
16. Belief in self and the almighty had brought a sense of peace within themselves and of brotherhood with all.
17. All members so happily participated that they would never miss a day of *satsang* despite their household duties or uncomfortable weather. They had clearly communicated to their family that this hour of day, they would like to spend with themselves and with their *satsang* mates, which all their family members understood and cooperated gradually. This also had enabled them in their own self-righteousness belief, and they learnt to be assertive and the significance of spending time with themselves. This should be understood in the context of the background that in India, conception of women has mostly been that of a provider than that of a receiver; she is expected to be present for all and at all times. Especially post-marriage, she naturally becomes her last priority. Self-neglect and multiple roles she plays in a family are more of a normal regime than "self-sabotage" in Indian rural communities.
18. Participation in *satsang*, women revealed, had allowed them to develop *sat vichar* (good and true thoughts). It had increased their knowledge and had most essentially made life easy and less burdensome for them (*zindagi bhojh nahi lagti*). Life now, they reported, felt like happiness and any sadness they

comprehended as a mere episode which they were able to circumvent or deal with maximum ease.

19. They got inspiration (*prerna*) to help others collectively. That is, development of pious brotherly thoughts helped them to reduce ego and promote benevolence.

20. It was observed that in *satsang* they also sang seasonal songs sometimes. They reported that it was a frequent activity in the village and evoked the feelings of love and liking in them, together with devotion and faith towards God.

21. Women participants included *bahu* (daughter-in-law) and *saas* (mother-in-laws). Most shared an amicable relationship, but few were frank in expressing their disagreements and conflicts. However, they admitted that participation in *satsang* has helped them to mellow down their conflicts as to develop altruism and tolerance.

22. In addition, reviews about *satsang* were compared between younger and senior participants, in terms of the time spent in the activity and duration of membership. For example, if *satsang* was more beneficial for people who have been attending it for more than 5 years, as compared to people who have been attending it for 2 years or less, and if so, then in what ways. All groups consisted of members attending satsang for 2–5 years as well as people attending for 25 years. All of them had similar experiences to share and differed only, if at all, in terms of the degree of benefit they received from the attribute, *satsang*. None denied the gains they received from *satsang* as a positive practice. One of the participants who was also the senior-most member of a group happened to be a widow of approximately 60 years. Hers was a child marriage who lost her husband at a very early age and at present had been staying with her brother's family. She shared that *satsang* had helped her to evolve and to abstain from adversities that she had been facing since early childhood.

23. Participants were also asked how they compared *satsang*'s effectiveness to other modalities (like meditation and *pravachan* (religious discourse)). All members collectively agreed that *satsang* was equally effective and in some ways better, owing to its collective nature, for promoting positive well-being.

5.5   General Discussion

In a nutshell, analyzing all three studies, an emerging pattern can be seen: all rural women felt much more empowered and free from stressors after participating in *satsang*. It is a common notion that music in any form is therapeutic and heals people mentally, physically, emotionally, and socially (Chiang 2008) and the same holds true for satsang as the results indicate. Repetitive participation in groups and singing songs carrying religious messages and positive virtues led to enhancement of well-being in the participants. Folk songs or regionally message-driven religious songs transmit beliefs and values to its members. The association of songs with specific places meant that composition is often linked with regional identity like through the celebration of local events, characters, and landscapes (Storey 2001). Additionally, various researches evaluating music as a therapeutic modality also observed it to be a source of positive emotions and well-being (Gilboa and Sagit 2009; Hills and Argyle 1998; Laukka 2007). Folk music plays a central role in the social construction of identity, and music engages people in emotional ways (Yarwood and Charlton 2009). Our findings of psychological well-being are also in confirmation with findings of Greitemeyer (2009b) who mentioned that listening to songs with pro-social message increased the accessibility of pro-social thoughts and lead to more helping behavior as compared to neutral lyrics. Moreover, it was noted that collective singing in an unconditional setting facilitated women's well-being and enabled reducing negative emotions especially in *satsang* (Singh and Singh 2010), where it acted as an agent of reinforcing system of positive beliefs and a medium of catharsis. It presents a community's overall perception and cognition and is essentially a reflection of collectivistic culture. Comparing collectivistic to individualistic cultures, Diener and Oishi (2000) proposed that though extended families in collectivistic societies could be more interfering at one end, they, at the same time, tend to provide greater social support in difficult times and individuals are seldom "left to fend for themselves."

Across all three studies, participants in unison testified that they felt free from stressors during singing, and *satsang* helped them nurture healthier interpersonal relations, bolstering strong family ties, and in building social support. Several studies support the fact that as compared to any other factor influencing well-being, social support is the most necessary factor for happiness and subjective well-being (Diener and Seligman 2002). It was also observed that participating in *satsang* which principally involved "group work," activities performed therein like active pro-social spending (group donations for welfare of deprived), sharing with same age group, and participation in religious activities all collectively enhanced well-being. Pro-social altruistic spending was observed to be contributing to well-being and happiness (Dunn et al. 2008). It has been debated that emergence of altruistic behavior and attitude has resulted in far-reaching social collaboration that has allowed human groups to flourish (Henrich and Henrich 2006; Tomasello 2009). Punia and Punia (2004) reported that folk songs helped in understanding the sociocultural sphere and the adjustment of an individual to his/her culturally constituted world.

Participants in the present study also reported that *satsang* was the "entertainment of the day" activity for them; this is in synchronization where it was studied that recalling the good event would make people happy (Seligman et al. 2005). "Positive mood and feelings" do not simply indicate current good health but also lead to further positive health (Fredrickson 2001).

Participating in *satsang* enabled rural women to visit "outside" their restricting familial boundaries, sought acceptance for individuality from significant family members, and to find time and space to reach "within" and search for meaning and purpose of their lives. Positive relationships and purpose of life were among the key identified dimensions of well-being (Ryff 1995; Seligman 2011). Following *guru pratha* and the path of spirituality were also noteworthy observations from *satsang* which resulted in furthering of subjective well-being. Accross all healing institutions like *Pir of Patteshah Dargah, Balaji, Shamana, Lama of Mcleodganj, Radha Soami sect,* and *Mata Nirmala Devi* along with the Ayurveda and *tantra* systems, role of sacredness were observed to be of prime importance (Kakar 1978). Company of enlightened people (*gurus*) radiates positive or spiritual energy which accelerates member's spiritual enhancement (Goel 2008).

Traditionally, considering the "oriental philosophy of life" and the partial industrialization and simultaneous robust family relations, present as protective factors, prevalence of mental illness in India was supposed to be much less than in the western countries (Prabhu and Raghuram 1987). Biomedical approach to mental health relied heavily on somatic and psychological factors in forming their diagnosis, completely ignorant of the influence of sociocultural and sociodemographic factors (Haslam 2000). Hence, several issues go unreported and underreported in India. Another factor contributing to this is poor self-esteem; lack of perceived control and hopelessness (Srivastava and Misra 2003) that prevent people from reaching out for help. Such an indigenous practice as *satsang* that is already existing in the society, if effectively regulated and augmented, can facilitate a form of "unspecified" therapeutic reform and reach the "unreachable" otherwise.

5.6 Conclusion

Music as a therapy has been acknowledged as culturally specific. Regional musical healing is variable in terms of its beliefs, religions, and messages. The success of traditional healing also strengthens the religious faith and beliefs that are centered in such cultures (Moreno 1995). India is rich and diverse in its culture and religious practices. Application of western therapies directly on eastern population is bound to have colored and nonspecific results. Moreover, in India, accessibility and affordability are important considerations especially for rural population. Health models should be rooted in culturally shared assumptions, ethical values, reasoning patterns, and sensibilities (Khare 1996). Also, while considering rural background's population, interventions involving less of language dependency, reading and writing skills efficiency, as well as cognitive mindedness should be considered to enhance well-being. Vella-Brodrick (2009) noted that there continues to be dearth of research on such interventions appropriate for populations such as children or those with limited writing skills. In this context, as supported by the abovementioned studies, *satsang* proved to be a powerful tool in promoting well-being in Indian rural women as analyzed. It was observed that *satsang* was not just a mere group activity where music, distraction, focused concentration, or group cohesion had its therapeutic effect, but the spiritual essence therein paved the way for connectivity with oneself and with their own higher self, whether it was represented as *guru* or idolized as God.

References

Alexander, C. N., Langer, E. J., Newman, R. I., Chandler, H. M., & Davies, J. L. (1989). Transcendental meditation, mindfulness, and longevity: An experimental study with the elderly. *Journal of Personality and Social Psychology, 57*(6), 950–964.

Banth, S., & Talwar, C. (2012). Anasakti, the Hindu ideal, and its relationship to well-being and orientations to happiness. *Journal of Religion and Health, 51*(3), 934–946. doi:10.1007/s10943-010-9402-3.

Bhawuk, D. P. S. (2010). Methodology for building psychological models from scriptures: Contributions of Indian psychology to indigenous and universal psychologies. *Psychology and Developing Societies, 22*, 49–93.

Brown, K. W., & Ryan, R. M. (2003). The benefits of being present: Mindfulness and its role in psychological well-being. *Journal of Personality and Social Psychology, 84*(4), 822–848.

Chiang, M. M. (2008). *Research on music and healing in ethnomusicology and music therapy.* Unpublished Master's thesis.

Chilton, G., & Wilkinson, R. A. (2009). Envisioning the intersection of art therapy and positive psychology. *Australian New Zealand Journal of Art Therapy, 4*(1), 27–35.

Cook, P. M. (1997). Sacred music therapy in North India. *The World of Music, 39*, 61–84.

Dalal, A. K. (2007). *Folk wisdom and traditional healing practices: Some lessons for modern psychotherapies.* New Delhi: Pearson.

Das, R. C. (1991). Standardization of the Gita inventory of personality. *Journal of Indian Psychology, 9*(1&2), 47–54.

Davar, B. (2001). *Mental health from a gender perspective.* New Delhi: Sage.

Delle Fave, A., Brdar, I., Freire, T., Vella-Brodrick, D., & Wissing, M. P. (2011). The eudaimonic and hedonic components of happiness: Qualitative and quantitative findings. *Social Indicators Research, 100*, 185–207.

Diener, E. (1984). Subjective well-being. *Psychological Bulletin, 95*(3), 542–575.

Diener, E., & Diener, M. (1995). Cross-cultural correlates of life satisfaction and self-esteem. *Journal of Personality and Social Psychology, 68*, 653–663.

Diener, E., & Oishi, S. (2000). Money and happiness: Income and subjective well-being across nations. In E. D. E. M. Suh (Ed.), *Culture and subjective well-being* (pp. 185–218). Cambridge, MA: MIT Press.

Diener, E., & Seligman, M. E. P. (2002). Very happy people. *Psychological Science, 13*, 81.

Diener, E., Oishi, S., & Lucas, R. E. (2003). Personality, culture, and subjective well-being: Emotional and cognitive evaluations of life. *Annual Reviews of Psychology, 54*, 403–425.

Duggal Jha, S., & Singh, K. (2011). An analysis of individualism-collectivism across Northern India. *Journal of the Indian Academy of Applied Psychology, 37*(1), 149–156.

Dunn, E. W., Aknin, L. B., & Norton, M. I. (2008). Spending money on others promotes happiness. *Science, 319*(5870), 1687–1688.

Feldman, G., Greeson, J., & Senville, J. (2010). Differential effects of mindful breathing, progressive muscle relaxation, and loving-kindness meditation on decentering and negative reactions to repetitive thoughts. *Behaviour Research and Therapy, 48*, 1002–1011.

Fredrickson, B. L. (2001). The role of positive emotions in positive psychology: The broaden-and-build theory of positive emotions. *American Psychologist, 56*, 218–226.

Gilboa, A., & Sagit, B. (2009). Sowing seeds of compassion: The case of a music therapy integration group. *The Arts in Psychotherapy, 36*, 251–260.

Gilman, R., & Huebner, E. S. (2000). Review of life satisfaction measures for adolescents. *Behaviour Change, 17*, 178–205.

Goel, M. S. (2008). *Devotional Hinduism: Creating impressions for God.* Bloomington: iUniverse.

Greitemeyer, T. (2009a). Effects of songs with pro-social lyrics on pro-social behavior: Further evidence and a mediating mechanism. *Personality and Social Psychology, 35*, 1500–1511.

Greitemeyer, T. (2009b). Effects of songs with prosocial lyrics on prosocial thoughts, affect and behavior. *Journal of Experimental Social Psychology, 45*, 186–190.

Grosswald, S. J., Stixrud, W. R., Travis, F., & Bateh, M. A. (2008). Use of the transcendental meditation technique to reduce symptoms of Attention Deficit Hyperactivity Disorder (ADHD) by reducing stress and anxiety: An exploratory study. *Current Issues in Education, 10*(2).

Hadi, N., & Hadi, N. (2007). Effects of hatha yoga on well-being in healthy adults in Shiraz, Islamic Republic of Iran. *East Mediterranean Health Journal, 13*(4), 829–837.

Halbfass, W. (1997). Happiness: A Nyaya-Vaisesika perspective. In P. Bilimoria & J. N. Mohanty (Eds.), *Relativism, suffering, and beyond: Essays in memory of B.K. Matilal* (pp. 150–163). Delhi: Oxford University Press.

Haslam, N. (2000). Psychiatric categories as natural kinds: Essentialist thinking about mental disorder. *Social Research, 67*(4), 1031–1058.

Henrich, J., & Henrich, N. (2006). Culture, evolution and the puzzle of human cooperation. *Cognitive Systems Research, 7*(2–3), 220–245.

Hills, P., & Argyle, M. (1998). Musical and religious experiences and their relationship to happiness. *Personality and Individual Differences, 25*, 91–102.

Hwang, K. (2004). The epistemological goal of indigenous psychology: The perspective of constructive realism. In B. N. Setiadi, A. Supratiknya, W. J. Lonner, & Y. H. Poortinga (Eds.), *Ongoing themes in psychology and culture*. Melbourne: International Association for Cross-Cultural Psychology.

Jain, A. (2007). Reformation of psyche through yogic discipline. *Yoga Varsha, 4*, 28–29.

Kakar, S. (1978). *The inner world: A psychoanalytic study of childhood and society in India*. Delhi: Oxford University Press.

Kamat, J. (2013, February 20). Swastika In Indian Culture. *Indian Culture*. Retrieved July 15, 2009.

Kapur, R. L. (2011). Yoga and the state of mind. In A. K. Dalal & G. Misra (Eds.), *New directions in health psychology* (pp. 249–258). New Delhi: SAGE.

Keyes, C. L. M. (1998). Social well-being. *Social Psychology Quarterly, 61*, 121–140.

Keyes, C. L. M. (2002). The mental health continuum: From languishing to flourishing in life. *Journal of Health and Social Behavior, 43*, 207–222.

Khare, R. S. (1996). Dava, daktar and dua: Anthropology of practiced medicine in India. *Social Science & Medicine, 43*, 837–848.

Kitayama, S., Markus, H. R., & Kurokawa, M. (2000). Culture, emotion, and well-being: Good feelings in Japan and the United States. *Cognition & Emotion, 14*, 93–124.

Krishnan, L. (2005). Concepts of social behavior in India: Daan and distributive justice. *Psychological Studies, 50*, 21–31.

Kumar, S. K. K. (2010). Indian indigenous concepts and perspectives: Developments and future possibilities. In G. Misra (Ed.), *Psychology in India: Theoretical and methodological developments* (Vol. 4). New Delhi: Dorling Kindersley (India) Pvt. Ltd.

Larsen, B. (2007). Room for 2000 philosophers. Many volunteers keep the faith on huge project. *The Peace Arch News*, 3.

Laukka, P. (2007). Uses of music and psychological well-being among the elderly. *Journal of Happiness Studies, 8*(1), 215–241.

Lindberg, D. A. (2005). Integrative review of research related to meditation, spirituality, and the elderly. *Geriatric Nursing, 26*(6), 372–377.

Lu, L., Gilmour, R., & Kao, S. (2001). Cultural values and happiness: An eastwest dialogue. *The Journal of Social Psychology, 141*, 477–493.

Malathi, A., Damodaran, A., Shah, N., Patil, N., & Maratha, S. (2000). Effect of yogic practices on subjective well being. *Indian Journal of Physiology and Pharmacology, 44*(2), 202–206.

Menon, S. (1998). The ontological pragmaticity of karma in Bhagvad Gita. *Journal of Indian Psychology, 16*(1), 44–52.

Misra, G. (1990). *Applied social psychology in India*. New Delhi: Sage.

Misra, G., & Paranjpe, A. C. (2012). Psychology in modern India. In *Encyclopedia of the history of psychological theories* (pp. 881–892). New York: Springer Science, Business Media, LLC.

Moreno, J. J. (1995). Ethnomusic therapy: An interdisciplinary approach to music and healing. *The Arts in Psychotherapy, 22*, 1–10.

Nastasi, B. K. (1998). A model for mental health programming is schools and communities: Introduction to the mini-series. *School Psychology Review, 27*, 165–174.

Outlook. (2005, January 10). Kya hai khusi ka khazana (What is the secret of happiness). *Outlook*.

Pande, N., & Naidu, R. K. (1992). Anasakti and health: A study of non-attachment. *Psychology and Developing Societies, 4*, 89–104.

Pargament, K. I., & Mahoney, A. (2002). *Spirituality*. New York: Oxford University Press.

Park, N., & Huebner, E. S. (2005). A cross-cultural study of the levels and correlates of life satisfaction among children and adolescents. *Journal of Cross-Cultural Psychology, 36*(4), 444–456.

Park, N., Peterson, C., & Seligman, M. E. P. (2006). Character strengths in fifty-four nations and the fifty US states. *The Journal of Positive Psychology, 1*(3), 118–129.

Patel, V., Ricardo, d. L., Mauricio, L., & Ana, T. C. (1999). Women, poverty and common mental disorders in four restructuring societies. *Social Science & Medicine, 49*, 1461–1471.

Perry, B. (2008). *Lecture*. Paper presented at the The American Art Therapy, Cleveland.

Prabhu, G. G., & Raghuram, A. (1987). Mental health in India. In *Encyclopaedia of social work in India* (Vol. 2, pp. 188–189). New Delhi: Ministry of Welfare.

Puchner, L. (2003). Women and literacy in rural Mali: A study of the socio-economic impact of participating in literacy programs in four villages. *International Journal of Educational Development, 23*, 439–458.

Punia, D., & Punia, R. K. (2004). Gender discrimination in Haryanvi folk songs. In B. Rama Raju (Ed.), *Folklore*. New Delhi: The New Millennium Research India Press.

Rauscha, S. M., Gramlinga, S. E., & Auerbacha, S. M. (2006). Effects of a single session of large-group meditation and progressive muscle relaxation training on stress reduction, reactivity, and recovery. *International Journal of Stress Management, 13*(3), 273–290.

Research Programme Framework: Action R&D on body, c. a. t. i. i. a. f. o. i. l. (2012). Retrieved September 3, 2012. http://www.sriaurobindoashram.org/research/research.php

Ryff, C. D. (1989). Happiness is everything, or is it? Explorations on the meaning of psychological well-being. *Journal of Personality and Social Psychology, 57*, 1069–1081.

Ryff, C. D. (1995). Psychological well-being in adult life. *Current Directions in Psychological Science, 4*(4), 99–104.

Ryff, C. D., & Keyes, C. L. M. (1995). The structure of psychological well-being revisited. *Journal of Personality and Social Psychology, 69*, 719–727.

Sachdev, N. (2001). The Radha Soami way of god realization. *The Times of India*, January 2001.

Sand, R. (1993). Of faith, hope & charity. *The Times of India*.

Seligman, M. E. P. (2011). *Flourish: A visionary new understanding of happiness and well-being*. New York: Free Press.

Seligman, M. E. P., Steen, T. A., Park, N., & Peterson, C. (2005). Positive psychology progress: Empirical validation of interventions. *American Psychologist, 60*(5), 410–421.

Singh, K. (2009). Intervention module for restructuring socio- cultural issues in Indian framework. In G. Sankar (Ed.), *Psychotherapy & yoga traditions* (pp. 180–194). Sagar: Pranjal Prakashan.

Singh, K., & Choubisa, R. (2009). Effectiveness of self focused intervention for enhancing student's wellbeing. *Journal of the Indian Academy of Applied Psychology, 35*(Special issue), 23–32.

Singh, K., & Dangi, S. (2011). Married migrant women in Haryana: A pilot study. *The Journal of Psychosocial Research, 6*(2), 265–273.

Singh, K., & Singh, D. (2010). *Development and socio-cultural changes in rural areas of Haryana*. Paper presented at XX annual convention of National Academy of Psychology, New Delhi: JNU.

Sinha, D. (2002). Culture and psychology: Perspective of cross-cultural psychology. *Psychology and Developing Societies, 14*(11), 11–25.

Sinha, D. (2011). Concept of psycho-social well-being: Western and Indian perspectives. In A. K. Dalal & G. Misra (Eds.), *New directions in health psychology* (pp. 95–107). Delhi: Sage.

Smith, S. (2000). Geography of music. In R. Johnston, D. Gregory, G. Pratt, & M. Watts (Eds.), *The dictionary of human geography* (pp. 530–531). Blackwell: Oxford.

Smith, C., Hancock, H., Blake-Mortimer, J., & Eckert, K. (2007). A randomised comparative trial of yoga and relaxation to reduce stress and anxiety. *Complementary Therapies in Medicine, 15*(2), 77–83.

Srivastava, A. K., & Misra, G. (2003). Going beyond the model of economic man: An indigenous perspective on happiness. *Journal of Indian Psychology, Andhra University, 21*, 12–29.

Srivastava, A. K., & Misra, G. (2011). In A. K. Dalal & G. Misra (Eds.), *New directions in health psychology* (pp. 109–131). New Delhi: Sage.

Storey, D. (2001). *Territory: The claiming of space*. Harlow: Prentice Hall.

Tomasello, M. (2009). *Why we cooperate*. Cambridge, MA: MIT Press.

Varjas, K., Nastasi, B. K., Moore, R. B., & Jayasena, A. (2005). Using ethnographic methods for development of culture-specific interventions. *Journal of School Psychology, 43*(3), 241–258.

Vella-Brodrick, D. T. (2009). *Interventions for enhancing well-being: The role of person-activity fit*. In Workshop presented at the First World Congress on Positive Psychology, Philadelphia.

Verma, S. K., & Verma, A. (1989). *Manual of P.G.I. general well-being measure*. Lucknow: Ankur Psychological Agency.

Wig, N. N. (1990). Indian concepts of mental health and their impact on care of the mentally ill. *International Journal of Mental Health, 18*, 71–80.

Wolfe, R. (2002). Spiritual lessons at service. *The Press Democrat*.

Yarwood, R., & Charlton, C. (2009). Country life? Rurality, folk music and "show of hands". *Journal of Rural Studies, 25*, 194–206.

Chapter 6
Cocurricular Activities and Student Development: How Positive Nations Encourage Students to Pursue Careers in Psychology

Mercedes A. McCormick, Grant J. Rich, Deborah Harris O'Brien, and Annie Chai

In Positive Nations and positive communities, college students learn both inside and outside the classroom through cocurricular activities. Since 1929, Psi Chi, the International Honor Society in Psychology, has grown into the world's largest honor society by developing a growing number of cocurricular programs to benefit the development of psychology students across the USA and internationally since 2009. This chapter reviews the following: (1) the background and value of cocurricular activities and their relation to positive psychology; (2) the mission and growth of Psi Chi, which now includes 600,000 life members in 1,100 chapters worldwide; (3) an overview of the diversity of Psi Chi's cocurricular programs; and (4) how these cocurricular programs benefit a nation by benefitting the development of students who go on to careers in psychology (Denmark and Heitner 2000) or other related fields (Takooshian and Landi 2011).

M.A. McCormick (✉)
Department of Psychology, Pace University, New York, NY, USA
e-mail: mmccormick2@pace.edu

G.J. Rich
APA Division 52 International Psychology,
American Psychological Association, Juneau, AK, USA
e-mail: optimalex@aol.com

D.H. O'Brien
Trinity Washington University, Washington, DC, USA
e-mail: harris-obriend@trinitydc.edu

A. Chai
Psychology Department and the United Nations International Council
of Psychologists, Pace University, New York, NY, USA
e-mail: annie.chai5@gmail.com

H. Águeda Marujo and L.M. Neto (eds.), *Positive Nations and Communities*, Cross-Cultural 101
Advancements in Positive Psychology 6, DOI 10.1007/978-94-007-6869-7_6,
© Springer Science+Business Media Dordrecht 2014

6.1   Introduction

"In Positive Nations and positive communities, how do psychology students' cocurricular psychology activities contribute to their future careers?" In this chapter, after
placing the topic within the context of positive psychology, we address this question
with four points: (1) the value of cocurricular activities (CCA), (2) Psi Chi as the
single largest source of promoting cocurricular activities, (3) examples of Psi Chi
cocurricular programs, and (4) how this likely impacts students' later careers in
psychology and other fields.

Since its inception in the late 1990s, positive psychology has aimed to balance the
attention psychology has historically devoted to the exploration of human weaknesses
with a "science of positive subjective experience, positive individual traits, and positive
institutions" that "promises to improve quality of life and prevent the pathologies that
arise when life is barren and meaningless" (Seligman and Csikszentmihalyi 2000, p.
5). As positive psychology enters its second decade, ample research has focused upon
positive subjective experience and traits. In fact, scholars have even developed what
may be termed as a DSM for the positive psychology movement, Peterson and
Seligman's (2004) *Character Strengths and Virtues: A Handbook and Classification*,
which classifies 24 specific strengths under six virtues that are argued to be consistently
found across cultures: wisdom, courage, humanity, justice, temperance, and transcendence. As such, the handbook may be viewed, as it is by its authors, as a "manual
of the sanities" (p. 3), and as a complement to the American Psychiatric Association's
Diagnostic and Statistical Manual of Mental Disorders (DSM), which, with a deficits
approach, categorizes mental disorders and offers their diagnostic criteria. Research
has documented these character strengths in youth as well (Steen et al. 2003).
Theoretically at least, any of the 24 strengths could be utilized and developed in cocurricular activities. From creativity, curiosity, and open-mindedness to love of learning,
perspective, and persistence, cocurricular activities seem to lend themselves to the
practice of these strengths. Likewise, strengths, such as integrity, virtue, and kindness,
and social intelligence, fairness, and hope may be enhanced through student participation in cocurricular activities.

Cocurricular activities, in the experience of the chapter authors, who have been
involved with Psi Chi and service learning, may especially be hypothesized to support development of the character strengths purported by the field of positive psychology such as citizenship, leadership, and gratitude. Even strengths such as
bravery, humor, and love may be potentially increased through cocurricular activities, as when, for instance, an English-as-a-second-language student courageously
overcomes a fear of public oral presentation or when students respond to an embar-
rassing moment with humor that does not diminish others but bonds them together
or when students develop a sense of loyalty, affection, and care for their classmates
and community members. Although current research does not explicitly explore
each of these 24 strengths as they each relate to cocurricular activities, substantial
research does exist now that documents the efficacy of such youth activities for
many of them, as will be discussed later in this chapter.

While much research has been produced over the past 10 years or so on the first
two pillars of positive psychology – positive subjective experience and positive

traits – there is a relative paucity of research on the third pillar, positive institutions. For instance, a survey of recent positive psychology textbooks (Rich 2011) found that though all six available classroom textbooks had chapters on happiness (a positive subjective experience) and positive emotions/traits, only one textbook devoted at least one full chapter to positive culture, and just three of the six textbooks devoted a chapter to positive institutions (Compton 2005; Peterson 2006; Snyder and Lopez 2007).

Although the value of positive institutions and concept of the moral character of society were noted even at the founding of positive psychology, positive psychologists have been slow to respond to the call to research on this topic for several reasons. First, psychologists have historically focused upon the examination of the individual person, while disciplines such as sociology tended to focus on institutions and group processes. Second, the study of collective processes that occur in groups and institutions poses a number of methodological challenges not always easily met with the standard analytical tools and research designs utilized by psychologists. Third, not all psychologists agree about the value and utility of quantitative tools as the exclusive methods for best illuminating the questions posed by positive psychologists. For instance, as early as 2001, Rich posed the question, "How should psychologists approach the examination of positive subjective experience, positive traits, and positive institutions?" Rich continues: "Will traditional quantitative methods suffice? Can we understand creativity via ANOVAs, happiness with regression, or the good life through structural equation modeling? Or are there topics that positive psychology cannot comprehend without the use of qualitative methods such as interviews, observations, and intense fieldwork? … such a [quantitative] approach seems … limited when one examines many of the phenomena of interest to positive psychologists" (2001, p. 9).

Psi Chi and its cocurricular activities may be described as an institution which aims to be positive, and certainly such cocurricular activities may be described as collective processes. With both the lack of research on positive institutions in general and the potential value for building Positive Nations and communities of identifying and understanding the strength building potential of cocurricular activities in particular, a careful examination of Psi Chi and related activities is a worthwhile endeavor for psychologists. Such an exploration, with ample attention to culturally sensitive processes, is even more valuable as Psi Chi continues to expand internationally.

6.2 Background and Value of Cocurricular Activities

Cocurricular activities, also known as extracurricular activities, are provided by educational institutions for students and are meant to supplement the institution's standard curriculum. Such activities are vital in that research has demonstrated that 50 % of students reported that their classes were boring (Steinberg et al. 1996), yet student engagement and enjoyment have been linked with school academic achievement (e.g., Csikszentmihalyi and Schneider 2000). Some research, using a national youth sample from the USA, indicates that youth are more likely to be psychologically engaged in extracurricular activities than in regular school curricular activities, such as with conventional classroom instruction. One reason may be that youth tend to perceive structured extracurricular activities, such as clubs and sports teams, as simultaneously work and play. By contrast, most school work is viewed as work, important to one's future goals, but not enjoyable. Informal socializing may be viewed as fun and play-like but of little relevance to one's future (Schmidt and Rich 2000). One analysis of student engagement in the classroom, using several hundred youth and an experience sampling method technique to explore the phenomenology of situated cognition, found that students were more engaged in group work in the classroom than when listening to lectures or watching videos (Shernoff et al. 2003). Further supporting evidence for the added engagement involved with groups comes from an examination of college student volunteers playing paddleball. Walker (2010) found that youth reported more enjoyment – what Csikszentmihalyi (1990) has termed "flow" – performing with others than alone.

One form of learning that may be termed cocurricular is service learning, which is becoming increasingly popular (Colby et al. 2003). This form of education aims to promote civic engagement and to develop a sense of social responsibility through community service, which is typically connected to other classroom learning through academic readings, lectures, and discussions. While service-learning projects can be solo, such as one student tutoring a child, they may also be group efforts, such as a class volunteering together at a soup kitchen. Some positive psychology seminars have successfully integrated both individual and group service-learning activities with academic work. In one such seminar, where a group of college students worked together with children from a range of racial, ethnic, national, and religious affiliations, the students reported an increased awareness of multicultural issues, an increased appreciation of the value of diversity, enhanced self-esteem, development of leadership skills and social intelligence, as well as enjoyment, deep engagement, and flow (e.g., Rich 2002). Some students in the seminar also reported increased interest in career exploration in psychology and related fields, such as counseling and social work. Notably, while the positive psychology movement is little over a decade old, the strengths-based perspective in social work is considerably more established, and its practical approach to enhancing well-being of individuals and communities seems to complement well the research approach of the new positive psychology (Saleeby 2002). Other research has indicated that service-learning participation is associated with better school grades, increased self-esteem, and an increased probability of future volunteering (Hart et al. 2008). In fact, one study of African-American and Latino youth in the USA found that service-learning participation could have a significant, substantial effect on preventing dropping out of school (Bridgeland et al. 2008). While some research indicates over one in four U.S. high schools require service learning (Metz and Youniss 2005), such required service learning is less common at the college and university level. In addition, there has been some debate concerning whether or not students gain the same benefits from "required volunteering" as they do from non-required service learning for which they truly volunteered. However, the authors write that both types of service learning – required and voluntary – "have the potential for yielding benefits when service is viewed as providing youth with opportunities to learn about systems of meaning through participatory action." The study authors continue by noting that "From the viewpoint of educational policy, schools can help students most when they organize service strategically and integrate service into the academic curriculum" (McLellan and Youniss 2003, p. 47).

There have been few research studies specifically on the impact of student engagement in extracurricular activity on student learning and leadership. Pascarella and Terenzini (2005) commented that success in college is determined by individual involvement in the academic, interpersonal, and extracurricular offerings provided by the academic institution. Toyokawa and Toyokawa's (2002) study of Japanese students studying in the USA found that engagement in extracurricular activities was positively related to students' levels of academic involvement and overall life satisfaction.

In Krause's (2008) study of retention among Australian university students, it was found that students at risk of dropping out in the first year of college showed no interest in extracurricular activities. Students she termed "persisters," who did not indicate they were considering leaving the university, felt they were a part of a group of students, felt they belonged to the university community, and were actively involved in college-based extracurricular activities. Similarly, Bringle et al. (2010) found that service learning by first-semester freshmen increased retention rates to the next semester and following year. Krause's study (2008) also found that students who were at a higher risk for potential dropout engaged in more hours of paid work, were working to meet their basic needs, and were from lower SES backgrounds than the students at lower risk of dropping out. Financial pressures may therefore be a mediator in that students with fewer resources have to work to support themselves and may not have time to participate in extracurricular activities. Cocurricular activities at universities need to take these types of constraints on students into account and help students see that their involvement in cocurricular experiences results in the development and the acquisition of skills and abilities that are often transferable to future leadership and work-related experiences in students' professional careers. Thus, there is responsibility on the part of leaders of cocurricular activities to show students the benefits of participation as well as scheduling meetings and activities in ways that allow the students who are also working to participate.

Students report improved self-confidence, personal organization, improved time management skills, and a sense of maturity, flexibility, adaptability, and well-being as a result of being engaged in satisfying cocurricular activities (Harvey et al. 1992). As Rich (2009) notes, "recently, more work has been directed at evaluation of organized youth activities, in addition to the work on service learning." Moreover, Rich (2009) compared informal socializing with peers to formal learning in academic classes. His findings demonstrated that organized youth activities may be the preferred context for exploring identity, acquiring anger and stress management skills, and developing teamwork and leadership skills.

Importantly, a social element is embedded in cocurricular activities. Cocurricular activities are often student-led under faculty sponsorship, allowing students to gain valuable leadership experience for the future. Cocurricular activities play a significant role in fostering academic and personal growth within students. Such growth is vital in achieving future career goals. A study conducted in 2003 and reported in the

Journal of Adolescent Research indicates that students who participate in cocurricular activities from grades 8 through 12 are likely to have successful academic careers and prosocial behaviors later on in life (Zaff et al. 2003). Students should be encouraged to consistently participate in cocurricular activities at all levels of their education in order to benefit themselves in the future. Consistent with prior findings on civic engagement, research reveals that participation in school clubs and political activities predicts higher involvement in political and social causes in young adulthood (e.g., Youniss et al. 1997).

Youniss and Yates (1997) hypothesize that cocurricular activities with structure expose students to the norms and values of the organization, which promotes networking and interpersonal connections for later on in life. Cocurricular activities have the potential to introduce students to political and philosophical ideas. Cocurricular activities allowed students to learn interpersonal and leadership skills which are likely to bring forth continued participation in political or civic issues (Glanville 1999; Hanks and Eckland 1978). Furthermore, some research indicates that extracurricular activities facilitate connection to the school institution and provide a social resource and place to belong (Eccles et al. 2003). Involvement with cocurricular activities can cultivate student connections to school by linking them to like-minded peers and competent adults and lead students to identify themselves as members of the school community (Eccles and Barber 1999; Eccles et al. 2003). Furthermore, Jordan and Nettles (1999) found that adolescents in cocurricular activities were more connected and committed to school and therefore more motivated to excel.

The focus on how students learn best is now spread worldwide. We see extracurricular activities branching out internationally. For example, in the late 1980s and early 1990s, satisfaction surveys were developed at the University of Central England in Birmingham. These surveys were based on focus group discussions with students about their learning experiences. Outcome information from these focus groups indicated the importance of extracurricular, and certainly cocurricular, activities.

Countries around the world have adopted new learning approaches based on asking students "What do you learn outside the classroom?" Peixoto (2004) studied the effects of extracurricular activities in a Portuguese school system where such type of activities, usually sports, existed but were not necessarily valued for character building. Peixoto (2004) analyzed the effects of these extracurricular activities on such factors as academic adjustment, self-concept, attitude toward school, and academic achievement. The findings indicated that underachievers benefited positively from participation in cocurricular activities with improvement in self-concept and school achievement.

Other countries have applied outcome findings from the Birmingham surveys to understand more fully the benefits of cocurricular activities on learning and character development in students during adolescence and young adulthood. Internationally, places such as Bologna, Italy, Singapore, China, and Lisbon, Portugal, have encapsulated cocurricular activities into the educational policies of their respective countries. Available information indicates that cocurricular activities foster teamwork that requires precision, management, and organizational skills that prepare students for careers in the outside world while building students' self-concept, self-esteem, confidence, and leadership skills.

College literary societies and Greek letter sororities and fraternities were the first cocurricular activities to be established in colleges across the USA and are still in existence. Subsequent cocurricular activities have developed throughout the twentieth century including sports teams, honor societies, and a multitude of interest-related clubs such as art history clubs. In the twenty-first century, cocurricular activities promote academic, personal, and career growth among psychology students as demonstrated by the cocurricular activities of Psi Chi, the International Honor Society in Psychology.

Over the past 60 years, psychology education has shown a stunning growth in US colleges, as psychology has emerged as the most popular major on US campuses (Takooshian and Landi 2011). In the USA, comparing enrollments in 1950 and 2008, the number of psychology baccalaureates increased 967 %, from 9,569 in 1950 to 92,587 in 2008; for master's degree, a 1,628 % increase from 1,316 in 1950 up to 21,431 in 2008; and for doctorates, a 1,871 % increase, from 283 in 1950 up to 5,296 in 2008. Once US high school psychology Advanced Placement (AP) courses were introduced in 1992, they showed an even faster growth rate of 3,858 %, from 3,914 in 1992 up to 151,006 in 2010. Moreover, since 1990, psychology education has been growing even faster outside the USA (Stevens and Gielen 2007). The US psychology honor society Psi Chi grew over 400 % in 25 years, from 157,812 members in 1985 up to 605,000 in 2010. In 2009, the Psi Chi Executive Board voted to "go global" and is now expanding to chapters outside North America.

Along with this growth of psychology courses in the USA and internationally, there has been a parallel growth of cocurricular activities to accompany these courses. Cocurricular activities, sponsored by Psi Chi, the International Honor Society in Psychology, benefit students within the USA and internationally, by encouraging student excellence, leadership opportunities, and the pursuit of careers in the field of psychology (Takooshian and Landi 2011).

Even before psychologist Theodore Newcomb's classic Bennington College studies in the 1930s, we knew that most of students' learning in college occurs outside the classroom (Newcomb 1943), and that this has a lifelong impact (Alwin et al. 1991). As Thomas Merton (2009) correctly noted, "The least of learning is done in the classroom." As much as students learn about psychology in their classes, they learn more through their fieldwork, research, and other cocurricular activities outside the classroom. Psi Chi has much to offer much in terms of such activities.

6.3 Psi Chi: The International Honor Society in Psychology

6.3.1 The Mission and Growth of Psi Chi

It was back on September 4, 1929, at Yale University that Psi Chi was founded by two students – Edwin Newman and Fred Lewis – during the historic Ninth International Congress of Psychology (Hogan and Takooshian 2004). In the past eight decades, Psi Chi has grown into the world's largest honor society, with over

600,000 members at 1,100 campuses across the USA, with several international chapters, including representation in Canada, the Caribbean, Russia, Ireland, Egypt, and New Zealand. The Central Office receives requests from universities/colleges around the world every month about how to become an international chapter. It is the primary source of cocurricular psychology programs of all sorts, including conferences, publications, awards, grants, service activities, and more. Psi Chi works as a federation of chapters based at each college or university, and its Central Office is in Chattanooga, Tennessee, in the southern part of the USA.

Since its founding, Psi Chi has grown into the world's largest psychology honor society by developing a growing number of cocurricular programs to benefit the development of psychology students across the USA and internationally. In 2009, Psi Chi became an international honor society in psychology, with the number of international chapters increasing each semester. Thirty-one famous psychologists have been honored with the designation of Distinguished Member of Psi Chi, reflecting their national or international reputations based upon their contributions to psychology and Psi Chi in teaching, research, and/or service. Among these Distinguished Members are leaders such as Past APA Presidents Philip Zimbardo, Florence Denmark, and Raymond D. Fowler; creativity researchers including Rollo May, Robert Sternberg, and J.P. Guilford; and scholars such as Canada's Albert Bandura, Puerto Rico's Guillermo Bernal, and Jerome Bruner, Elizabeth Loftus, and John Cacioppo of the mainland USA.

Psi Chi's key goals are to provide academic recognition to its members and for each of the Psi Chi chapters to nurture the motivation to accomplishment by offering a supportive climate to members for creative development. To reach these goals, Psi Chi chapters deliver opportunities to encourage professional development through programs and cocurricular activities designed to expand the regular curriculum and to provide realistic experiences and camaraderie through connection with the chapter. In addition, Psi Chi's international organization develops programs to help reach these goals. Annually Psi Chi holds regional conventions held in connection with psychological associations, research award competitions, and certificate recognition agenda. Quarterly Psi Chi publishes the *Psi Chi Journal of Research*, which presents an invaluable opportunity for graduate and undergraduate students to acquire skills in research, publishing, and the process of scholarly peer review. Also, the society publishes quarterly the *Eye on Psi Chi* magazine which features current news and recognizes accomplishments of its chapters and members.

To begin a Psi Chi chapter, universities, departments, and students must meet certain criteria. While the specific details of these criteria are available from the Psi Chi Central Office (also visit the following website: www.psichi.org), in general, colleges and universities must be fully accredited as a 4-year or senior-level institution and offer baccalaureate and/or graduate degrees in psychology. Undergraduate students must meet certain class rank and overall GPA (grade point average) requirements and be psychology majors or minors meeting a minimum GPA in their psychology courses. Psi Chi recognizes that grading systems and psychology programs vary considerably internationally. Thus, the Psi Chi Executive Director will assist international faculty advisors at universities outside the USA to discuss how eligibility requirements may be achieved.

6.3.2   Activities of Psi Chi Chapters

Psi Chi aims to positively encourage and foster growth among students through various cocurricular activities. The Psi Chi International Honor Society of Psychology offers many cocurricular activities, including conferences, publications, awards, grants, and service-learning experiences. Such cocurricular activities inspire students to seek field/internship experiences that have the potential to inspire them to pursue careers in psychology.

What kinds of specific activities do Psi Chi chapters do? These activities often are educational in nature. These activities include the following: inviting speakers who speak on a psychological issue/topic, listening as a group to a home institution professor's lectures on research or together attending campus symposiums, participating in workshops on graduate school and/or GRE (Graduate Record Examination) preparation, reviewing submissions for student research poster sessions, or field trips to psychological points of interest in the campus community. Other popular educational activities include inviting guest speakers to describe careers in psychology and offering workshops on psychology-related internships and jobs available to students with the bachelor's degree in psychology.

Psi Chi chapter activities include service-learning projects to help individuals and groups in the community. For instance, noted activities in service learning include mentoring younger students; participating in environmental activities, such as a beach cleanup; and organizing and leading activities such as clothing drives, blood donation drives, and toy and book drives for children in homeless shelters (especially at holidays). Other popular activities include service as research assistants, leading fund raisers for charities, and group volunteering with *Habitat for Humanity*, an organization which promotes building simple, affordable housing for the needy. Psi Chi especially has designated three activities as National Service Projects: food drives, *Habitat for Humanity,* and Adopt-A-Shelter, as ways of chapters serving their local communities. Psi Chi chapters have ample opportunities for volunteering, and popular sites have been nursing homes for the elderly, drug rehabilitation centers, children's hospitals, homeless shelters, prisons, and shelters for high-risk children and adolescents. Some chapters have become involved with the *Big Brothers Big Sisters* organization in the USA, whose mission is to help children reach their full potential through the support of one-on-one mentoring relationships. *Big Brothers Big Sisters* is among the largest youth mentoring groups in the USA.

Psi Chi chapters engage in a full range of activities, and in addition to the educational, service, and volunteering examples already noted, student groups often also participate in team-building activities that promote social bonding, friendships, and group unity. Such activities may include picnics or barbeques, film nights (often featuring movies with psychological themes), and mindfulness exercises. In addition to promoting social cohesion, such activities are fun. Some Psi Chi chapters have found it worthwhile to engage in activities with other student organizations. For instance, chapters may participate in diversity retreats with other student groups (such as those aimed at particular ethnic groups), an activity that enhances multicultural understanding and builds communication skills.

6.3.3   The Role of the Psi Chi Advisor

Each chapter of Psi Chi is led by a faculty advisor whose mission is to mentor student members toward academic excellence and leadership competency in the field of psychology. The faculty advisors and co-advisors for each chapter form vital links to each chapter's psychology department, institution, and community and to other Psi Chi chapters and to the discipline of psychology as a whole. Leaders are especially important for Psi Chi, as they offer experience, continuity, and advice to all student members. As noted earlier, a faculty chapter advisor must hold a doctoral degree in psychology (such as a Ph.D., Ed.D., or Psy.D.) and needs to be a member of Psi Chi. The Central Office of Psi Chi has many resources for advisors on a range of topics, from details about awards, conventions, and publications to policies and suggestions of service activities.

While responsibilities of Psi Chi chapter advisors may vary according to their chapter's needs, a number of tasks are commonly encountered. Faculty advisors ensure appropriate selection of qualified members and facilitate positive peer culture and supportive group dynamics. Advisors need to keep careful records of members and report chapter activities regularly to the Central Office. Of course, attending and participating in chapter meetings and other Psi Chi activities is also vital. Importantly Psi Chi encourages service activities by requiring a chapter to engage in them to receive the model chapter award, which involves not only honor but a monetary award.

Faculty advisors serve an important role as they guide student members toward the development of leadership skills and a maturing understanding of the profession of psychology. As part of this role, advisors may model professional behavior in applied practice, by sharing their own leadership and academic work with students or by working to coauthor research presentations and/or publications with students. Many successful faculty advisors in Psi Chi adopt a strengths-based positive psychology approach to their leadership role. For instance, in encouraging students to become professional through applying for Psi Chi research grants, developing chapter service projects, or participating in chapter and association professional conventions, such leaders will strive to create environments conducive to intrinsic motivation and flow. Students are encouraged to participate in Psi Chi and chapter activities to learn about the field of psychology and the pursuit of psychology for intrinsic personal gains, such as the joy of intellectual stimulation and the personal satisfaction a student finds in conducting research and the improved sense of well-being that emerges participating in a service-learning project or volunteering one's time to mentor another to improve in school or another life skill.

As societies welcome prosperity, in comparison to past generations, some students tend to focus more on the need for a high-paying job, or for prestige, than on the pursuit of questions of personal meaning, values, or philosophy. Yet positive psychology research indicates that although societies and individuals have increased in prosperity, they have not tended to increase in happiness and in life satisfaction (Peterson 2006). Faculty advisors well versed in positive psychology can help young people better understand how activities that promote character strengths and virtues (Peterson and Seligman 2004) will result in long-term life satisfaction compared to the consumerist mentality promoted in many Western cultures. For instance, will the latest iPhone, plasma screen TV, digital device, or application make one happy and for how long? Will the pleasure derived from binge drinking or illicit drug use offer much life satisfaction or meaning? Or will such activities lead to emptiness rather than to the "good life," as many positive psychologists have suggested, as a person needs ever more and better technological gadgets or drugs to achieve ever less interesting emotional effects? (Seligman 2011).

Positive psychology research supports Psi Chi's implementation of cocurricular activities that enhance student engagement, mentorship, building of character strengths, encouragement of flow, intrinsic motivation, and sense of well-being. These Psi Chi outcomes are linked to achievement, creativity, and academic and professional excellence. For instance, adolescents who received high marks in science and math subjects reported that they did not enjoy these subjects and were significantly less likely to pursue these subjects several years later as assessed in longitudinal research on this topic (Csikszentmihalyi and Schneider 2000; Rich 2003). Furthermore, these positive psychologists noted that young people often pursue their career choice for the personal satisfaction it affords not for external recognition or financial gain (Csikszentmihalyi 1996; Csikszentmihalyi and Rich 1997).

Thus, the importance of a Psi Chi academic advisor leadership style needs to be emphasized as influential in the psychosocial development of student members, chapter flow, and intrinsic motivation of students for future career pursuits. In addition, scholarship on the positive psychology of leadership, creativity, and talent development suggests that one role of an effective leader is to help connect the right person with the right domain or project. For instance, multiple intelligences work by Howard Gardner (2011) and work on the systems model of creativity by Mihaly Csikszentmihalyi and others indicate that one role of a mentor/leader is to facilitate entry into the field (Csikszentmihalyi 1996; Nakamura et al. 2009). For a Psi Chi mentor, this research may indicate that advisors should introduce students to field leaders, such as eminent psychologists, and/or to faculty colleagues with lab openings or research opportunities. The connections that are made with community leaders and organizations can also be very important to the students who may use these ties for networking in the future.

Just as important, however, is the commitment to service of others modeled by the Psi Chi advisor and fostered by group projects in the community. Of course, not only are effective leaders an asset to Psi Chi as faculty advisors, it is also important to remember that Psi Chi develops leadership in its student members. Leadership positions offered in Psi Chi empower students and endow them with the skills required to become a successful and competent leader. These skills are transferable and will benefit students throughout their careers. Psi Chi student leaders can be chapter officers, positions that allow ample opportunity to develop skills including negotiation, conflict resolution, moderating group discussion, and consensus building. Other leadership opportunities for Psi Chi students often emerge in the course of service activities as previously mentioned, such as Psi Chi groups involved with

Habitat for Humanity projects or with organizing food drives and fund raisers for charitable groups.

The importance of cocurricular activities, especially in encouraging students to pursue careers in the field of psychology, can hardly be overstated. Even those students who opt not to pursue further formal education and training in psychology often find that their Psi Chi activities benefitted them in numerous ways, such as linking them with careers in related helping professions or academic disciplines or developing leadership skills and insights into people that endure a lifetime. Such cases should also be viewed as successes for Psi Chi, as they reflect its commitment to foster leadership development and positive personal values, as well as academic excellence.

6.4 Conclusion

In sum, it is clear that Psi Chi, the International Honor Society in Psychology, has much to offer Positive Nations and communities. College students learn not only inside the classroom but beyond its walls, in the community. Since its founding in 1929, Psi Chi has grown into the world's largest honor society by developing a growing number of cocurricular programs to benefit the development of psychology students across the USA. Since 2009, Psi Chi has expanded internationally, with chapters in Canada, the Caribbean, Ireland, and New Zealand, with more being added at an increasing pace.

This chapter described research and evidence relating to the background and value of cocurricular activities, such as those offered by many Psi Chi chapters. Particular attention was devoted to research from positive psychology and strengths-based approaches. Then, one stellar example of an organization that utilizes cocurricular activities, Psi Chi, the International Honor Society in Psychology, was described. The history, mission, and growth of Psi Chi were detailed, including some explanation of the requirements for starting a chapter and for becoming a member or faculty mentor. Descriptions of sample activities engaged in by a number of Psi Chi chapters clearly show the value placed by the organization on service activities in local communities. Finally, the role of the Psi Chi advisor was discussed, and positive psychology research was presented relating to positive leadership in both faculty mentors and Psi Chi students. Special attention was devoted to the importance of intrinsic motivation, flow, and engagement as positive psychology concepts that impact the Psi Chi and cocurricular activity experience.

The collective processes involved with Psi Chi's cocurricular activities benefit a nation by benefitting the development of students who go on to careers in psychology (Denmark and Heitner 2000) and related fields in the helping professions (Takooshian and Landi 2011). Research and experience indicate that cocurricular programs of the type offered by Psi Chi encourage students to pursue careers in psychology and other related service professions. Presentation and participation at professional conferences and writing and receiving research grants give students a positive learning experience, which may foster an appreciation for the science of psychology. Service projects offered via Psi Chi chapters allow students to gain valuable experience in applied group settings, engaging the interest of students in careers in the helping professions. In this way, these cocurricular activities can begin to create Positive Nations and positive communities, by encouraging students to pursue psychology careers. While there is ample evidence documenting the value of cocurricular activities in promoting student engagement and professional development, future directions for research ought to examine more systematically how the collective processes involved may vary cross-culturally and cross-nationally. In this respect, the recent expansion of Psi Chi internationally promises to offer student members assistance on the path to academic excellence, exciting research possibilities, leadership opportunities, mentorship for career advancement, and opportunities to provide service to their communities.

Appendix

Definitions

Cocurricular student activities encourage positive growth among students in order for them to become socially, morally, emotionally, and cognitively competent.

Optimal human functioning (OHF) is a science of that makes people flourish and thrive. OHF is a branch of psychology that focuses on "building what's strong" as opposed to "fixing what's wrong."

Empowerment: To give or delegate power or authority to another. Empowerment increases the spiritual, political, social, or economic strength of individuals and communities. The outcome of empowerment enables an individual to gain insight and build confidence in his/her capacities.

Enhancement: An improvement that makes something more agreeable.

Enrichment: To make better or improve in quality.
   Note: Enhancement and enrichment are listed as synonyms for each another and may be used interchangeably.

Positive communities: Local regions which encourage, foster, and support the growth of its individuals on a smaller scale through positive institutions, including universities, schools, and local honor society chapters.

Positive Nations: Global regions which encourage, foster, and support the growth of its individuals through positive institutions.

Positive psychology: A research approach promoted by Martin Seligman and Mihaly Csikszentmihalyi that focuses on the empirical study and support of positive emotions, traits, and institutions.

Positive universities/colleges/schools: Academic environments which focus on positive growth and development, particularly in the youth population.

References

Alwin, D. F., Cohen, R. L., & Newcomb, T. M. (1991). *Political attitudes over the life span: The Bennington women after fifty years*. Madison: University of Wisconsin Press.

Bridgeland, J. M., Dilulio, J. J., & Wulson, S. C. (2008). *Engaged for success*. Washington, DC: Civic Enterprises.

Bringle, R. G., Hatcher, J. A., & Muthiah, R. N. (2010). The role of service learning in the retention of first year students to second year. *Michigan Journal of Community Service Learning, 16*, 38–49.

Colby, A., Erhlich, T., Beaumont, E., & Stephens, J. (2003). *Educating citizens: Preparing America's undergraduates for lives of moral and civic responsibility*. San Francisco: Jossey-Bass.

Compton, W. C. (2005). Positive institutions. In W. C. Compton (Ed.), *Positive psychology* (pp. 217–249). Belmont: Wadsworth.

Csikszentmihalyi, M. (1990). *Flow*. New York: Harper & Row.

Csikszentmihalyi, M. (1996). *Creativity*. New York: Harper Collins.

Csikszentmihalyi, M., & Rich, G. (1997). Musical improvisation: A systems view. In K. Sawyer (Ed.), *Creativity in performance* (pp. 43–66). Greenwich: Ablex.

Csikszentmihalyi, M., & Schneider, B. (Eds.). (2000). *Becoming adult*. New York: Basic Books.

Denmark, F. L., & Heitner, E. (2000). The impact of Psi Chi on eminent psychologists. *Eye on Psi Chi*. Psi Chi, The National Honor Society in Psychology. Retrieved from http://www.psichi.org/awards/winners/hunt_reports/heitner.aspx

Eccles, J. S., & Barber, B. L. (1999). What kind of extracurricular involvement matters? *Journal of Adolescent Research, 14*, 10–43.

Eccles, J. S., Barber, B. L., Stone, M., & Hunt, J. (2003). Extracurricular activities and adolescent development. *Journal of Social Issues, 59*, 865–889.

Gardner, H. (2011). *Leading minds*. New York: Basic Books.

Glanville, J. L. (1999). Political socialization or selection? Adolescent extracurricular participation and political activity in early adulthood. *Social Science Quarterly, 2*, 279–291.

Hanks, M., & Eckland, B. (1978). Adult voluntary associations and adolescent socialization. *The Sociological Quarterly, 19*(481–490), 509–520.

Hart, D., Matsuba, M. K., & Atkins, R. (2008). The moral and civic effects of learning to serve. In L. Nucci & D. Narvaez (Eds.), *Handbook of moral and character education*. New York: Psychology Press.

Harvey, L., Burrows, A., & Green, D. (1992). *Total student experience: A first report of the QHE national survey of staff and students' views of the important criteria of quality*. Birmingham: University of Central England QHE.

Hogan, J. D., & Takooshian, H. (2004). Psi Chi, the National Honor Society in Psychology: 75 years of scholarship and service. *Eye on Psi Chi*. Psi Chi, The National Honor Society in Psychology. Retrieved from http://www.psichi.org/Pubs/Articles/Article_432.aspx

Jordan, W., & Nettles, S. (1999). *How students invest their time out of school: Effects on school engagement, perceptions of life chances, and achievement* (Report No, 29). Baltimore: Center for Research on the Education of Students Placed at Risk. [ERIC Document Reproduction Service No. ED 428 174].

Krause, K. L. (2008). *Student engagement and retention in the first year: Challenges and opportunities!* Presentation for the Moving Forward Project. Glasgow Caledonian University. Retrieved from http://www.academy.gcal.ac.uk/movingforward/docs/GCUkrause2008.pdf

McLellan, J. A., & Youniss, J. (2003). Two systems of youth service: Determinants of voluntary and required youth community service. *Journal of Youth and Adolescence, 32*(1), 47–58.

Merton, T. (2009). *Bridges to contemplative living*. Bethany Spring: The Merton Institute for Contemplative Living.

Metz, E. C., & Youniss, J. (2005). Longitudinal gains in civic development through school-based required service. *Political Psychology, 26*, 413–437.

Nakamura, J., Shernoff, D. J., & Hooker, C. H. (2009). *Good mentoring*. San Francisco: Jossey-Bass.

Newcomb, T. M. (1943). *Personality and social change: Attitude formation in a student community*. Fort Worth: Dryden Press.

Pascarella, E., & Terenzini, P. (2005). *How college affects students: A third decade of research* (Vol. 2). San Francisco: Jossey-Bass.

Peixoto, F. (2004). *What kind of benefits students have from participating in extracurricular activities?* Lisbon: Higher Institute of Applied Psychology (ISPA).

Peterson, C. (2006). Enabling institutions. In J. Rappaport (Ed.), *A primer in positive psychology* (pp. 275–304). New York: Oxford.

Peterson, C., & Seligman, M. E. P. (2004). *Character strengths and virtues*. Oxford: Oxford University Press.

Rich, G. (2001). Positive psychology: An introduction. *Journal of Humanistic Psychology, 41*(1), 8–12.

Rich, G. (2002). *Teaching positive psychology: A seminar.* Poster presented at National Institute on the Teaching of Psychology, St. Petersburg, FL.

Rich, G. (2003). The positive psychology of youth and adolescence. *Journal of Youth and Adolescence*. doi:10.1023/a10210-17-4214-13.

Rich, G. (2009). Character education. In S. J. Lopez (Ed.), *The encyclopedia of positive psychology*. London: Blackwell Publishing.

Rich, G. (2011). Teaching tools for positive psychology: A comparison of available textbooks. *The Journal of Positive Psychology, 6*(6), 492–498.

Saleeby, D. (Ed.). (2002). *The strengths perspective in social work practice* (3rd ed.). Boston: Allyn & Bacon.

Schmidt, J., & Rich, G. (2000). Images of work and play. In M. Csikszentmihalyi & B. Schneider (Eds.), *Becoming adult: How teenagers prepare for the world of work* (pp. 67–94). New York: Basic Books.

Seligman, M. E. P. (2011). *Flourish*. New York: Free Press.

Seligman, M. E. P., & Csikszentmihalyi, M. (2000). Positive psychology: An introduction. *American Psychologist, 55*, 5–14.

Shernoff, D. J., Csikszentmihalyi, M., Schneider, B., & Shernoff, E. S. (2003). Student engagement in high school classrooms from the perspective of flow theory. *School Psychology Quarterly, 18*(2), 158–176.

Snyder, C. R., & Lopez, S. J. (2007). Positive environments. In C. R. Snyder & S. J. Lopez (Eds.), *Positive psychology* (pp. 377–472). Thousand Oaks: Sage.

Steen, T. A., Kachorek, L. V., & Peterson, C. (2003). Character strengths among youth. *Journal of Youth and Adolescence, 32*(1), 5–16.

Steinberg, L. D., Brown, B. B., & Dornbusch, S. M. (1996). *Beyond the classroom*. New York: Simon & Schuster.

Stevens, M. J., & Gielen, U. P. (2007). *Toward a global psychology: Theory, research, intervention, pedagogy*. Mahwah: Erlbaum.

Takooshian, H., & Landi, G. (2011). Psychological literacy: An alumni perspective. In J. Cranney & D. Dunn (Eds.), *The psychologically literate citizen: Foundations and global perspectives* (pp. 306–321). New York: Oxford University Press.

Toyokawa, T., & Toyokawa, N. (2002). Extracurricular activities and the adjustment of Asian international students: A study of Japanese students. *International Journal of Intercultural Relations, 26*(4), 363–379.

Walker, C. J. (2010). Experiencing flow: Is doing it together better than doing it alone? *The Journal of Positive Psychology, 5*(1), 3–11.

Youniss, J., & Yates, M. (1997). *Community service and social responsibility in youth*. Chicago: The University of Chicago Press.

Youniss, J., McLellan, J. A., & Yates, M. (1997). What we know about engendering civic identity. *American Behavioral Scientist, 40*, 620.

Zaff, J. F., Moore, K. A., Papillo Romano, A., & Williams, S. (2003). Implications of extracurricular activity participation during adolescence on positive outcomes. *Journal of Adolescent Research*. doi:10.1177/074355-840-3254-779.

Part III
Realization: From Individual to Collective

Chapter 7
The European Football Championship as a Positive Festivity: Changes in Strengths of Character Before, During, and After the Euro 2008 in Switzerland

René T. Proyer, Fabian Gander, Sara Wellenzohn, and Willibald Ruch

Positive psychology can briefly be defined as the study of what is best in people and of traits, institutions, and conditions that allow people to flourish (see Seligman and Csikszentmihalyi 2000). Within this field, sport psychology is a comparatively understudied area. Brent and Leslie-Toogood (2009) argue that there is a similarity between positive psychology and sport psychology as "the primary focus is on building human strengths and striving for optimal experience" (p. 932; Gould 2002). For example, helping people to find meaning and engagement (flow) facilitates their personal growth toward better performance (cf. Newburg et al. 2002). In this study, we argue that not only pursuing sport but also following sport (a football [soccer] tournament) may have an impact on the strengths of people.

There is much literature suggesting that watching sports has an impact on the spectators, for example, the experience of positive affect in spectators with high identification with a winning team or increased negative affect in high identification with a losing team (Wann et al. 1994). Greater levels of team identification have been associated with various aspects of positive psychological functioning such as social well-being, higher vigor (energy), or openness (for an overview see Wann et al. 2011). Additionally, these findings remain stable after controlling for general interest in sport (Wann et al. 2003).

There are further data from the *Fédération Internationale de Football Association* (FIFA) World Cup, which was held in 2006 in Germany, demonstrating that emotional stress seemed to increase during games of the German team, as indicated by an increase in cardiac emergencies on these days in comparison with a control period (by a factor of 2.66; Wilbert-Lampen et al. 2008). Furthermore, there is empirical

---

The preparation of this chapter has been facilitated by a research grant of the Swiss National Science Foundation (SNSF; 100014_132512).

R.T. Proyer (✉) • F. Gander • S. Wellenzohn • W. Ruch
Department of Psychology, University of Zurich, Zurich, Switzerland
e-mail: r.proyer@psychologie.uzh.ch; f.gander@psychologie.uzh.ch;
s.wellenzohn@psychologie.uzh.ch; w.ruch@psychologie.uzh.ch

evidence that hosting a football tournament boosts happiness in the host country at a national level (tested in countries where football is the dominant sport)—at least for a short term; the effects were also shown to be large by comparison to some sociodemographic factors (Kavetsos and Szymanski 2010); however, Kavetsos and Szymanski also note that an error in measurement for some (socioeconomic) factors may have underestimated their influence. Interestingly, the performance of the home country team at the event was of lesser importance than hosting the event itself. Potential causes for such effects may be seen in "the enjoyment of attending events, of being involved as a volunteer organizer, enjoyment of the proximity of the events even if one does not attend, cultural showcases, and national pride" (Kavetsos and Szymanski 2010, p. 159). Hence, people seem to be affected by the event in many different ways, even if not following the matches themselves.

7.1 Character Strengths in the Face of Adversity

In the present study, it was tested whether there are any effects of a football tournament on character strengths in a society (the host country). Peterson and Seligman (2004) revived psychology's long abandoned interest in character. They see character strengths as morally positively valued traits and developed a classification of 24 character strengths (e.g., curiosity, zest, or self-regulation; see Table 7.1 for an overview of all strengths) and six universal virtues (i.e., wisdom and knowledge, courage, humanity, justice, temperance, and transcendence; *Values in Action classification*, VIA). The VIA classification allows studying the "good character." By definition (Peterson and Seligman 2004), each of the strengths is fulfilling and has a potential for contributing positively to the well-being of individuals. The *Values in Action Inventory of Strengths* (VIA-IS) allows the subjective assessment of these strengths (Peterson et al. 2005). Studies using the VIA-IS provide broad evidence for a positive relation between character strengths and various indicators of subjective well-being (e.g., Brdar et al. 2011; Gander et al. 2012; Güsewell and Ruch 2012; Littman-Ovadia and Lavy 2011; Park and Peterson 2006a, b; Park et al. 2004; Peterson et al. 2007; Proyer et al. 2011; Ruch et al. 2010a, b; Weber and Ruch 2012).

Positive psychology addresses positive experiences in people. Nevertheless, research has also dealt with adversity and the role character strengths may play in such an environment. For example, there are studies on the role of strengths in posttraumatic growth and in the recovery from physical illness or psychological disorders (Peterson et al. 2006, 2008; see also Wadey et al. 2011). In the aftermath of the terror attacks of September 11 in the USA on 2001, Peterson and Seligman (2003) were interested in whether this dramatic event had an impact on character strengths. They compared mean scores in the VIA-IS of participants completing the questionnaire online before 9/11 ($n=906$) and at 1 month ($n=295$) and 2 months ($n=195$) after the attacks (cross-sectional). The strengths of gratitude, hope, kindness, leadership, love, spirituality, and teamwork increased at both time periods. Peterson and Seligman related their findings to so-called theological virtues (i.e., faith, hope, and charity [love]; Aquinas trans. 1966). When analyzing these strengths in a total score together, the authors found a significant increase in the mean scores at time periods of 0–2, 2–4, and 4–10 months after the event. This score decreased in the latter 3 months in size numerically with the score from the final interval being significantly different from the first one. Although these data were not longitudinal, the authors argued that they reflected mean-level changes as the demographics of people visiting to the website were similar at all times.

One of the main findings of this study was that strengths can reflect changes and incidents in the "real world." However, the question arises if strengths do only change in the face of adversity or whether there is also an impact of positive events. Thus far, this question has not been addressed empirically. Positive events should be a "natural home" for the study of the good character. It is argued that flourishing and cultivating positive traits are facilitated in positive environments. The prime aim of the present study is to test whether strengths at a national level are subjected to changes due to positive events, in comparison with changes in the face of adversity such as the 9/11 terror attacks.

7.2   The European Football Championship as a "Positive Festivity"

When thinking about potential positive "candidate events" for such a study, one has to conclude that there are not many events that might have had an impact on a whole nation. One might think of achievements such as man's first landing on the moon or other events such as a political change toward democracy and an economic upturn (cf. Inglehart et al. 2008). However, even events of comparatively less importance on a community (e.g., because they are limited in time or appeal to people differently) might have a potential in impacting people.

One such event could be the *UEFA* (*United European Football Associations*) *European Football Championship* (Euro 2008), which was held in Switzerland and Austria (June 7–29, 2008). This event is held every 4 years in a different country (or countries), and teams had to qualify in a sequential set of games prior to the championship starting from August 2006 (16 out of 52 teams are allowed to participate). The European Football Championship is considered the biggest sporting event in Europe, and it was, until now, the largest sport event organized in Switzerland; e.g., the capital (Berne) has 120,000 inhabitants and hosted one million visitors over the course of the tournament (cf. Martinolli et al. 2011). Being selected as the host country is a competitive process (14 nations applied and provided plans, and Switzerland and Austria won the elections at the UEFA). There is extensive media coverage guaranteed for this event; e.g., according to official figures from the broadcast companies, the drawing of the teams to four groups held in Lucerne (Switzerland) has been broadcasted in 138 countries (37 live) and has been seen by approximately 120 million people.

It is argued that even people, who were not interested in football, were nonetheless affected by the event. For example, major Swiss cities (where games were played, i.e., Basel, Bern, Geneva, and Zurich) were decorated to celebrate the event; public screening of all matches were held in numerous places; people decorated their cars with flags of their favored team; headlines of the newspapers were occupied by the event to a large extent; the Swiss and Austrian team also participated; media reported extensively about the event (all 31 games were broadcasted in national TV [and worldwide] plus additional coverage); advertisements in TV, radio, or newspaper were adjusted to the event; companies offered special prices related to the tournament or special activities (e.g., for each goal scored by the Swiss team, a reduction of prices in a certain percentage); and people talked about the event in the workplace or when out with friends. Furthermore, politicians and representatives of the economy highlighted the relevance of the tournament for political (e.g., representation of Switzerland to a worldwide audience) and economical reasons (e.g., expectancy of a positive effect on tourism). A further example would be that, according to press releases from broadcast companies, the TV broadcast of the first game of the Swiss team has been seen (on the average) by 1.6 million people in Switzerland (a country with close to eight million inhabitants), which was a market share of 79.2 %. The official slogan of the UEFA Euro 2008 was "Expect emotions," which refers to the potential of the games evoking emotional reactions in supporters as well as in a larger audience. Thus, it is argued that this event had an impact on both football supporters and people who were not interested in the games themselves. In this study, the Euro 2008 is seen as a "positive festivity," which included not only the football games themselves but had also an impact on the hosting country.

7.3   Character Strengths in the Face of a "Positive Festivity"

In the present study, we were interested in whether the VIA scores changed over the course of a potentially positive event, the Euro 2008 (in comparison of measurement periods before, during, and after the tournament). The VIA-IS allows the assessment of strengths at different levels: (1) at the level of the 24 *single strengths*, (2) at the level of 5 broader *strengths factors* (i.e., interpersonal, emotional, restraint, intellectual, and theological strengths) that typically emerge in factor analyses of the VIA-IS (e.g., Güsewell and Ruch 2012; Littman-Ovadia and Lavy 2011; Müller and Ruch 2011; Peterson 2006; Peterson and Seligman 2004; Ruch et al. 2010a), and (3) at the level of two dimensions retrieved from factor analyses of ipsative scores (Peterson 2006; Ruch et al. 2010a), namely, *strengths of the mind* (e.g., open-mindedness, self-regulation) vs. *heart* (e.g., gratitude, love) and *self* (e.g., curiosity, creativity) vs. *other-directed* (e.g., teamwork, fairness) strengths.

Peterson and Seligman (2004) suggest that character strengths are ubiquitous, fulfilling, morally valued, trait-like, distinct, and measurable individual differences. Peterson and Seligman (2004) postulate that strengths are malleable (under specific conditions such as sustained practice). There is evidence that character strengths can be altered by external events (e.g., Peterson and Seligman 2003; Peterson et al. 2006, 2008) but also by means of deliberate interventions (e.g., Proyer et al. 2013;

Seligman et al. 2005). We expected that the tournament (as an external event) had potential for increasing emotional, interpersonal, and intellectual strengths.

Emotional strengths (such as love, social intelligence, or humor) relate to the amount of time spent with others (Peterson and Seligman 2004; Ruch et al. 2010a). Given that the tournament is a social event (e.g., when joining public screenings or talking with friends and colleagues about the games and the tournament in general), emotional strengths were expected to increase. A preference for watching sports was also found to be positively associated with gregariousness (Appelbaum et al. 2012). Interpersonal strengths are strengths that are highly valued in football (or in team sports in general), such as fairness, teamwork, or kindness (cf. Lee and Cockman 1995). Furthermore, there are specific rituals in football to cultivate these strengths, e.g., shaking hands and exchanging gifts (e.g., exchanging team pennants between competing teams before a game) or praising the fairest teams or players at the end of a season or a tournament. Furthermore, during the game a referee punishes players violating the regulations of the game or for misconduct (e.g., foul play). Typically this is followed by media coverage discussing the violations (e.g., deliberately taking into account hurting other players). Overall, this could be seen as a model for fair interactions with others. Additionally, such an event allows for engaging with others in many different ways (e.g., meeting with supporters of other teams). Overall, it was expected that interpersonal strengths increase over the course of the tournament.

Sharing experiences with other people along with learning more about foreign people and customs (e.g., when meeting supporters from other countries in the cities or following media coverage about the countries involved in the tournament) was expected to have an impact on the expression of intellectual strengths such as curiosity or open-mindedness. If translating this into the broader two strengths factors, an increase in strengths of the heart and other-directed strengths was expected. Data was also analyzed at the level of single strengths. While it was expected that changes would be mainly reflected in the broader strengths factors, strengths that could be seen as indicative for these factors such as fairness, zest, or authenticity were also expected to increase over the course of the tournament.

The main aim of this study was to test whether there were mean-level changes in character strengths in terms of the period before, during, and after the UEFA Euro 2008 in Switzerland.

7.4 Method

7.4.1 Participants

The total sample consisted of $N = 1{,}253$ adults aged between 18 and 84 years with a mean age of $M = 42.13$ ($SD = 13.80$). One-third of the sample was male (33.8 %), and about two-thirds were female (66.2 %); all were Swiss. In the first time period 51–26 days prior to the UEFA Euro 2008, $n = 97$ participants completed the VIA-IS (35.1 % men), $n = 258$ completed the survey 26–0 days prior to the championship

(29.5 % male), $n = 128$ during the championship (28.1 % male), $n = 134$ 0 to 1 month after the championship (34.3 % male), and 636 participants completed the survey 1–2 months after the UEFA Euro 2008 (36.5 % male).

7.4.2 Instruments

The *Values in Action Inventory of Strengths* (VIA-IS; Peterson et al. 2005; in the German adaptation by Ruch et al. 2010a) consists of 240 items (10 per strength) for the assessment of the strengths of the VIA classification. Answers are given on a 5-point Likert scale (1 = *"very much unlike me,"* 5 = *"very much like me"*; sample item: "I never quit a task before it is done," persistence). Ruch et al. (2010a) reported high internal consistencies and test-retest correlations (6, 9 months). Additionally, they provided information on the factorial as well as convergent validity of the German form, which has already been used in several other studies (e.g., Gander et al. 2012; Güsewell and Ruch 2012; Proyer and Ruch 2009, 2011; Proyer et al. 2011; Ruch et al. 2010b). Alpha-coefficients in this sample ranged between .71 and .90 (median = .78).

7.4.3 Procedure

Participants completed the VIA-IS on a research website hosted by the institution conducting the study. The website was initiated 51 days before the Euro 2008 started (but independently from it) and was advertised broadly in newspapers and via different sources over the Internet (e.g., mailing lists). We analyzed Swiss individuals, who completed the VIA-IS till two months after the tournament. Usage of the website is free of charge and an automated feedback on the individual strengths of the participant is given. The participants provided basic demographic information and could choose among several instruments from positive psychology (e.g., on humor, work satisfaction, and life satisfaction) with the VIA-IS being one of them. The completion of the VIA-IS takes about 35–45 min depending on the working speed. All questionnaires were administered in German. In the literature, collecting data in online studies has been criticized (e.g., for possible biases of the collected samples). However, there is empirical evidence that data collected via the Internet is comparable to data collected in more conventional ways (see, e.g., Gosling et al. 2004). The study has been planned and conducted in accordance with the guidelines for "good practice" in Internet-delivered testing (Coyne and Bartram 2006).

Data on character strengths were available for Switzerland starting from the 17th of April 2008, and the time period before the championship (51 days) was split in two periods of 26 and 25 days. Since data collection only started on this website 51 days before the first game in the tournament, this starting point was a rather pragmatic decision. A further time period was available during the tournament

(23 days), and two time periods after the tournament (in each case 1 month) also entered the study. The data collection on the online platform that was used for this study started only 51 days before the tournament. Therefore, we were not able to fully parallel the time periods before and after the period of the games.

7.5   Results

7.5.1   Preliminary Analyses

The men:women ratio was comparable across all time periods ($\chi^2_{[4, N = 1.253]} = 6.14$, $p = .19$). However, there were differences in the age of the participants across the time periods (F [4, 1284] = 15.63, $p < .001$). Therefore, age was controlled in the subsequently conducted analyses for ruling out any age effects in the data.

As in Ruch et al. (2010a), we conducted a principal component analysis (for the full sample) and six factors exceeded unity (eigenvalues were 9.10, 2.50, 1.85, 1.22, 1.14, 1.05, and 0.77). In accordance with the findings for self- and peer-rated strengths with the German VIA-IS (Ruch et al. 2010a), five factors were extracted and rotated to the varimax criterion. The results converged very well with those reported for the German VIA-IS (Tucker's Phi coefficients between Ruch et al.'s solution and the one in the present sample were .99, .99, .99, .99, and .89), and we labeled the factors accordingly (i.e., *emotional strengths* [e.g., zest, hope], *interpersonal strengths* [e.g., leadership, teamwork], *strengths of restraint* [prudence, persistence], *intellectual strengths* [e.g., love of learning, creativity], and *theological strengths* [e.g., religiousness, gratitude]). Additionally, a two-factor solution using ipsative data was considered. Again, the results converged well with the Ruch et al. (2010a) study, and the two factors were labeled as *mind* (e.g., open-mindedness, prudence) vs. *heart* (e.g., kindness, gratitude) and *focus on self* (e.g., creativity, zest) vs. *others* (e.g., fairness, leadership). These factors were used for the data analysis along with the 24 scales of the VIA-IS.

7.5.2   Mean-Level Differences at the Level of Strengths Factors

An overall multivariate analysis of covariance with five broader strengths factors as dependent variables, the five time periods as factors, and the age as covariate was conducted. The analysis yielded a significant result for the covariate ($V = 0.07$, F [5, 1243] = 17.98, $p < .001$, $\eta^2 = .07$) and the factor ($V = 0.04$, F [20, 4984] = 2.25, $p < .01$, $\eta^2 = .01$). Coefficients for the subsequently conducted univariate analyses of variance (controlled for age) as well as means and standard deviations for all time periods are shown in Table 7.1.

The Table shows that mean scores differed among time periods for three out of the five strengths factors (i.e., emotional strengths, interpersonal strengths, and

Table 7.1 Adjusted mean scores, standard deviations, and analyses of covariance of character strengths as a function of time periods, with participants' age as covariate

VIA-IS		Time periods					ANCOVA	
		−2	−1	0	+1	+2	$F\,(4,\,1247)$	Post hoc
Scales								
Creativity	M	3.50	3.50	3.62	3.60	3.60	1.53	–
	SD	0.65	0.66	0.70	0.71	0.63		
Curiosity	M	4.06	4.02	4.03	4.03	4.08	0.78	–
	SD	0.50	0.50	0.60	0.49	0.50		
Open-mindedness	M	3.84	3.82	3.88	3.89	3.84	0.53	–
	SD	0.55	0.53	0.49	0.48	0.44		
Love of learning	M	3.90	3.79	3.83	3.86	3.89	1.44	–
	SD	0.62	0.59	0.68	0.60	0.54		
Perspective	M	3.51	3.56	3.58	3.56	3.55	0.25	–
	SD	0.53	0.50	0.46	0.47	0.45		
Bravery	M	3.57	3.58	3.61	3.65	3.59	0.62	–
	SD	0.53	0.54	0.51	0.54	0.49		
Persistence	M	3.64	3.53	3.58	3.49	3.49	1.80	–
	SD	0.50	0.57	0.59	0.65	0.59		
Authenticity	M	3.74	3.85	3.89	3.89	3.84	2.06[+]	−2<0, +1, +2[a]
	SD	0.45	0.45	0.41	0.37	0.44		
Zest	M	3.63	3.71	3.64	3.67	3.66	0.51	–
	SD	0.54	0.54	0.66	0.56	0.53		
Love	M	3.92	3.86	3.81	3.85	3.81	1.29	–
	SD	0.53	0.57	0.56	0.57	0.49		
Kindness	M	3.75	3.83	3.85	3.90	3.84	1.55	–
	SD	0.51	0.49	0.45	0.47	0.44		
Social I	M	3.76	3.69	3.75	3.76	3.72	0.89	–
	SD	0.48	0.45	0.45	0.41	0.42		
Teamwork	M	3.51	3.59	3.64	3.60	3.64	1.79	–
	SD	0.57	0.49	0.47	0.50	0.46		
Fairness	M	3.84	3.94	3.98	3.99	4.00	2.79[*]	−2<0, +1, +2
	SD	0.55	0.50	0.39	0.47	0.42		
Leadership	M	3.63	3.66	3.69	3.68	3.71	1.14	–
	SD	0.54	0.49	0.45	0.45	0.45		
Forgiveness	M	3.53	3.56	3.57	3.57	3.63	1.57	–
	SD	0.57	0.54	0.57	0.53	0.50		
Modesty	M	3.25	3.24	3.21	3.32	3.35	2.93[*]	−1, 0<+2
	SD	0.60	0.54	0.56	0.57	0.56		
Prudence	M	3.34	3.33	3.40	3.40	3.40	0.97	–
	SD	0.53	0.50	0.54	0.54	0.52		
Self-regulation	M	3.29	3.26	3.23	3.32	3.33	1.49	–
	SD	0.52	0.56	0.54	0.58	0.52		

(continued)

Table 7.1 (continued)

VIA-IS		Time periods					ANCOVA	
		−2	−1	0	+1	+2	F (4, 1247)	Post hoc
Beauty	M	3.65	3.64	3.68	3.73	3.70	0.91	–
	SD	0.51	0.55	0.56	0.56	0.53		
Gratitude	M	3.73	3.77	3.79	3.79	3.78	0.22	–
	SD	0.55	0.55	0.54	0.54	0.53		
Hope	M	3.60	3.66	3.60	3.60	3.59	0.61	–
	SD	0.60	0.58	0.65	0.62	0.57		
Humor	M	3.53	3.70	3.67	3.62	3.62	1.61	–
	SD	0.54	0.60	0.62	0.60	0.59		
Religiousness	M	2.98	3.17	3.03	3.00	3.19	2.74*	−2, +1 < +2
	SD	0.94	0.91	0.87	0.90	0.85		
5-factor solution								
Emotional strengths	M	−0.01	0.12	0.12	0.07	−0.09	2.71*	−1, 0 > +2
	SD	1.03	1.05	1.04	1.05	0.95		
Interpersonal strengths	M	−0.26	−0.11	−0.02	0.05	0.08	3.57**	−2 < +1, +2; −1 < +2
	SD	1.19	1.01	0.90	1.09	0.95		
Strengths of restraint	M	0.07	−0.02	0.02	0.02	−0.01	0.18	–
	SD	0.93	0.99	1.02	1.12	0.99		
Intellectual strengths	M	−0.03	−0.15	0.00	0.02	0.06	2.14^{+}	−1 < +2
	SD	1.06	1.09	1.11	0.98	0.93		
Theological strengths	M	0.00	0.06	−0.19	−0.15	0.05	2.43*	0 < −1, +2; +1 < +2
	SD	1.11	1.01	1.08	1.09	0.93		
2-factor solution								
Self vs. others	M	−0.20	−0.06	−0.01	0.03	0.05	–	–
	SD	1.05	1.00	1.06	1.13	0.95		
Heart vs. mind	M	−0.08	0.08	−0.04	−0.03	0.00	–	–
	SD	1.00	0.98	1.05	1.16	0.96		

Note: $N=1,253$ ($n_{−2}=97$, $n_{−1}=258$, $n_0=128$, $n_{+1}=134$, $n_{+2}=636$). Beauty = appreciation of beauty and excellence; time periods: −2 = 51–26 days prior, −1 = 26–0 days prior, 0 = during the championship (23 days), +1 = 0–1 month after. +2 = 1–2 months after

Effect size (partial eta squared) was .01 for all significant ANCOVAS. Post hoc tests differed at $p < .05$ (LSD)

$^{+}p < .10$, $*p < .05$, $**p < .01$

[a]The mean level at time period −2 (1–2 months prior) was significantly lower than the mean levels at the time periods 0, +1, and +2 (i.e., during the championship, 0–1 month after, and 1–2 months after)

Social I = Social intelligence

theological strengths). Additionally, changes in the mean scores in intellectual strengths approached significance (F [4, 1247] = 2.14, $p = .07$). Emotional strengths increased numerically before the championship and decreased again after the end of the championship. Post hoc tests confirmed that the time period directly before the championship, and the period during the championship, differed from the last period. Interpersonal strengths were higher at both time periods after the championship compared with the first time of measurement. Intellectual strengths increased from the time period directly before the championship to the last time period, and theological strengths *de*creased first as the championship started but increased at the last time period coming back to the level measured before the tournament.

The factor scores for the two-factor solution were also used as dependent variables in a multivariate analysis of covariance, with time periods as factors and age as covariate. The analysis yielded nonsignificant results for both the covariate ($V=0.00$, F [2, 1246] $=0.65$, $p=.52$) and the dependent variable ($V=0.01$, F [8, 2494] $= 1.06$, $p=.39$).

7.5.3 Mean-Level Differences at the Level of Single Strengths

The analysis of the data followed the same procedure as used for the broader strengths factors. The 24 character strengths were subjected to a multivariate analysis of covariance as dependent variables, with the time periods as factors, and age as covariate. Results revealed that the covariate was significantly related to character strengths (Pillai's trace, $V=0.13$, F [24, 1224] $=7.43$, $p<.001$, $\eta^2=.13$). When controlling for effects of age, time had a significant effect on the character strengths ($V=0.13$, F [96, 4908] $=1.66$, $p<.001$, $\eta^2=.03$). The subsequently conducted univariate analyses of variance (see Table 7.1) showed that three out of the 24 character strengths differed between time periods regarding their mean levels, i.e., *fairness*, *modesty*, and *religiousness*. As a fourth strength, authenticity approached significance (F [4, 1247] $=2.06$, $p=.08$). Post hoc tests revealed that scores for the strengths of authenticity and fairness were higher during and after the UEFA Euro 2008 compared to both time periods before the championship. Modesty was higher at the time period 2 months after the tournament compared with the periods directly before and during the championship. Religiousness was higher at the last follow-up in comparison with the first time period and compared with the time period directly after the championship.

7.6 Discussion

Peterson and Seligman (2003) tested the impact of a dramatic and shocking event, which affected a whole nation (the 9/11 terror attacks in the USA), on the expression of character strengths before and after that event. The main ambition behind the present study was to test whether a positive event with a national impact (the Euro 2008) also has the potential for impacting character strengths at a national level. The present study shows an increase in emotional, interpersonal, and, to a lesser extent, intellectual strengths (approached significance) during/after the tournament compared to the measurements before the tournament. Furthermore, there were changes in theological strengths over the course of time. At the level of single strengths, changes in mean levels in authenticity, fairness, modesty, and religiosity were reported.

In more detail, there was an increase in emotional strengths immediately before and during the tournament. It seems reasonable that a factor set together of strengths such as zest and hope increases in the advance of such an event. People feel enthusiastic and energetic about the time ahead. This might also have been facilitated by observing the supporters of the different nations not only during the games but also while celebrating in the cities (e.g., at public screenings of the games). Similar arguments have been put forward for increases in well-being due to football tournaments (Kavetsos and Szymanski 2010).

Interpersonal strengths increased over time and intellectual strengths also tended to increase. Such a sport event is a good opportunity for practicing interpersonal strengths like teamwork and kindness in everyday behavior, be it by helping visitors to find their way or by organizing activities as a group. Intellectual strengths such as love of learning and curiosity can also easily be trained, e.g., when learning more about a country that is part of the tournament or when talking to people from this country visiting the own hometown. Theological strengths were lowest during the tournament and were about the same directly after the tournament. This seems to be contradictory to the findings reported earlier for the religiosity scale. One might argue that the aspect of moral behavior is less pronounced in this factor and that it focuses more strongly on truly theological virtues. People might focus on them less during the tournament (due to the great distractions); however, they then come back to the initial level after the tournament.

Interestingly, religiosity (spirituality) was also among the strengths that increased in the face of adversity in the Peterson and Seligman study, whereas the other strengths were different. In the present study, there was no steady increase for religiosity, but in comparison of the longest time periods before and after the tournament, the strength increased. Peterson and Seligman (2004) define this strength as "having coherent beliefs about the higher purpose and meaning of the universe and one's place within it. People with this strength have a theory about the ultimate meaning of life that shapes their conduct and provides comfort to them. Furthermore, spirituality and religiousness are linked to an interest in moral values and the pursuit of goodness" (p. 533). Football is a game with strict rules that are controlled by several officials (referees), whose head is allowed to immediately punish violations of the rules (e.g., by sending a player off the field without allowing him to be replaced by a different player and, thus, weakening the team—*red card*). Also, negative incidents such as foul play or cheating are extensively discussed and debated (e.g., in the sport section in newspapers). Thus, one might argue that this conveys a sense of moral behavior and adhering to rules (of the game). Also, many teams have rules of conduct for players and other team members while being at the tournament (e.g., regulating behavior toward supporters, consumption of alcoholic beverages, or behavior during public statements). Supporters who appreciate and applaud good moves from the opposing team (as a sign of fairness) and who cheer for their team in a positive and/or funny way are usually positively discussed in the media. Strengths such as fairness and religiosity (in the sense of a morally positively valued behavior) might be cultivated by such examples.

In their introduction of the VIA classification, Peterson and Seligman (2004) state in the chapter on authenticity: "We think that sports are popular not just because they allow us to thrill in vicarious victory and agonize in vicarious defeat but also because they allow an ultimately innocuous form of public discussion of honesty" (p. 208; honesty is one of the synonyms [along with integrity] the authors use for authenticity). It is argued that events such as the UEFA Euro 2008 do not only allow for the public discussion of honesty but is also a place where it can be observed in real life. One of the most remarkable examples of such a discussion among those interested in football is the one about Diego Maradona's (Argentina) goal in the final of the 1986 *FIFA* (*Fédération Internationale de Football Association*) *World Cup* in Argentina's 2:1 victory over England. Maradona scored one goal with his hands, which entered football history as the "Hand of God." His action was not penalized by the referee and caused heated discussion in the aftermath of the game—the debate got even more complicated as, only minutes later, Maradona scored a second goal in this match, which is considered by some as the "Goal of the Century" and an example of his genius at play. As said before, usually cheating and misbehavior is sanctioned quickly and directly in a football game. This example shows how football may serve as basis for the discussion of honesty and authenticity in action. The refusal of the British swimmer Rebecca Adlington (Olympic gold medalist) to use a new (and legal) swimsuit, because she thought it was cheating, is yet another example of how an athlete's behavior might elicit a public discussion of strengths like fairness and honesty—the English newspaper *The Times* published a report on Adlington entitled "Fair play to Rebecca, a champion of honesty" (Broadbent 2009).

For modesty, one might argue that the aftermath of the enhanced attention that has been brought to Switzerland (e.g., extensive media coverage not only of the games but also of the country in general) could have led to a reconciliation of modest and more withdrawn behavior, away from the spotlight of the attention, or as Peterson and Seligman argue: "This character strength is a quiet one" (p. 435). This also seems to relate to the perception of national identities (e.g., valuing modesty in Switzerland; see, e.g., Schmid Mast et al. 2011), which has also been addressed by the local media coverage (e.g., Kneidinger 2010; see also Nüesch and Franck 2009). This can also be related to a specific way of dealing with the accomplishment and contribution of people to such an event (e.g., the athletes, the [voluntary] helpers, organizers). It is argued that this perception has a potential for fostering and contributing to self-evaluations (e.g., modest self-presentations during this period) and reflections of one's role in a broader context, regarding ones strengths and limitations.

This study has several limitations. First, all data are cross-sectional, as we could not gather longitudinal data in this study. Unlike Peterson and Seligman's (2003) study, we found differences in the demographic factors of the people, who visited our research website. Although we controlled for the impact of age, it cannot be ruled out that people differed in other characteristics that could also have impacted the findings and may cause problems when comparing the different measurement times. Additionally, different sample sizes (e.g., 97 at time 1 but 636 at time 5) need to be acknowledged. Furthermore, we had more women in our sample than men—given that more men follow football than women, this may have an impact on the findings. It would also have been desirable if data from other countries could have been added as an additional control. However, these data were not available. Finally, the generalizability of the samples to the Swiss society in general can be debated (e.g., educational level). Therefore, further studies of the contribution of positive events (e.g., sport events such as the Euro or the World Cup) would be needed. Unfortunately, such events are rather rare and it is impossible to replicate the findings in Switzerland in the next decades. However, similar studies could be carried out in other countries with a more elaborate design (e.g., longitudinal data with the same individuals completing the measures on repeated occasions but also the inclusion of further data such as different indicators of well-being or more information on the personal perception of the event).

It is difficult to provide empirical support for the assumption that even those people not interested in football were also affected by the tournament. When scanning the websites from large newspapers, it is evident that they have a large number of entries about the UEFA Euro 2008 in this time span, which decreases considerably afterward. Nevertheless, people might have been less affected by the event than was assumed. One might even argue that people who really were interested in the football event were in turn less interested in accessing the website to fill in questionnaires. However, the number of positive events that potentially could have a national appeal is rather limited and the Euro 2008 seemed to be a good approximation to us. It also needs to be considered that the Swiss team was eliminated early from the tournament after the preliminary rounds, which could have had an impact on the findings. Unfortunately, there are only very few data from Austria to allow for a cross-validation of the findings.

It also needs to be acknowledged that the idea of a game as a model and athletes as models of moral behavior needs to be discussed at different levels. For example, the competitiveness and high pressure of the event may produce negative outcomes among the athletes themselves. If winning for the sake of winning (even if it is "winning dirty") becomes more important than the game itself, moral standards (the "sportsmanship orientation"; Priest et al. 1999) could be lowered for acquiring the win (see Howe 2004). The European Football Championship is a sport event at the highest level of professionalism and, of course, important for the careers of the athletes. However, given the high media attention and media coverage, the cheating athlete has to deal with negative reports for misbehavior. However, while single players could misbehave (without being penalized), it is argued that the sport itself and the example it provides are rather morally driven.

The effects reported in the present study were relatively small and caution in their interpretation is warranted. However, it is argued that there is a substance in the findings. Overall, this line of research gave preliminary hints that strengths might be malleable at the national level—as a consequence of negative as well as positive events. In general, sport events such as Football Championships may have a potential for a positive impact in communities. Positive psychology can provide a framework for studying such changes. Furthermore, research in strengths of character (at an individual level) may be a topic following for researchers in the field of sport psychology. One might argue that strengths facilitate the performance of athletes in various ways. For example, a strengths-based coaching model could help uncovering yet untapped potentials and support peak performance. Recently, studies from work psychology have further supported the notion that signature strengths are important for positive behavior at work (e.g., Harzer and Ruch 2012, in press), and this may provide ground for follow-up studies in the realm of sport psychology. However, more research in this area is needed, and the study argues for more attention to topics from sport psychology within the field of positive psychology.

References

Appelbaum, L. G., Cain, M. S., Darling, E. F., Stanton, S. J., Nguyen, M. T., & Mitroff, S. R. (2012). What is the identity of a sports spectator? *Personality and Individual Differences*. doi:10.1016/j.paid.2011.10.048.

Aquinas, T. (1966). *Treatise on the virtues* (J. A. Oesterle, Trans.). Englewood Cliffs: Prentice-Hall.

Brdar, I., Anić, P., & Rijavec, M. (2011). Character strengths and well-being: Are there gender differences? In I. Brdar (Ed.), *The human pursuit of well-being: A cultural approach* (pp. 145–156). Dordrecht: Springer. doi:10.1007/978-94-007-1375-8_13.

Brent, M. E., & Leslie-Toogood, A. (2009). Sport psychology. In S. J. Lopez (Ed.), *The encyclopedia of positive psychology* (pp. 932–935). Oxford: Blackwell.

Broadbent, R. (2009, July 21). Fair play to Rebecca, a champion of honesty. *The Times*, 4.

Coyne, I., & Bartram, D. (Eds.). (2006). ITC guidelines on computer-based and internet-delivered testing. *International Journal of Testing*. doi:10.1207/s15327574ijt0602_3.

Gander, F., Proyer, R. T., Ruch, W., & Wyss, T. (2012). The good character at work: An initial study on the contribution of character strengths in identifying healthy and unhealthy work-related behavior and experience patterns. *International Archives of Occupational and Environmental Health*. doi:10.1007/s00420-012-0736-x.

Gosling, S. D., Vazire, S., Srivastava, S., & John, O. P. (2004). Should we trust web-based studies? A comparative analysis of six preconceptions about Internet questionnaires. *American Psychologist*. doi:10.1037/0003-066X.59.2.93.

Gould, D. (2002). Sport psychology in the new millennium: The psychology of athletic excellence and beyond. *Journal of Applied Sport Psychology*. doi:10.1080/10413200290103455.

Güsewell, A., & Ruch, W. (2012). Are only emotional strengths emotional? Character strengths and disposition to positive emotions. *Applied Psychology: Health and Well-Being*. doi:10.1111/j.1758-0854.2012.01070.x.

Harzer, C., & Ruch, W. (2012). When the job is a calling: The role of applying one's signature strengths at work. *The Journal of Positive Psychology*. doi:10.1080/17439760.2012.702784.

Harzer, C., & Ruch, W. (in press). The application of signature character strengths and positive experiences at work. *Journal of Happiness Studies*. doi:10.1007/s10902-012-9364-0.

Howe, L. A. (2004). Gamesmanship. *Journal of the Philosophy of Sport, 31*, 212–225.

Inglehart, R., Foa, R., Peterson, C., & Welzel, C. (2008). Development, freedom, and rising happiness: A global perspective (1981–2007). *Perspectives on Psychological Science*. doi:10.1111/j.1745-6924.2008.00078.x.

Kavetsos, G., & Szymanski, S. (2010). National well-being and international sports events. *Journal of Economic Psychology*. doi:10.1016/j.joep.2009.11.005.

Kneidinger, B. (2010). Die Konstruktion nationaler Identität in der österreichischen und Schweizer Sportberichterstattung—eine qualitative Inhaltsanalyse zur Fußball-Europameisterschaft 2008 (National identity construction in Austrian and Swiss sports media coverage—A qualitative content analysis of the European Football Championship 2008). *SWS-Rundschau, 50,* 164–186.

Lee, M. J., & Cockman, M. (1995). Values in children's sport: Spontaneously expressed values among young athletes. *International Review for the Sociology of Sport.* doi:10.1177/101269029503000307.

Littman-Ovadia, H., & Lavy, S. (2011). Character strengths in Israel: Hebrew adaptation of the VIA Inventory of Strengths. *European Journal of Psychological Assessment.* doi:10.1027/1015-5759/a000089.

Martinolli, L., Tanyelli, E., Hasler, R. M., Burkhardt, P., Bähler, H., Neff, F., Rupp, P., Zimmermann, H., & Exadaktylos, A. K. (2011). 1.000.000 Fußballfans in einer Stadt mit 120.000 Einwohnern—ein notfallmedizinischer Albtraum? Die Euro 2008 und das "Oranje-Wunder von Bern" (One million football fans in a city of 120,000 inhabitants—A nightmare for emergency medicine and disaster management? Euro 2008 and the "Oranje wonder of Berne"). *Unfallchirurg.* doi:10.1007/s00113-009-1736-5.

Müller, L., & Ruch, W. (2011). Humor and strengths of character. *The Journal of Positive Psychology.* doi:10.1080/17439760.2011.592508.

Newburg, D., Kiemiecik, J., Durand-Bush, N., & Doell, K. (2002). The role of resonance in performance excellence and life engagement. *Journal of Applied Sport Psychology.* doi:10.1080/10413200290103545.

Nüesch, S., & Franck, E. (2009). The role of patriotism in explaining the TV audience of national team games—Evidence from four international tournaments. *Journal of Media Economics.* doi:10.1080/08997760902724472.

Park, N., & Peterson, C. (2006a). Character strengths and happiness among young children: Content analysis of parental descriptions. *Journal of Happiness Studies.* doi:10.1007/s10902-005-3648-6.

Park, N., & Peterson, C. (2006b). Moral competence and character strengths among adolescents: The development and validation of the Values in Action Inventory of Strengths for Youth. *Journal of Adolescence.* doi:10.1016/j.adolescence.2006.04.011.

Park, N., Peterson, C., & Seligman, M. E. P. (2004). Strengths of character and well-being. *Journal of Social and Clinical Psychology.* doi:10.1521/jscp.23.5.603.50748.

Peterson, C. (2006). *A primer in positive psychology.* New York: Oxford University Press.

Peterson, C., & Seligman, M. E. P. (2003). Character strengths before and after September 11. *Psychological Science.* doi:10.1111/1467-9280.24482.

Peterson, C., & Seligman, M. E. P. (2004). *Character strengths and virtues: A handbook and classification.* Washington, DC: American Psychological Association.

Peterson, C., Park, N., & Seligman, M. E. P. (2005). Assessment of character strengths. In G. P. Koocher, J. C. Norcross, & S. S. Hill III (Eds.), *Psychologists' desk reference* (2nd ed., pp. 93–98). New York: Oxford University Press.

Peterson, C., Park, N., & Seligman, M. E. P. (2006). Greater strengths of character and recovery from illness. *The Journal of Positive Psychology.* doi:10.1080/17439760500372739.

Peterson, C., Ruch, W., Beermann, U., Park, N., & Seligman, M. E. P. (2007). Strengths of character, orientations to happiness, and life satisfaction. *The Journal of Positive Psychology.* doi:10.1080/17439760701228938.

Peterson, C., Park, N., Pole, N., D'Andrea, W., & Seligman, M. E. P. (2008). Strengths of character and posttraumatic growth. *Journal of Traumatic Stress.* doi:10.1002/jts.20332.

Priest, R. F., Krause, J. V., & Beach, J. (1999). Four-year changes in college athletes' ethical value choices in sports situations. *Research Quarterly for Exercise and Sport, 70,* 170–178.

Proyer, R. T., & Ruch, W. (2009). How virtuous are gelotophobes? Self- and peer-reported character strengths among those who fear being laughed at. *Humor: International Journal of Humor Research.* doi:10.1515/HUMR.2009.007.

Proyer, R. T., & Ruch, W. (2011). The virtuousness of adult playfulness: The relation of playfulness with strengths of character. *Psychology of Well-Being: Theory, Research and Practice.* doi:10.1186/2211-1522-1-4.

Proyer, R. T., Gander, W., Wyss, T., & Ruch, W. (2011). The relation of character strengths to past, present, and future life satisfaction among German-speaking women. *Applied Psychology: Health and Well Being*. doi:10.1111/j.1758-0854.2011.01060.x.

Proyer, R. T., Ruch, W., & Buschor, C. (2013). Testing strengths-based interventions: A preliminary study on the effectiveness of a program targeting curiosity, gratitude, hope, humor, and zest for enhancing life satisfaction. *Journal of Happiness Studies*. doi:10.1007/s10902-012-9331-9.

Ruch, W., Proyer, R. T., Harzer, C., Park, N., Peterson, C., & Seligman, M. E. P. (2010a). Adaptation and validation of the German version of the Values in Action Inventory of Strengths (VIA-IS) and the development of a peer-rating form. *Journal of Individual Differences*. doi:10.1027/1614-0001/a000022.

Ruch, W., Proyer, R. T., & Weber, M. (2010b). Humor as character strength among the elderly: Empirical findings on age-related changes and its contribution to satisfaction with life. *Zeitschrift für Gerontologie und Geriatrie*. doi:10.1007/s00391-009-0090-0.

Schmid Mast, M., Frauendorfer, D., & Popovic, L. (2011). Self-promoting and modest job applicants in different cultures. *Journal of Personnel Psychology*. doi:10.1027/1866-5888/a000034.

Seligman, M. E. P., & Csikszentmihalyi, M. (2000). Positive psychology: An introduction. *American Psychologist*. doi:10.1037//0003-066X.55.1.5.

Seligman, M. E. P., Steen, T. A., Park, N., & Peterson, C. (2005). Positive psychology progress: Empirical validation of interventions. *American Psychologist*. doi:10.1037/0003-066X.60.5.410.

Wadey, R., Evans, L., Evans, K., & Mitchell, I. (2011). Perceived benefits following sport injury: A qualitative examination of their antecedents and underlying mechanisms. *Journal of Applied Sport Psychology*. doi:10.1080/10413200.2010.543119.

Wann, D. L., Dolan, T. J., McGeorge, K. K., & Allison, J. A. (1994). Relationships between spectator identification and spectators' perceptions of influence, spectators' emotions, and competition outcome. *Journal of Sport & Exercise Psychology, 16*, 347–364.

Wann, D. L., Dimmock, J. A., & Grove, J. R. (2003). Generalizing the team identification-psychological health model to a different sport and culture: The case of Australian rules football. *Group Dynamics: Theory, Research, and Practice*. doi:10.1037/1089-2699.7.4.289.

Wann, D. L., Waddill, P. J., Polk, J., & Weaver, S. (2011). The team identification-social psychological health model: Sport fans gaining connections to others via sport team identification. *Group Dynamics: Theory, Research, and Practice*. doi:10.1037/a0020780.

Weber, M., & Ruch, W. (2012). The role of a good character in 12-year-old school children: Do character strengths matter in the classroom? *Child Indicators Research*. doi:10.1007/s12187-011-9128-0.

Wilbert-Lampen, U., Leistner, D., Greven, S., Pohl, T., Sper, S., Volker, C., Güthlin, D., Plasse, A., Knez, A., Küchenhoff, H., & Steinbeck, G. (2008). Cardiovascular events during World Cup Soccer. *The New England Journal of Medicine*. doi:10.1056/NEJMoa0707427.

Chapter 8
Positive Psychology and Interpersonal Forgiveness Within Cultures

Júlio Rique Neto, Robert Enright, Bruna Seibel, and Silvia Koller

This chapter examines Enright's theory on "the socio-moral development of forgiveness" into the paradigm of positive psychology presenting the following: firstly, a social psychology model of attitudes for interpersonal forgiveness; secondly, a process model of forgiving; and thirdly, a socio-cognitive developmental model of forgiveness. Then, the following questions will be addressed by research findings: "What generally is the case of perceived unfair treatment for most people across cultures?" "What is the degree at which people forgive by affect, behavior, and judgments?" "How people go about forgiving another person?" "What are the necessary conditions for forgiveness?" "Are the necessary conditions for forgiving culture specific?". Finally, the chapter proposes how positive psychology can promote forgiveness in schools.

J. Rique Neto (✉)
Center for Research and Studies on Sociomoral Development (NPDSM),
Universidade Federal da Paraíba – UFPB, João Pessoa, Brazil
e-mail: julio.rique@uol.com.br

R. Enright
Department of Educational Psychology, University of Wisconsin-Madison,
859 Education Sciences, 1025 W. Johnson St, Madison WI 53706-1796, USA
e-mail: renright@wisc.edu

B. Seibel
Center for Psychological Studies CEP-RUA, Universidade Federal do Rio
Grande do Sul, Porto Alegre, Brazil
e-mail: brunaseibel@gmail.com

S. Koller
Department of Psychology, Federal University of Rio Grande do Sul, Institute
of Psychology, Rua Ramiro Barcelos 2600, 104, Porto Alegre 90035 003, Brazil
e-mail: silvia.koller@gmail.com

H. Águeda Marujo and L.M. Neto (eds.), *Positive Nations and Communities*, Cross-Cultural   135
Advancements in Positive Psychology 6, DOI 10.1007/978-94-007-6869-7_8,
© Springer Science+Business Media Dordrecht 2014

8.1   Introduction

Interpersonal forgiveness was introduced into positive psychology as a portal for compassion and ego strength, a door that once opened can take one far from unnecessary suffering (Snyder and Lopez 2009). Furthering this approach, one can say that forgiving for the right reasons takes one from suffering and prepares him or her to influence communities and societies to function on a positive ethic of justice and compassion.

Enright's theory of interpersonal forgiveness (Enright and The Human Development Study Group 1991) was conceived within the cognitive developmental approach, which Snyder and Lopez (2009) cited in their overview of theories on positive psychology as one important theoretical framework for the study of human development. The cognitive developmental approach has to do with descriptions of patterns on how people perceive their social world and themselves. The approach is cognitively based, but it recognizes that every developmental conception of the self and the social world has affectivity and behavioral components present in the social psychology of attitudes and in the individual assessment of socio-moral reasoning and, finally, that people grow toward greater adaptation in the world (Kohlberg 1984).

Enright's theory of interpersonal forgiveness (Enright and The Human Development Study Group 1991) has provided robust psychological models empirically supported across cultures: a social-psychological model of attitudes for forgiving, a process model of forgiving, and a socio-cognitive developmental model of forgiveness reasoning (Enright and Fitzgibbons 2000). According to Klatt and Enright (2009), psychology and education can integrate these empirically supported theoretical models and educational practices for the promotion of forgiveness into the paradigm of positive youth development.

This chapter will guide the reader to examine Enright's theory of interpersonal forgiveness presenting, firstly, the social-psychological model of attitudes for interpersonal forgiveness. This model has been researched internationally and addressed the following questions: "What generally is the case of perceived unfair treatment for most people across cultures?" "What is the degree at which people forgive by affect, behavior, and judgments?" Secondly, the socio-cognitive developmental model of forgiveness is introduced and the following questions have been addressed by research findings: "What are the necessary conditions to best resolve conflicts after unfair treatment via forgiveness?" "Are the necessary conditions for forgiving culture specific?" And, thirdly, a process model of forgiving that has examined how people forgive another person after injustices is posed. Finally, the chapter will address how positive psychology can promote the moral development of forgiveness in schools.

8.2   The Socio-moral Development of Forgiveness

Enright and Fitzgibbons (2000) defined interpersonal forgiveness from the perspective of the offended person as follows:

> People, upon rationally determining that they have been unfairly treated, forgive when they willfully abandon resentment and related responses (to which they have a right), and endeavor to respond to the wrongdoer based on the moral principle of beneficence, which may include compassion, unconditional worth, generosity and moral love (to which the wrongdoer by nature of the hurtful act or acts, has no right). (p. 24)

This definition implies that every person has a sense of justice that is central to morality, but after injustice, the offended person can voluntarily choose to forgive by decreasing his or her negative thoughts, affect, and behavior and increasing or returning to think, feel, and behave positively toward an offender.

According to Enright, forgiveness requires a sense of justice and relates to specific context situations of injustices. Justice is a duty, a prescriptive judgment in which a person wants to think about "what should be done" in absolute terms. On the other hand, for forgiveness, a person asks "under what conditions forgiveness is possible after an injustice."

Still according to Enright, "identity" is the cognitive element that motivates an offended person to forgive by judging the offender's act without losing humane values (Enright and The Human Development Study Group 1994). "Identity" and "ideal reciprocity" are cognitive operations that require reversibility, which is best known as the Golden Rule (one should treat others as one would like others to treat oneself). These kinds of reasoning are used to resolve conflicts of justice. However, the thought of ideal reciprocity requires a kind of reversibility in which injustice would be undone, a fact that is logically impossible. Thus, identity is the cognitive operation required by forgiveness. For that, an offended person should first acknowledge the injustice; then, he or she should see the other for who he/she is and come to understand that despite the wrong committed, the other is still a person worth of dignity. In other words, the forgiveness process leads a person "to understand that the offending person is more than the offense (or offenses) committed" (Enright and Rique 1999). This operation requires a different kind of cognitive reversibility that is to take the perspective of the offender, see the other as human and equal to the "self," who is also a person capable of committing wrong.

8.2.1 The Social Psychology Model of Attitudes for Interpersonal Forgiveness

Enright's operational definition for forgiving, that is, the offended person can voluntarily choose to forgive by decreasing his or her negative thoughts, affect, and behavior and increasing or returning to think, feel, and behave positively toward an offender, defined the social-psychological model of interpersonal forgiveness. To verify this model, Enright and colleagues operationalized this definition in an objective measure: the Enright Forgiveness Inventory – EFI (Subkoviak et al. 1995).

The EFI asks participants to think of the most recent experience of someone hurting you deeply and unfairly. In the front page, participants rate their degree of hurt on a 5-point scale (1 = no hurt, 5 = a great deal of hurt), report who the offender was and how long before the offense happened, and write a brief description of the offense. Next, participants are asked to keep the offense and the offender in mind and rate the presence of positive affect (e.g., I feel love toward him/her) and the absence of negative affect (e.g., I feel resentment toward him/her), the presence of positive behavior (e.g., I would help him or her) and the absence of negative behavior (e.g., I avoid him or her), and the presence of positive thinking (e.g., I think he/she is worthy of respect) and the absence of negative thinking (e.g., I think he/she is a bad person). The sum of the positives and negatives in each subscale allows one to obtain a score of affect, behavior, and judgment toward the offender, and the sum of the subscale scores gives the overall score of the degree to which a person has forgiven the other person after injustice. The results should be interpreted as "the presence of positive affect, behavior, and judgment" and "the absence of negative affect, behavior, and judgment" toward an offender. The EFI does not use the word forgiveness during the inventory. After the inventory, participants are asked to answer an independent scale: the "1-Item Forgiveness Scale." This item asks the person to rate on a 5-point scale how much he/she has forgiven the person that was evaluated in EFI.

What Generally Is the Case of Perceived Unfair Treatment for Most People Across Cultures?

The original validation study for the EFI was carried out among American adolescents and their parents (Subkoviak et al. 1995). The authors observed that the most reported area of conflicts and contexts of injustices by age group were conflicts in the family and among friends. For example, they selected young adults experiencing a great deal of hurt in romantic relationships and verified that those who had forgiven via their feelings (i.e., reduced negative affect and increased positive affect) had significantly lower anxiety than those who kept residual resentment and anger toward the significant other who committed the offense. The same trend appeared to happen when the authors looked at parents reporting conflicts in parent–child relationships or between spouses. Participants distributed their forgiving scores on the EFI (i.e., EFI total score) and on the 1-Item Forgiveness Scale in relation to the perceived degree of hurt, that is, the higher the intensity of hurt, the lower was the degree of forgiveness, and also to the degree of social proximity with the offending person, offenders who were close (i.e., spouses, children, friends, romantic partners) received higher degrees of forgiveness than offenders who were less intimate.

In conclusion, according to the authors, developmental issues or what they called "developmentally appropriate contexts of hurt" should be on focus if forgiveness is to be used as a coping strategy promoted in education and the helping professions. How often is that the case when we look at different cultures?

An international project on forgiveness invited guest researchers to use the same methodological procedures used in the USA and the back-translation procedure for adaptation and validation of EFI in their cultures. Currently, the EFI has been adapted to seven cultures, Austria, Brazil, Israel, Korea, Norway, Taiwan, and the

Table 8.1 Psychometric results of the EFI in seven nations

Nation	Sample (N)	Cronbach's ∝	1-item forgiveness (r)
Austria	376	.98	.78
Brazil	599	.98	.72
South Korea	326	.97	.68
United States	394	.98	.68
Israel	164	.98	.71
Norway	141	.98	.68
Taiwan	321	.97	.68

Note: From Enright and Fitzgibbons (2000)

United States, and six languages, English, Portuguese, Hebrew, Chinese, German, and Norwegian. The EFI is administered to participants with paper and pencil and has to be answered individually. Table 8.1 shows that the EFI maintains a high level of internal reliability and significant positive correlations with the 1-Item Forgiveness across Cultures.

To verify contexts of hurt across cultures, Rique et al. (2007) and Rique and Enright (1998) examined findings from the EFI in samples of adolescents, young adults, and adults from Austria, Brazil, Israel, Norway, South Korea, Taiwan, and the United States. The analysis supported the findings of Subkoviak et al. showing that people most often report hurt in developmentally appropriate relationships. Adolescents and young adults reported lack of care in family relationships, lack of trust in romantic partners, betrayal among same-sex friends, etc. Adults reported verbal and physical aggression from spouses, infidelity, and injustices perpetrated by coworkers or employers in the work environment, among others.

Thus, evidence has accumulated that people are hurt a great deal in their daily life by conflicts in the family and among friends. Yet, people are more willing to forgive significant others, indicating that they take into consideration how meaningful the relationship is before forgiving the other.

What Is the Degree at Which People Forgive by Affect, Behavior, and Judgments?

Another aspect of findings from people reporting spontaneous forgiving in the EFI has to do with the degree of forgiveness by the dimensions of affect, behavior, and judgment. Research has found that most people forgive primarily by judgments (e.g., he/she is a good person) than behaviors (e.g., I help him or her) or affect (e.g. I love him or her). Looking at the findings from people who forgive a great deal (i.e., score ≤4 on the 1-Item Forgiveness Scale), a significant pattern emerged across the seven cultures mentioned previously (see Fig. 8.1). People forgive mostly by restoring their judgments toward offenders than developing love and friendship for them.

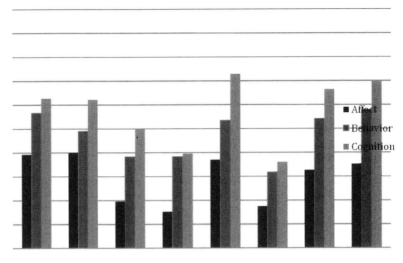

Fig. 8.1 Pattern of responses to the EFI by subscales of affect, behavior and cognition

This pattern confirmed Subkoviak's findings and it calls attention to his statement which says that it is affective forgiveness that has a negative relation to anxiety (Subkoviak et al. 1995). Therefore, the process of forgiveness is still left undone or incomplete even for those who forgive the most, because affective forgiving is still lower than the other dimensions of forgiveness. Consequently, the perception of unfair treatment still leads the relationship to engage in a cycle of conflicts. This issue on how to forgive others in close relationship would be better accomplished if parents and schools could work together as a community for positive socialization. Therefore, positive psychology would assert in agreement with Subkoviak that a good measure of personal development and healthy forgiving is the degree to which people affectively forgive others.

8.2.2   The Process Model of Forgiveness

How People Go About Forgiving Another Person?

The process model of forgiveness is the most commonly used model for forgiveness in education (Enright and Fitzgibbons 2000; Enright and Rique 1999; Al-Mabuk et al. 1995; Helb and Enright 1993). The forgiveness process has four phases, with wide individual differences within them, which form a developmental progression. Not everyone goes through the process in the same way or at the same speed. Within each phase there are a series of units most people seem to go through. See Table 8.2 for a brief overview of the process.

Enright highlights that this four-phase model of forgiving is not a rigid, stepwise model in which people must start with the first phase and proceed following the

Table 8.2 A process model of interpersonal forgiveness

Uncovering Phase. This first phase describes the person's insight about whether the injustice and subsequent injury have compromised his or her life. This can be an emotionally painful time. Yet, if the person concludes that he or she is suffering emotionally because of someone else's injustice, this can serve as a motivator to change. The emotional pain can be a motivator to think about and try forgiveness. This phase involves examining psychological defenses, remaining anger, guilt, and/or shame, etc.

Decision Phase. This is when the person thinks about what forgiveness is and is not. A decision to forgive is a cognitive process, not one in which forgiveness is completed. The person must distinguish what a commitment to forgive is and all that is involved in the process. Otherwise, upon committing to forgive, the person may conclude that most of the work is over. On the contrary, it is only the beginning. This phase involves a change of heart or the development of new insights or resolution strategies, considers forgiveness as an option, and makes a commitment to forgive the offender

Work Phase. Here the participant begins to understand that the offending person is more than the offense (or offenses) committed. The one forgiving begins to experience some compassion toward the offender. The focus shifts from self, where most of the attention was centered in the Uncovering Phase, to the offending person. This phase requires the offended person to exercise empathy, and role-taking, and to begin viewing the other in his or her context

Deepening Phase. Insights about an offender often stimulate other thoughts: Have I needed their forgiveness in the past? What was it like for me when I was forgiven? Is there any sense in all of the pain I endured? Am I motivated to interact in new ways with the offender and with people in general? The answers may lead to a recycling through the other phases, this time in a deeper, more insightful way. This phase involves giving meaning for the self and the others, developing new purposes in life because of the injustice suffered

Note: From Enright and Rique (1999, p. 7) with adaptation

order to the end. The process guides educational and therapeutic strategies. It is possible, for example, for one to feel empathy (Work Phase) for an offender right in the beginning of the process, which requires counselors first to examine whether or not a person has overcome important milestones (e.g., he or she has overcome psychological defenses), then follow the process as needed in a case-by-case situation.

8.2.3 The Socio-cognitive Developmental Model of Forgiveness

Spontaneous forgiveness, that is, people forgive by intuitive strategies, is usually confounded by justice, forgetting, or a defense mechanism. Therefore, the theory may be incomplete without understanding people's proper reasoning for forgiving.

What Are the Necessary Conditions for Forgiveness?

Enright et al. (1989) interviewed adolescents and adults to know under what conditions forgiveness is possible after an injustice. Their results showed six ways of thinking about forgiveness related to age development and justice reasoning

Table 8.3 The socio-moral developmental pattern of forgiveness

Stage	Pattern	Characteristic
1 and 2	*Revengeful*	*Strategies*: Get back at the offender
		Manifestations: External and behavioral; internal hostility remains
		Conditions: Forgiving is offered only after the offender having suffered greater than the pain inflicted upon the victim. Or victims receive compensation for what was lost or stolen
3 and 4	*External*	*Strategies*: Passive coping, anger remains
		Manifestation: External and behavioral; defense mechanisms; suppression of anger
		Conditions: Pressures from social groups (family, friends) and institutions (e.g. church and law)
5 and 6	*Internal*	*Strategies*: Perspective taking gives meaning for the event from the perspectives of the self and the other (reframing)
		Manifestation: Internal transformations lead to external behavioral expressions. Significant reduction of anger and increase of positive feelings
		Conditions: Understand the principles of love and compassion

Note: From Park and Enright (1997, p. 395)

(Kohlberg 1984). The earliest form of thought of forgiveness was related to the use of forgiveness as revenge (Stage 1) or compensation (Stage 2). Then, forgiving is related to social pressures from family and friends (Stage 3) and/or institutional, community, or religious conventions (Stage 4). Finally, more mature ways of thinking about forgiveness consider the consequences of forgiving for society, forgiveness becomes a function of social harmony (Stage 5), and the most advanced thought is when the person understands forgiveness as an ethic based on identity, love, and unconditional compassion for humanity (Stage 6). Later, Park and Enright (1997) combined Enright et al. (1989) model of six stages of forgiveness reasoning with Trainer's (1981) patterns of strategies and manifestation of forgiving, that is, (a) role-expected forgiveness (forgiveness is behaviorally demonstrated but internally absent), (b) expedient forgiveness (forgiveness is offered with condescension and hostility), and (c) intrinsic forgiving (forgiveness implies internal psychological transformation). In this way, Enright developed a parsimonious model of three patterns on the development of forgiveness as shown in Table 8.3.

Are the Necessary Conditions for Forgiving Culture Specific?

Park and Enright (1997) examined the socio-cognitive model of forgiveness reasoning in South Korean high-school and college students who suffered a great deal of hurt from close friends. Participants of the research were screened to match the criteria of having experienced a serious unfair conflict of physical, moral, emotional, or monetary implications caused by a close same-gender friend in the previous 5–6 months. A selected sample of 30 high-school and 30 college students, with equal number of males and females in each group, all self identified as Christians participated in the study. Participants responded a forgiveness interview that was an adaptation of the Heinz Dilemma (Kohlberg 1984) and a Friendship Dilemma (Selman 1980), a Restoring Friendship Strategy scale, and a Degree of Forgiveness scale adapted from previous work by Trainer (1981) and Lazarus and Cohen (1977). Results showed that forgiveness was moderately related to age, that is, college students showed significantly higher understanding of forgiveness than high-school students, and the higher was one's understanding of forgiveness, the more he or she used strategies for the restoration of friendship. Finally, the authors found no correlation between participants' actual degrees of forgiveness and their understanding of forgiveness. In other words, a person's degree of forgiveness is unrelated to a proper understanding of the value. Therefore, the pattern of spontaneous forgiving across cultures shown in Fig. 8.1 may not imply proper understanding of forgiveness. Thus, education within communities should provide contexts for people to think about forgiveness as a match of cognitive, affective, and behavioral attitudes. That is the promotion of one's understanding of forgiveness related to positive emotional and behavioral development, that is, low anger and positive behaviors, after unfair treatment.

In a carefully delineated quasi-experimental study, Huang and Enright (2000) interviewed 1,427 male and female Taiwanese from four age groups using an Objective Scale of Forgiveness (OSF), which asked them to choose from pairs of sentences representing levels of forgiveness reasoning and strategies for forgiving. To assess forgiveness reasoning, participants had to consistently choose one specific kind of reasoning from several pairs. Results from the large screening sample showed significant age differences indicating a linear trend from seventh graders to adults on the means of the OSF. Then, the authors selected 60 Taiwanese adults for participation in the study to test whether the quality of understanding of forgiveness is related to more affective forgiving, that is, low anger, low blood pressure, and other measures of healthy emotional development. Participants in the selected sample contributed further by answering measures of anger expression, and facial expression and also blood pressure were measured during certain intervals of time throughout the experimental procedures. Results showed no differences on the level of anger expression among participants who think of forgiveness as social expectation versus participants who favored internal motivation and transformation for forgiving. On the other hand, participants who thought of forgiveness as unconditional showed more consistent performance across all measures than participants who thought of forgiveness as social expectation. They varied across measures of blood pressure and the observation of facial expressions indicating residual anger. Unfortunately, the authors did not compare participants' actual degree of forgiveness with their understanding of forgiveness and behavioral forgiveness.

While Enright and colleagues examined victim's reasons for forgiving conflicts in family and schools, Rique and Lins-Dyer (2003) used a dilemma situation to examine the quality of teachers' reasoning on forgiveness. Would teachers endorse (a) forgiveness for conflict resolution between the students in schools and (b) schools' pardon of the offender's behavior? The vignette was as follows:

> John and Marc are both 13-year-olds. They are good friends, but normally harass each other. One day, their behavior escalates into a physical fight. They violate rules and policies against violence in school. Although the boys resolve the conflict using forgiveness, they still have

to deal with the violation of school rules. Considering that the boys took responsibility for their personal actions, they asked the teacher to intervene supportively in the process by asking the school to pardon their behavior. (p. 239)

Interpersonal forgiveness was examined apart from institutional pardon. Teachers who supported interpersonal forgiveness reported that forgiveness should be part of a school community expectation, an attitude of care and humanitarian response to interpersonal conflicts (i.e., forgiveness should be part of social conventions). On the other hand, they believed that institutional pardon would not be advisable in education because pardoning students would favor recidivism and put others at risk for repeated wrongdoing. Prudence and justice were virtues preferred by teachers for orienting institutional conflict resolution. On the other hand, teachers who viewed their role as figures of authority or disciplinarians did not support either interpersonal forgiveness or institutional pardon for conflict resolution.

8.3   Positive Psychology and Forgiveness in Schools

In the introduction of this chapter, forgiveness was presented as a moral attitude that for the right reasons takes one from suffering and prepares an offended person to influence communities and societies to function on a positive ethic of justice and compassion. The approach is cognitively based but has affectivity and behavioral components present in the process of growth from suffering to a new and positive form of adaptation in the world. Positive psychology can create forgiveness education programs in schools to help children, adolescents, young adults, and adults in the family assimilate forgiveness as a positive asset and coordinate their attitudes to resolve conflicts and overcome injustices living a life of hope, at full potential for happiness. The models and research findings on forgiveness can be integrated into one developmental framework to guide different education programs tailored at specific themes or real-life experiences. The field already knows that across cultures forgiveness is used as a coping strategy; people forgive spontaneously. Characteristically, forgiving occurs in developmentally appropriated relationships with a high level of meaning and a high level of commitment in contexts of the family and schools. To forgive others in close relationship would be better accomplished if parents and schools work together as a community for positive socialization. A community for positive socialization should involve norms, the economic status of its members, socialization types, values, and psychological attributes. Such a program can work first at the levels of social norms, that is, making forgiveness part of social expectations in the school and community of families. Positive norms for forgiveness can be cultivated in schools by authoritative styles of communication that should be beyond the school walls including counseling and education for families supporting parenthood and careful supervision of the community members, allowing forgiveness to be viewed as part of positive assets and values. Such a context of norms and values would lead people to understand the role of forgiveness in close relationships and in society, help them to generalize forgiving from family and friends to humanity, and to match affect and judgment in their degree of forgiveness for actual events in the community. The community should know that the perception of unfair treatment still leaves the relationships prone to engage in a cycle of conflicts. Finally, positive psychology programs would assert that forgiveness is good for personal and social development. Programs can help a culture of schools and families to assimilate forgiveness as a positive moral asset, promoting societal, familial, and/or religious norms that would foster the moral development of forgiveness.

Healthy forgiving is the degree to which people affectively forgive others. On the other hand, it is often easier to understand an offender than it is to feel empathy or compassion for him or her (Fitzgibbons 1986). Educational programs can aim at promoting cognitive reframing, which is part of the Work Phase of the forgiving process. Reframing can lead the process of emotional transformation providing new insights about the other via exercises such as thinking about what the context of the case situation is, who the other person who offended is, what the relationship means to him or her (the offended person), and, finally, what are the necessary conditions for forgiving.

The Enright Forgiveness Inventory (EFI, Subkoviak et al. 1995) has shown to be valid across cultures and can be used as a tool for education. The EFI measures the degree of forgiveness given to a specific situation of injustice. Rique et al. (1999) suggested the use of the EFI in educational programs for positive community socialization. They considered that a key issue on forgiveness is the feeling of resentment. While education can work with children, adolescents, young adults, and adults on reducing the resentment they feel, the EFI can assess what effect an education program has on participants' thoughts and behaviors toward the person who hurt them. Asking participants to complete the EFI on separate occasions, with sufficient time between assessments to avoid response-set bias, can assess whether helping youth to forgive a particular person for a particular event leads to a more generalized forgiveness of the same person across other events. If children and adolescents showed generalization across situations with the same person and across different people, forgiveness has become a valued asset in the community. Also, being able to forgive people across different situations of injustices shows that adolescents' moral identity has assimilated the virtue of forgiveness into their world view.

In *The Adolescent as Forgiver*, Enright et al. (1989) position a person thinking at the center of the judgment process looking for meaning from unfair treatment (or injustices). In this case, an offended person should not allow his or her attitudes to be guided by affect, that is, anger and resentment. After injustices, negative affect is working against one's judgment process. Education can help one to find internal strength (perspective taking, empathy, values, etc.) and external support (i.e., social norms, counseling, and education for forgiveness) to let compassion work its way into cognition to help one's judgments with mercy. It is no surprise to find that across cultures people forgive close ones but are left with residual anger and anxiety. The risk here is that anger and anxiety are cumulative emotions that will surface in other occasions of unfair treatment misleading one to perceive independent events in close relationships as a cycle of recurring unfairness.

Theory and research indicates that forgiving actual events of injustices is related to age and the way people have spontaneously thought and used strategies for forgiveness. Park and Enright's (1997) results showed how much age is important for student's understanding of forgiveness. Programs in schools should be age related and give the means to have students using strategies for the restoration of friendship.

Rique and Lins-Dyer's (2003) study verified that schools do not have norms that allow students to use them on their side for the restoration of friendship conflicts. Huang and Enright's study that showed reasoning for forgiveness as social expectation is one and the same as reasoning of forgiveness as unconditional, perhaps showing that social harmony is not a condition for forgiveness but a necessary value within the person. It is necessary to mention that participants were from a society where respect and compassion for others in the community are broadly supported in Confucian philosophy as well as Christian views. The degree of internalization of protecting harmony in society may vary between Taiwan, Brazil, and the United States. Therefore, it is possible that schools as positive communities help to challenge different levels of thinking about forgiveness toward the protection of social harmony. Emphasis on moral identity as Enright claims (Klatt and Enright 2009; Enright and The Human Development Study Group 1994) should come first as it is developmentally appropriate for early age, then one's identity should be challenged to rise to the next level via the promotion of cognitive decentering where moral identity takes new social perspectives. Social harmony is integrated into peace that comes through unconditional forgiveness.

If a school community expects youth to learn how to resolve conflicts in a positive ethic, forgiveness should restore meaning to relationship, provide social harmony, and see how the moral functioning of a community happens on a different set of social norms. One can expect that society will change for better justice, more tolerance, more compassion, etc., if schools promote positive ways to resolve conflicts. Thus, it is a task for positive psychology.

In conclusion, positive education for forgiveness can help people to (a) coordinate attitudes with proper understanding of social conflicts, injustices, and forgiveness and (b) work on feelings as well as judgments and behaviors. Nevertheless, this is only a starting point because this kind of education can go further to promote a community in which social norms follow pedagogical and psychological orientations for positive social development where interpersonal forgiveness relates to norms, politics, the collective, and peace.

References

Al-Mabuk, R., Enright, R. D., & Cardis, P. (1995). Forgiveness education with parentally love-deprived college students. *Journal of Moral Education, 24*, 427–444.

Enright, R. D., & Fitzgibbons, R. (2000). *Helping clients forgive: An empirical guide for resolving anger and restoring hope*. Washington, DC: APA.

Enright, R. D., & Rique, J. (1999). *The moral development of forgiveness: Research and education*. In Symposium conducted at the meeting of the annual conference of The Association for Moral Education, Minneapolis, MN.

Enright, R. D., & The Human Development Study Group. (1991). The moral development of forgiveness. In W. M. Kurtines & J. Gewirtz (Eds.), *Handbook of moral behavior and development* (Vol. 1, pp. 123–152). Hillsdale: Erlbaum.

Enright, R. D., & The Human Development Study Group. (1994). Piaget on the moral development of forgiveness: Identity or reciprocity? *Human Development, 37*, 63–80.

Enright, R. D., Santos, M. J. O., & Al-Mabuk, R. H. (1989). The adolescent as forgiver. *Journal of Adolescence, 12*, 95–100.

Fitzgibbons, R. P. (1986). The cognitive and emotional uses of forgiveness in the treatment of anger. *Psychotherapy, 23*, 629–633.

Helb, J. H., & Enright, R. D. (1993). Forgiveness as psychotherapeutic goal with elderly females. *Psychotherapy, 30*, 658–667.

Huang, S. T., & Enright, R. D. (2000). Forgiveness and anger-related emotions in Taiwan: Implications for therapy. *Psychotherapy, 37*, 71–79.

Klatt, J., & Enright, R. D. (2009). Investigating the place of forgiveness within the positive youth development paradigm. *Journal of Moral Education, 38*(1), 35–52.

Kohlberg, L. (1984). *Essays on moral development: Vol. 2. The psychology of moral development*. San Francisco: Harper & Row.

Lazarus, R. S., & Cohen, J. (1977). *Coping questionnaire*. Unpublished research.

Park, Y. O., & Enright, R. D. (1997). The development of forgiveness in the context of adolescent friendship conflict in Korea. *Journal of Adolescence, 20*, 393–402.

Rique, J., & Enright, R. D. (1998, November). Contexts of hurt in relation to forgiveness: An empirical analysis in four cultures. In L. Walker (Chair.), *Cross-cultural perspectives on moral development*. Symposium conducted at the meeting of the XXIV annual conference of The Association for Moral Education, Hanover, NH.

Rique, J., & Lins-Dyer, M. T. (2003). Teacher's views of forgiveness for the resolution of conflicts between students in school. *Journal of Moral Education, 18*, 641–655.

Rique, J., Waltman, M., Sarinopoulos, I., Lin, W., Wee, D., Engstrand, E. A., & Enright, R. D. (1999). The tools of forgiveness education: Validity studies of the Enright Forgiveness Inventory. In *The moral development of forgiveness: Research and education*. Symposium conducted at the meeting of the annual conference of The Association for Moral Education, Minneapolis, MN.

Rique, J., Camino, C., Enright, R. D., & Queiroz, P. (2007). Perdão interpessoal e contextos de injustiça no Brasil e Estados Unidos [Interpersonal forgiveness and the contexts of injustices at Brazil and the United States]. *Psico, 38*(2), 185–192.

Selman, R. (1980). *The growth of interpersonal understanding*. New York: Academic.

Snyder, C. R., & Lopez, S. J. (2009). *Psicologia positiva. Uma abordagem científica e prática das qualidades humanas* (Tradução de Roberto Cataldo Costa). Porto Aleger: ARTMED.

Subkoviak, M., Enright, R. D., Wu, C. R., & Gassin, E. (1995). Measuring interpersonal forgiveness in late adolescence and middle adulthood. *Journal of Adolescence, 18*, 642–655.

Trainer, M. (1981). *Forgiveness: Intrinsic, role-expected, expedient, in the context of divorce*. Unpublished doctoral dissertation, Boston University, Boston.

Chapter 9
South Africa's Truth and Reconciliation Process as Applied Positive Psychology in Nation Building

Marié P. Wissing and Q. Michael Temane

There is gap in positive psychology with regard to what is meant by a positive society and a positive nation. In this chapter we reflect on the functioning of South Africa's Truth and Reconciliation Committee (TRC), established as part of the transition to a more democratic government and recognition of human rights in the aftermath of the abolishment of the apartheid regime, in order to gain insights into processes facilitating a more positive society. We discuss TRC processes and outcomes through the lens of positive psychology, illustrating how implementation of character strengths and other positive psychosocial characteristics conceptualised in positive psychology was part of the process, and how it could have contributed to constructively building a more just and positive nation. It is analysed to what extent post-traumatic growth took place on an individual level and on a social and national level as manifested in reconciliation and coping with consequences. It is also argued how insights gleaned from the work of the TRC can enrich our understanding of phenomena described in positive psychology by taking also a more collectivist cultural perspective into account. The contribution of the TRC processes to nation building is evaluated, and challenges and opportunities for the road ahead are indicated.

9.1 Introduction

At the first Portuguese Positive Psychology Conference on Positive Nations, Helena Agueda Marujo and Luis Miguel Neto created a window of opportunity to reflect on 'Positive Nations' from the perspective of positive psychology and, in doing so,

M.P. Wissing (✉) • Q.M. Temane
School for Psychosocial Behavioural Sciences, North-West University,
Potchefstroom, South Africa
e-mail: Marie.Wissing@nwu.ac.za; Michael.Temane@nwu.ac.za

H. Águeda Marujo and L.M. Neto (eds.), *Positive Nations and Communities*, Cross-Cultural   149
Advancements in Positive Psychology 6, DOI 10.1007/978-94-007-6869-7_9,
© Springer Science+Business Media Dordrecht 2014

identify the best of the past century, and to co-create new visions and dreams for the future. The importance of this meeting is accentuated by the fact that there is currently a large gap in the still very individualistic-oriented positive psychology with regard to what is meant by a positive society and a positive nation. In this chapter we want to contribute to this debate and filling up this lacune by sharing reflections on South Africa's Truth and Reconciliation process as applied positive psychology in nation building. South Africa had developed miraculously through various processes in the past two decades, from being the scoundrel of the world with its apartheid regime into the so-called rainbow nation. Although the Truth and Reconciliation Commission's (TRC) work began in a ritual manner, it had an important impact on the process of national reconciliation, despite the fact that there are still many challenges ahead.

Up front we want to note that we focus in this chapter on the best from the past, but this does not mean that we are ignorant of the horrors, pain and human rights violations that were experienced under apartheid and that were revealed at the TRC's hearings, and it does not mean that we are blind to the current violent crimes and corruption taking place in our country, but it does mean that we note the positive aspects of the TRC's courageous and penetrating work in trying to uncover the truth and to facilitate growth towards reconciliation. Although the TRC process was flawed in many respects, it was nevertheless a psychologically powerful process.

9.2   Functioning of TRC

9.2.1   Background

South Africa's difficult past with its many grotesque human rights violations is well known to the world. And when former President Nelson Mandela came into office in 1994, he inherited a nation divided along racial lines and the challenge of what to do with those who committed the gross violations during the apartheid regime. He had three options (cf. Markel 1999, 2001): (1) Try to prosecute those responsible for the gross human rights violations in criminal courts (Nuremberg option), (2) provide blanket amnesty to the perpetrators, or (3) find something new – and this is where the TRC was born. This is referred to by some social commentators as *Faustian bargain* (sic) used in order to secure majority rule (see Blomfield 1985).

The first option of criminal prosecution was problematic because (1) without some immunity the security forces and supporters would probably have mounted a large-scale resistance; (2) the latter would especially be the case as Mandela and De Klerk had negotiated an interim Constitution in 1993 in which it was stated that to advance the rebuilding of society, amnesty will be given for offences with political aims that occurred in the past; (3) the new government had limited resources to investigate, prosecute and incarcerate the violators; (4) even with resources, many of the overwhelming number of claims could not have been proven without reasonable doubt, as many incidences happened long ago and evidence had been destroyed; and (5) if prosecution for violence with political aims would have to been extended to all races, some of the officials in the ANC would have been affected. The second option of blanket amnesty to close the book of the past was also problematic, because (1) the losses of victims of the past are not socially recognised, (2) perpetrators will not take responsibility and (3) no information and lessons will be gained from the past. The literature on the TRC has some examples of the challenges where blanket amnesty could have been a possibility (see Méndez 2005; Skaar 1999).

The third option was that the past will be re-examined and retold for purposes of social reconciliation. The late Mr Dullah Omar, a former minister of Justice suggested that '*a commission is a necessary exercise to enable South Africans to come to terms with their past on a morally accepted basis and to advance the cause of reconciliation*' (http://www.justice.gov.za/trc/). The Government of National Unity under the leadership of Nelson Mandela then established the Truth and Reconciliation Commission (TRC) through the promotion of the *National Unity and Reconciliation Act, No 34 of 1995*. Most importantly, this Act focused on restorative justice rather than retributive justice (Stein et al. 2008) which was more a political compromise as indicated. The objectives of the TRC were thus to '*promote national unity and reconciliation in a spirit of understanding which transcends the conflicts ... and divisions of the past*'.

The *mandate* of the TRC was to (1) establish a comprehensive picture and record the nature, causes and extent of crimes relating to human rights violations in the past, (2) to grant amnesty in cases under specified conditions (full disclosure about crimes committed), (3) to oversee reparation and rehabilitation to victims of abuse, (4) to compile a report on the activities and findings of the TRC and (5) to formulate recommendations to the president with regard to measures and creation of institutions that will foster a stable and fair society and prevent future human rights violations (see Gobodo-Madikizela 2002). In this way, according to Dr Alex Boraine (co-chairperson of the TRC) in a lecture on the TRC: '*South Africa has decided to say no to amnesia and yes to remembrance; to say no to full-scale prosecutions and yes to forgiveness*' (Boraine 1996, p. 7). To a large extent the ethos of the TRC is quite related to one of the freely paraphrased presuppositions of political psychology, namely, that knowledge promotes forgiveness and reconciliation flows from truth.

The TRC was viewed by many as a crucial component of the miraculous transition to full and free democracy in South Africa, on the one hand, and sceptically, on the other, for lack of rigour (such as used in the social sciences) in analysing its own findings (Chapman and van der Merwe 2008) and careful definition of some basic concepts such as the dichotomy between victim and perpetrator (Borer 2003) and reconciliation. However, the South African TRC was the first of about 19 internationally to stage public hearings, the first to individualise amnesty and the first to allow people from both sides of the conflict to testify as victims and perpetrators at the same forum (see Mamdani 2002) under various levels of public scrutiny and interest. The TRC received some 20,000 statements from victims and their families and approximately 7,000 applications for amnesty (information available from the TRC's website: www.truth.org.za).

9.2.2   Structure and Processes of the TRC

Structure

The TRC was a 17 member Commission, based in Cape Town, and conducted its work through three legalised committees (SATRC 1998):

1. *The Human Rights Violations Committee* – conducted public hearings throughout the country to investigate gross abuses that occurred between March 1960 and 11 May 1994 (gross rights violations were pragmatically narrowly defined to only include victims of killing, torture, abduction as well as severe ill treatment) (a shortcoming was thus that socio-economic disparities and sociopolitical marginalisation were not the focus of the inquiry).
2. *The Amnesty Committee* – considered applications of individuals who committed political crimes that occurred (i.e. crimes that were politically motivated, proportionate and fully disclosed by the person applying for amnesty).
3. *The Reparation and Rehabilitation Committee* – had to formulate proposals on how to implement a reparations policy and restore the victims' dignity.
4. An *Investigative Unit* was also established that conducted investigations to help the Commission to reach its goals.

Processes

The Human Rights Committee held hearings at many venues in South Africa, amongst others in Johannesburg (at the Central Methodist Mission), Cape Town (at the University of Cape Town) and Randburg (at the Rhema Bible Church). In rural areas the hearings attracted many people from the communities, whereas in the cities there were many other things occupying attention, except in the case of high-profile hearings when venues were packed. It is estimated that approximately 50 % of the population was in some way involved in TRC processes (as victims testifying, perpetrators explaining, attendance of public hearings or following processes via the radio, television and other media – Stein et al. 2008).

The strategy of the Commission was to invite victims and perpetrators to come forward and attest before the Commission, but they specifically started with the taking of statements of victims and from there uncover specific human rights violations. The core of the TRC's work was the victim hearings and that occupied most of the first year of hearings, whereas in the second year the emphasis was more on perpetrator findings.

The TRC appointed trained statement-takers, who were fluent in the local languages and used a standard protocol to document victim's stories. Emotionally distressed persons were supported and referred to mental health professionals. Statement-takers were recruited from nongovernmental organisations (NGOs), community-based organisations (CBOs), religious structures, etc., through which people were reached in remote rural areas and urban areas where public hearings were not held. Victim narratives were the moral core of the TRC process. Because of the overwhelming numbers of statements taken, only about 10 % of victims (approximately 2,000) had the opportunity to tell their stories at public hearings, but of course all people's narratives were recorded, analysed and included in some way in the final report which was a voluminous 3,500 pages long. The selection of people to tell their stories at public hearings was aimed at a reflection of the various types of human rights abuses, and to ensure that victims on all sides of the conflict were included and to be representative of gender, age and race. While the overwhelming majority of victims were black people who suffered under apartheid, also many white victims (e.g. from the church street bombings) told their stories, and white as well as black perpetrators applied for amnesty.

9.3 Processes and Outcomes of the TRC Through the Lens of Positive Psychology

Constructs from various theoretical perspectives in positive psychology will be used in this section as a lens to interpret processes in the TRC as manifestations of applied positive psychology. Or, put in another way, the TRC processes and outcomes manifested much of what we have learnt in positive psychology until now – most of it as applied to individuals, but also very relevant in enhancing well-being on social levels as shown in the current analysis. Fredrickson (2001, 2009) had hypothesised and empirically shown in laboratory experiments how individual positivity reflected in emotions such as gratitude, hope and inspiration can broaden perspectives and build well-being on a social level. Some theoretical models from which insights are drawn for the current analyses are amongst others the Broaden and Build model (Fredrickson 2001, 2009), the Values-in-Action (VIA) model of character strengths (Peterson and Seligman 2004), the social well-being model by Keyes that is also part of his Mental Health Continuum model (Keyes 1998, 2007), the Sense of Coherence model (Antonovsky 1987) and meaningfulness models (Baumeister 1991; Wong 2010). The various strengths and processes linked to becoming a more positive nation are illustrated by, firstly, referring to some evidence in the run up to the TRC; secondly, overarching processes and outcomes of the TRC are highlighted; and then more individual behaviours and processes that were part of the TRC endeavour are linked to social outcomes. Some remarks on the aftermath of the TRC's work will follow.

9.3.1 Towards the TRC...

Leadership

The political transition in South Africa was to a great extent peaceful because of the great leadership shown by Nelson Mandela and Willem de Klerk who led the negotiation process.

Leadership is a character strength in the cluster of civic strengths that underlie healthy community life as conceptualised in the Values-in-Action model of character strengths (Peterson and Seligman 2004). Negotiations for the transfer of power led by De Klerk and Mandela was a first step towards the possibility of a new future and the realisation of a more healthy and positive nation. Recognition of their leadership in this regard culminated in them being recipients of the Nobel Prize for Peace in 1993.

There were of course many other leaders in this process, for example, Archbishop Desmond Tutu who became the chairperson of the TRC, Dr Alex Boraine who was elected the deputy chair and the late former minister of Justice, Dullah Omar, who was the first to suggest that a commission is necessary for South Africans to come to terms with their past on a morally accepted basis and to advance the cause of reconciliation. This paved the way towards the establishment of the TRC.

Former President Nelson Mandela believed that the wrongs of the past cannot just be forgotten: They needed to be investigated, recorded and made known (Hay 1999). Therefore, he supported the establishment of the TRC. Mandela manifested all the characteristics of a good leader who could influence and direct behaviour towards a collective good. The strength of Mandela's *leadership* reverberates also in his *wisdom and perspective, integrity and social intelligence* with which the choice was made of options on how to deal with what happened under apartheid: The establishment of the TRC under his leadership was a choice of *balance, fairness, justice and kindness*.

Justice

Justice is conceptualised in the Values-in-Action model (Peterson and Seligman 2004) both as a virtue cluster of civic strengths that underlie healthy community life and as a specific psychological character strength in this cluster. As a character strength justice refers to giving everyone a fair chance and not letting personal feelings bias decisions about others. Justice as virtue and character strength is also linked to leadership, fairness and social responsibility.

Justice was shown in planning of the TRC's processes by the decision to put the victims of apartheid in the centre space – first of all, their stories of suffering and human rights violations would be heard. This process recognised the dignity of victims and communicated to them respect.

9.3.2   Overarching Outcomes and Processes

Several overarching outcomes, processes and strategies of the Truth and Reconciliation Commission can be seen as operating strengths and applied positive psychology facilitating a more positive nation.

Social Awareness and Recovery of a Lost History

Keyes (1998) described the social well-being facet 'social coherence' as the experience of seeing the world as intelligible, logical and predictable, with care about and interest in society and context. Mindfulness entails taking a step back and gaining a wider perspective (Fredrickson 2009). Brown and Ryan (2003) also describe the importance of mindfulness for well-being.

The TRC's overarching process of listening and recording experiences from both sides of the conflict, and from black and white victims and perpetrators from both sides at the same forum, facilitated a deeper understanding of what happened and created thereby a greater and fuller social awareness. Silenced or unrecognised histories were uncovered and integrated into a fuller common history and mindfulness of who we are. This shared history and mindfulness of who we are facilitated also social integration in the sense described by Keyes (1998), i.e. feeling part of a community and sharing commonalities with a community.

This was a powerful political action for victims who told their stories and whose voices were sought, a powerful process for perpetrators to take responsibility and a powerful process to build a common history shared by all included in this new, healthier nation that we were hoping to become. As a nation we dare not silence or forget the past again as that may allow the horrors of the past to repeat themselves. Thus, the historical facts uncovered also showed what must never happen again – it gave moral limits also to the new government. Thereby the distinction between pathology and well-being in a nation's functioning was highlighted.

Thus, the TRC, by uncovering repressed and unrecognised histories, paved the way for shared consciousness and awareness, and a new social coherence and order in which there may be a future for reconciliation between previous divides.

Meaning-Making and Social Contribution

There is a unique human need to seek and construct meaning (Antonovsky 1987; Baumeister 1991; Wong 2010), especially in a changing context. Meaning is constructed at both the individual and social levels, and can protect and empower people (Wong 2010). The construction of meaning is related to the capacity for imagination, responsible action, personal growth, purpose and hope (Wong 2010). Meaning is best understood, expressed and constructed in narratives which also provide the opportunity for re-authoring of life stories (Van der Merwe et al. 2009).

By recovering lost histories, filling in of gaps in knowledge of what happened to loved ones, by realising the consequences of own actions for others, by guidance towards a reconciled future, a greater picture came into awareness, a better understanding took place, and opportunities opened up to express and construct new meanings at individual and social levels during the TRC processes. The sharing of life experiences and contribution to a wider understanding provided the victims an opportunity to experience a new meaningfulness on a social level, i.e. they had something valuable to give to society and their contributions are valued by the community.

This is in line with what Keyes (1998) describes as 'making a social contribution' as one of the facets of social well-being. The TRC processes thus provided the opportunity for the construction of new meanings that enhanced the possibility of becoming a more positive nation.

Towards Harmony and Peace-Building

Peace-building started in the negotiations leading up to the 1994 transitions in SA, before the induction of the TRC. Although the TRC's efforts at peacemaking and peace-building had mixed results and impacts as viewed from various social positions, there is wide consensus that it played a significant role in the social transition from conflict to peace (Hay 1999; Statman 2000; Stevens 2005). The TRC created the space for further peacemaking and fuelled peace-building that is a continuous process to be nursed.

Harmony as facilitated by the TRC processes refers to both intrapersonal and interpersonal feelings of balance, acceptance and integration of opposites into a whole as conceptualised by Chenyang (2008), and it was linked to peacemaking and moves towards reconciliation. The TRC thus played a significant role in making peace and building peace, and balancing opposite factions into a whole for developing a new nation in the move towards reconciliation. This created more social acceptance and harmony. Keyes (1998) described 'social acceptance' as a facet of social well-being, characterised by acknowledgement of others and general acceptance of people despite their sometimes complex and perplexing behaviour.

Compassion

The TRC processes first and foremost focused on victims and their families. The TRC and audiences attending listened respectful, attentive and compassionate to the stories of victims and their families and recorded their experiences. As such then, compassion was inherently part of the TRC's processes: It intended to ease the suffering of victims and contribute to the healing of a broken nation.

Compassion as a phenomenon is related to others such as kindness, altruistic love, nurturance and generosity as conceptualised in the Values-in-Action model (Peterson and Seligman 2004). Such a nurturing, other-regarding attitude is the basis of moral and spiritual life in all the major religious orientations in the world (Peterson and Seligman 2004). Compassion, linked to the other strengths of humanity as shown at the TRC's hearings, became a model for growth towards a more humane society in the South African context.

Spirituality

Spirituality as character strength and religious orientation played an (unexpected) major role in the TRC processes. Spirituality is described as one of the character strengths in the VIA model (Peterson and Seligman 2004), forming part of the transcendence cluster. There was a strong spiritual and Christian *leitmotiv* in the work of the TRC shown in religious practices, the focus of content and the way processes were steered. Although also criticised in analyses by some, it was seemingly accepted by victims, Commission members and perpetrators alike. The inauguration of the TRC on 13 February 1996 was in the St Georges Cathedral and included the singing of inter-church songs, burning of candles and use of olive branches. Meetings of the TRC were also opened and closed with prayers. The Commission emphasised religious themes such as a search for truth, confession of guilt, forgiveness and the promise of redemption/amnesty, reconciliation and transformation. From this religious 'authority' the TRC suggested to victims and perpetrators on a personal level the road to be followed and thereby also curbed the expressions of revenge and hatred.

Former Archbishop Tutu, as chairperson of the TRC, explicitly said at the beginning of the hearings that religion is central to the process of healing, and that we need to reach deep into the spiritual wells of our different religious traditions in order to draw strength and grace with which to address the challenges of healing and nation building. This orientation might have contributed to the development of a more morally responsible nation.

Spirituality played a major role in the healing process guided by the TRC – not only as a character strength but especially as an ultimate concern (cf. Emmons 2003) or transcendental orientation focusing on something that refers to a greater good. Many South Africans are spiritually or religiously orientated and observing something greater than themselves. That might have helped us to reconcile and unite.

Facilitation of Hope and Optimism

The importance of hope in facilitating psychological well-being is described by Snyder (2000), and the importance of optimism is long known to scientists in positive psychology (e.g. Seligman et al. 1995). The future-orientated strategy of the TRC created hope and optimism for becoming a healed nation (cf. also Stevens 2005). Hope and optimism were especially important when obstacles were faced in the transitional period in SA.

Hope, future-mindedness, future orientation and optimism are indicative of an emotional, cognitive and motivational stance towards the future. By fulfilling its mandate to promote reconciliation and reconstruction, and formulate recommendations to the president with regard to measures and processes to foster a stable and fair society and prevent future human rights violations, the TRC was strongly future-minded in its processes and the creator of hope for a better future. This facilitated the sense of a positively evolving society where the world is becoming a better place for all – i.e. social actualisation as conceptualised by Keyes (1998) as a facet of social well-being.

9.3.3   Linking Individual and Social Processes

Telling the Truth

In the TRC's processes of telling the truth was a major component in cleaning wounds and healing hearts towards a possible better future and healthier nation (Stevens 2005; Statman 2000). It can be asked 'whose truth?' Various types of truths were witnessed at the TRC hearings: factual or forensic truth, personal or narrative truth, social or dialogue truth and healing truth. The latter goes further than the verifiable forensic truth, and the personal truth is a spiritual search for understanding, self-insight, acceptance of responsibility, healing, justice and reconciliation. Tutu said at a hearing in 1996 that the TRC listens to everyone, and that it is therefore important that everyone should be given a chance to say his or her truth as the person himself or herself sees it. True stories were sought from victims as well as perpetrators from both sides of the conflict alike.

Telling the Truth 1: Victims

Regaining Voices: Telling of Stories of Suffering and Showing Strengths

Victims regained their voices by sharing their painful experiences of suffering. They became survivors who had the power to grow and make a difference in creating a fuller history and a more humane society. In this process they showed strengths of courage, temperance and humanity as conceptualised in the VIA model (Peterson and Seligman 2004) – and beyond. Growth was shown in remarks about the experience of a fuller humanness.

As viewed in narrative theory (Van der Merwe et al. 2009), it is possible to create alternative stories to the dominant stories of people's lives. Dominant stories include only selected experiences, and these directed further interpretations and shaped lives. For many black people the dominant stories of their lives were that of trauma and hardships under apartheid. The TRC process allowed these stories to be heard and changed from victim-hood to survivorship, from helplessness and suffering to resilience and strength by taking the morally higher ground of forgiveness and being powerfully instrumental in promoting a greater good and developing a more humane society.

However, proportionally few statements of victims were recorded (21,298 – Statman 2000, p. 25; SATRC Report 1998, Vol. 1, Chap. 6, Appendix 2, 29), and it is hoped that witnessing the stories of others also brought vicariously relief to those not testifying.

Post-traumatic Growth

The narrative reconstruction of experiences in the socially supportive context of the TRC might have helped in the cognitive processing of past traumas. The appreciation and recognition thereof by the TRC, as well as the TRC's prompting towards forgiveness and possibilities of reconciliation, might have encouraged growth. For example, at a point during the hearings, Archbishop Tutu (MUFC hearings transcript, p. 2,383 – Statman 2000) proposed that the victims in the room be publicly acknowledged:

> …as an expression of our respect for people who have suffered… we all stand… and I just want to say that on behalf of our country, we hope that the pain and anguish of so many will be something that goes towards the healing of our land. We want them to know our very deepest sympathies for them for what they have suffered and we thank them and hope that they will have it in their hearts to reach out to those who may have caused them pain, to reach out in order for our land to be healed.

Post-traumatic growth was in a sense facilitated through TRC processes via its link with forgiveness as integration towards a greater wholeness. The possibility of growth that came out of talking about their pain and being compassionately embraced in their suffering by others during the TRC's processes is shown in remarks reflecting fuller humanness via forgiveness and repentance as part of interconnectedness (see later on). Post-traumatic growth in this sense can also be seen as transformational coping (cf. Aldwin 1994).

Although victims from both sides told their stories which might have provided moments of relief and feeling heard and affirmed, it is a question whether this was sufficient to heal wounds in the long term. For some yes, for others more are needed (Kagee 2006).

Telling the Truth 2: Perpetrators' Confessions

Taking of Responsibility: Growing in Integrity

Telling the truth by transgressors as operative in the TRC processes required a full disclosure of past violations. More than 7,000 perpetrators applied for amnesty. Some applications were withdrawn, 5,392 refused and 849 granted.

Truth-telling in the context of the TRC was an interpersonal and social honesty expression that required acceptance of responsibility. It provided the opportunity to grow in integrity – painful as this might have been. Although telling the truth in many instances might have only selfish aims, i.e. to be granted amnesty, it was also a positive and healing experience for others. Perpetrators who revealed the truth about their actions and confessed to the wrongs they did took responsibility, showed the strength of courage and could grow in integrity in this process. By opening up they became free to change.

Regret as Applied Mindfulness: Asking for Forgiveness

Although regret is a negative emotion, it may have positive consequences, depending on how it is acted upon (Kashdan 2010). To feel regret is to recognise the consequences of what had been done; it requires empathy from the wrongdoer for the victim (Gobodo-Madikizela 2008). Regret was shown by some of the perpetrators who told the full stories of their past human rights violations under the apartheid regime. Some of them begged forgiveness. Guilt feelings motivate to undo wrongs and offer an opportunity to learn and to grow. Showing regret by perpetrators was also a step towards social reconciliation.

Forgiveness

The TRC operated from the principle that reconciliation depends on forgiveness, and that forgiveness can only take place if the terrible violations of human rights are fully disclosed and recognised. Some evaluators critiqued the TRC processes as luring victims into forgiveness with a view to reconciliation and nation building, and providing too little space for their anger and desire for revenge (Statman 2000), and others even argued that forgiveness is not necessary to move on after the abolishment of apartheid (Alais 2007). Nevertheless, forgiveness played a crucial positive role in the TRC's processes towards building a more positive nation (Gobodo-Madikizela 2003; Hay 1999; Krog 2008). Tutu pointed out that the act of forgiveness opens a window on the future for both the forgiver and wrongdoer. Stories of forgiveness during the TRC processes did not only include the direct participants – the effect was much broader: By vicarious participation in stories of forgiveness, the nation began to heal itself.

A consensual definition of forgiveness is suggested by Peterson and Seligman (2004) referring to the work of McCullough et al. (2000). According to this, forgiveness 'represents a suite of prosocial changes *within an individual* (our italics), who has been offended or damaged by a relationship partner' (Peterson and Seligman 2004, p. 446). Forgiveness is stressed to be an intra-individual, prosocial change that includes cognitive, emotional and behavioural facets. Forgiveness is linked to mercy, self-regulation and also to kindness, compassion, leniency and harmony. Although forgiveness is often linked to repentance on the part of the transgressor as in Judaism and Hinduism, it is not the case in Christianity and Islam (Peterson and Seligman 2004). Most scholars distinguish between forgiveness and reconciliation and contend that they can exist separately.

From an African more collective perspective on forgiving, victims became the gatekeepers to what the transgressor desires, namely, reintegration into the human community (Gobodo-Madikizela 2003). Forgiveness does not overlook the awfulness of what happened but rises above it. '*This is what it means to be human, I cannot and will not return the evil you inflicted on me*' (Gobodo-Madikizela 2003, p. 117). Forgiveness, as shown in the TRC processes, is thus a generous gift to transgressors who are in no position to demand or deserve it. Forgiveness can only be given by an individual, is essentially interpersonal and cannot be given by a commission or organisation. Forgiveness spoken at the TRC hearings is, in view of the atrocious wrongs that preceded it, almost above human acts of kindness. As witnessed during the TRC processes, forgiveness is more a strength of transcendence than of temperance as conceptualised in the VIA model of Peterson and Seligman (2004).

This observation may have theoretical implications: Strengths may cluster differently in various contexts or in individual versus more collectivist cultural contexts as found by Wissing and Temane (2008).

Forgiveness as witnessed at the TRC hearings is, however, also a much broader and encompassing phenomena than described in the literature thus far. It is linked to more than repentance.

Forgiveness: An African Contribution

What transpired at the TRC with regard to forgiveness and growth is something that can enrich the understanding of the concept of forgiveness in the science of positive psychology from a cultural perspective. Forgiveness, in the African, more collectivist worldview, is not only an individual process but also a social process that includes reconciliation through which growth towards fuller humanness of both victim and transgressor becomes possible.

Gyekye (1997, p. 37) refers to Menkiti who said, '*as far as Africans are concerned, the reality of the communal world takes precedence over the reality of the individual life histories*'. Thus, the community defines the individual, and social values are deeply cherished. This allows for a broadening of the concept of forgiveness, in contrast to the traditional, more western descriptions thereof. 'Forgiveness' is more than an individual process; it is also a social and collective process integrating people towards becoming fuller human beings together when viewed from an African 'ubuntu' or communitarian perspective. Although some analysts of the TRC processes (e.g. Wilson, in Krog 2008) regarded the ubuntu idea as something superficial and part of an ANC agenda to legitimise the new government, others (such as Gobodo-Madikizela 2003 and Krog 2008) pointed out a much deeper meaning and importance. This meaning was manifested in the words and behaviour of former Archbishop Tutu and Commissioner Ntsebeza, references by victims, and as also found in African philosophy and theology (e.g. Gyekye 1987; Setiloane 1976; Soyinka 1976) and described by an African Psychologist Pumla Gobodo-Madikizela (2003). Krog (2008) argued that this worldview was the essence of the TRC process but came only visible to some via wrappings of Christianity and restorative justice. The perspective of ubuntu (being human through the humanness of others) helped to bring coherency that enabled the TRC to do its work while curbing revenge, and also instill politically and legally contaminated concepts with new meaning and possibility. Some Commissioners and ordinary black people attending the meetings of the TRC knew the possibility that '*one could only fully 'build' oneself within a caring reconciled community*', and it was this collective wisdom that drove the process rather than any political agenda or pact between elites (Van Binsbergen 2001).

Through the work of the TRC, we noticed that, from an African perspective, 'forgiveness' is an individual as well as a social process that includes reconciliation – which is a prerequisite for growth towards fuller humanness of victim, transgressor and society as a whole. Forgiveness as such an inclusive growth process was named '*interconnectedness-towards-wholeness*' by Krog (2008). Interconnectedness-towards-wholeness is more than a theoretical knowledge that everything in the world are linked; it refers to a physical and mental awareness '*that one can only 'become' who one is, or could be, through the fullness of that which is around one – both physical and metaphysical*' (Krog 2008, p. 355). Thus, wholeness is a process of becoming and the fullest self can only be reached through and with others.

Interconnectedness-towards-wholeness includes both forgiveness (letting go personally of resentment and moving away from victim-hood) and reconciliation (mutual commitment of former hostile parties to an improved ethical future and acceptance of the other). Forgiveness and reconciliation are mutually interdependent: Forgiveness opens up the process of becoming, via regret and gratitude on part of the transgressor, and reconciliation is the next step of becoming more humane – thus a process of including both the victim and the perpetrator.

A deep understanding of this interconnectedness as related to forgiveness was expressed in the words of one of the Gugulethu Seven mothers (Mrs. Ngewu) whose son was part of a group of seven men killed through an askari (i.e. a black guerilla fighter who secretly also worked for the SA police). The police involved in the killings as well as the askari had to testify before the TRC. After the hearings the askari asked for a private meeting – overseen by a TRC member – with the mothers to ask for forgiveness. This translation of Mrs. Ngewu's words after the meeting was broadcasted on SABC radio:

> This thing called reconciliation... if I am understanding it correctly... if it means this perpetrator, this man who has killed Christopher Piet, if it means he becomes human again, this man, so that I, so that all of us, get our humanity back... then I agree, then I support it all. (Krog 1998, p. 109)

Forgiveness can never be without reconciliation; reconciliation thus requires a fundamental change in the life of the one that forgave as well as the life of the one who is forgiven. Preferably the process should begin with the perpetrator who first asks for forgiveness, but the victim may also grow towards greater wholeness without the perpetrator asking. But after forgiveness the perpetrator must change and tries to restore. This reverberated in the words of Reverend Frank Chikane who after the trial of Wouter Basson (an apartheid chemical warfare expert) of whom he was a victim: Chikane said he forgave his tormentors, but '*until the perpetrator says 'I am sorry' and want to change and lead a different life, he becomes a prisoner forever, even if I have forgiven him. So my forgiveness does not liberate the perpetrator*' (Brand 2002, p. 19). After the former Minister of Police Adriaan Vlok washed the feet of Reverend Chikane in an act of asking forgiveness, the reverend said, '*I shared it with the congregation and people just broke down and cried. And there is no way that you can have that experience and keep it quiet*'.

This culturally embedded form of forgiveness may enrich the understanding of forgiveness as phenomenon studied in positive psychology. This kind of forgiveness and reconciliation as part of interconnectedness and growth to fuller humanness reverberates on a theoretical level also very well with Kinman's metaphor of Rhizome networks – we are all linked to each other in a vital manner where giving and grateful receiving are inherently part of mutual growth (cf. Kinman 2010).

Gratitude

Gratitude is conceptualised as a strength of Transcendence in the VIA model (Peterson and Seligman 2004) but also as a far more general psychological strength by Emmons and others (Emmons 2007; Emmons and McCullough 2004). In positive psychology much had been said about gratitude and its relationship with psychological well-being. In the African TRC context gratitude was, although not in the forefront, deeply linked with social processes and especially with forgiveness on an interpersonal level. There was gratitude on part of the transgressors for forgiveness and not only for amnesty where received. Therefore, there was a need to make restitution. Although many white South Africans did not understood the depth of the meaning of instances of forgiveness spoken at the TRC hearings, there was a general thankfulness by many South Africans, black and white, that we managed to steer towards greater peace and reconciliation, and not an intensified conflict situation. This general gratefulness and wonder united us and inspired more efforts towards reconciliation.

Gratitude as related to TRC processes is more a humble strength of Temperance than of Transcendence as hypothesised in the VIA model of Peterson and Seligman (2004). This indicates that context should be taken into consideration in theories of psychological strengths. Gratitude as linked to forgiveness in the TRC processes is part of a life orientation in which growth of one individual is linked to the growth of another and the communal good. Until now very little has been written on gratitude in analyses and evaluations of the TRC's processes – the opportunity to gain more insight into the unique manifestation of this very important strength as manifested in this specific context should be ceased.

9.4   Beyond the Miracle

The contribution (strengths and weaknesses) of the TRC processes to nation building will be evaluated in this section especially as they pertain to the opportunities for growth realised by victims of the *ancien regime*, on the one hand, and the perpetrators, on the other, and all South Africans. As indicated, the lens of positive psychology will be used to understand this process of the TRC.

9.4.1   Summary and Evaluation of TRC's Contribution to Nation Building

In the movement towards the TRC, the strengths and virtue of leadership and justice stood out. Telling of stories by victims in a supportive and compassionate environment, revelations from remorseful perpetrators and guidance by commissioners with a view to reconciliation created greater social awareness, meaning, balance and hope (see also Gobodo-Madikizela 2002).

The process of telling the truth of their sufferings gave victims a voice, restored their dignity, facilitated post-traumatic growth and empowered some of them to find it in their hearts to forgive their wrongdoers and thereby grow in fullness to being human (see Stein et al. 2008). Stein et al. (2008) compare the foregoing to the rubrics of 'testimony therapy' in terms of its cathartic healing and a possible *humanisation* (see Gobodo-Madikizela 2002) of the victim.

Telling the full stories of their human rights violations in the past, perpetrators took responsibility for the consequences of their actions, showed remorse and asked for forgiveness, and then grow in humanness together with those who forgave them – together building a more humane society. The story of Eugene de Kock quite often cited in relation to many horrid and unimaginable acts of cruelty is used in many instances to cast *rehumanisation* (see Gobodo-Madikizela 2002). Gratitude was experienced by all that we moved away from conflict to more harmony and becoming a new and more positive nation.

Strengths/Positives of the TRC Process

1. The TRC created a platform for victims to tell their story and help them to 'unburden' themselves of a past in the presence of an attentive and sympathetic audience characterised by compassion.
2. Victims gained control of their narratives and were not alone anymore in their suffering of not knowing the truth of what happened in the past.
3. The TRC helped South Africa as a nation to transcend the cycle of anger and vengeance, while daily facing the powers that produced it.
4. The TRC was essential to avoiding a civil war in an already spiked country on the precipice of an explosive backlash.

Weaknesses/Negatives of the TRC Process

1. The methodology followed by the TRC is faulted by many social commentators for lack of rigour.
2. Chapman and van der Merwe (2008), for example, indicate that although the TRC process was premised on honest dialogue, societal ills such as racism are avoided by the report of the TRC.
3. Victims were not properly compensated for pain and suffering (see Gibson 2002).
4. Some murderers and perpetrators who did not apply or were not granted amnesty were not brought to book or prosecuted.

However, in spite of its many shortcomings and opposition to the Commission from many sides, it can be pointed out that the positive effects of the TRC outweigh its limitations. Some victims of the *ancien regime*, in spite of their disillusionment with the TRC process, have expressed an interest in pursuing reconciliation with perpetrators (see Chapman and van der Merwe 2008). There is a widespread agreement that it played a tremendous role healing the social psyche of the nation.

9.4.2   Reflections on the Miracle

The TRC recognised that dignity is rooted in the notion that *justice* consists of the refusal to turn away from the ravages of suffering visited upon victims from many walks of life. In a sense, the work of the TRC can easily be likened to a *moral reawakening* premised on a common narrative and understanding of a chequered history. On the one hand, victims were given centre stage, a space in the justice system usually reserved for perpetrators. This lent substantial power to victims to tell their story. The final report of the TRC clearly attests to this: '*The Commission's quest for truth … had to do with helping victims become more visible and valuable citizens through public recognition and official acknowledgement of their experiences*' (SATRC 1998: Report, Vol. 1, Ch. 5, par. 1). Theoretical insights for understanding trauma very clearly indicate that traumatised people have a need to tell their stories on their own terms and have their experiences validated. On the other hand, perpetrators who could have been perceived as 'autonomous moral agents' who in spite of this acted on the orders of State also had the opportunity to tell their own story.

The Foucauldian concept of *positive power* is comparable to the TRC processes as it allowed everybody to talk, discuss and read about the work of the Commission. Positive power is rooted in society as a whole, with possible contributions emanating from everybody: victims, members of society and the Commission itself, to create a new narrative from various perspectives. Dignity is easily the centrepiece of the outcome of the TRC processes. Dignity has an interesting flipside as contained in Mandela's inaugural speech on the 10th of May 1994 and is often cited on this theme: '*Never, never and never again shall it be that this beautiful land will again experience the oppression of one by another and suffer the indignity of being the skunk of the world*' (South African Government Information 1994). Therefore, the supporting discourse of the TRC is precisely this *summum bonum*, the highest good of lending dignity to victims and disambiguate the ravages of the past and seek a new beginning.

There are many instances to cast South African society evolving out of its past: The myth of Orestes, the son of the tragic Agamemnon and Clytemnestra, is invoked as a reference point from how far the country has come. Aeschylus' tale of the relationship between Agamemnon and Clytemnestra will not be retold here but suffice to say that the movie 'The Browning Version' would be most useful in helping to understand the myth of Orestes who in this context is seen as a new beginning. Quite recently, the FIFA World Cup played in South Africa preceded by rugby matches in Soweto has seen South Africans rallying behind the country and supporting nation building. There are several images of these events that will remain permanently etched in people's memories for a long time. It is important to talk about the rugby matches in Soweto and the FIFA World Cup separately.

Rugby in South Africa has a specific identity as a sport played by white people only, but its history tells a different story. The events leading to the Soweto rugby matches were quite fortuitous as a venue for rugby was not available given the preparations for the FIFA World Cup were underway and a decision was taken to play the match in Soweto, a previously 'no-go' area to many white people. This was at once not an easy decision for many reasons, chiefly security, number of tickets that could be sold and readiness and orientation of a black township to host such a match. The success of the hosting is nothing but legend! In an uncanny sort of way, playing a rugby match would have been expected even by some optimists as a disaster in progress, but the outcome was a small miracle of unity for all. South Africans surprised even themselves about the outcome. Needless to say, many rugby matches are now planned to be played in predominantly black townships. Some manifestations of the new, more positive nation are evident not only in sport but also in the arts such as literature, music, theatre, films, poetry, and dance. These are snippets of some of the inadvertent effects of some of the work done by TRC in building the New South Africa which would otherwise have been impossible to imagine in this lifetime.

9.5   Our Dreams for the Future and Conclusions

The truth revealed by the TRC made it possible, despite its many limitations, to start the planning and development of a new social order in a society that cares for all its people and acknowledges the virtue of universal human rights, a society that in its social practices fosters *temperance* and sensitivity to the poor in the face of consumerism and new class struggles, a society that makes it possible for dialogue about social challenges in a depoliticised atmosphere. These virtues need to be reflected in the everyday life experiences of ordinary people and not just that of the elite or those with political connections. Service delivery to all South Africans need to be equitable; socio-economic practices of the *ancien regime* should be entirely eliminated so that the positive nation that South Africa was meant to become should be realised. Although these virtues did not formally inform the processes of the TRC, they can nevertheless guide a society that will lead the world in terms of how to survive a challenging past.

In a response to the report of the TRC, former President Thabo Mbeki (April 2003) said to Parliament: *'The TRC built a people's contract for a better SA'*, and also *'The road we have traveled and the advances we have made convey the firm message that we are moving towards the accomplishment of the objectives we set ourselves. They tell us that, in the end, however long the road that we still have to travel, we will win'*. He also contended, *'The pain and the agony that characterized the conflict among South Africans over the decades, so vividly relived in many hearings of the Commission, planted the seed of hope – of a future bright in its humanity and its sense of caring'* (Government Communications 2003, p. 8). These insights have guided the roots for the building of the positive nation that South Africa aspires to be.

Quite undoubtedly, more social cohesion is needed to sustain efforts at nation building with a climate of trust and peace. Secondly, efforts need to be made to deal with the anger and frustration of some of the black and white youth who may feel sidelined by mainstream society. Social challenges such as poverty, unemployment and corruption need to be handled. Finally, the main challenge for the future is how to build on the positive gains of the miraculous political transition and the work of the TRC, and prevent the past history from repeating itself. Intentional application on community and national levels of knowledge from the domain of positive psychology may contribute to further the building of a positive nation. Therefore, scientists, community leaders, politicians and ordinary lay people need to take hands.

In conclusion, various psychosocial strengths and specifically *character strengths* from all virtue clusters (cf. the VIA model) could be identified in the TRC processes and outcomes and have been used as a lens to understand the TRC process as applied positive psychology. Such analyses may contribute to a knowledge base for Positive Nations.

Now, more than a decade later, South Africa still has many social, economic and political challenges to meet but also many individual, group and societal strengths to be utilised in the process of building a more positive nation. In South Africa, we have a long and very painful history, but now also a promising new road as a nation. This was envisioned by Mandela in his inauguration speech, saying, '*We know it well that none of us acting alone can achieve success. We must therefore act together as a united people, for national reconciliation, for nation building, for the birth of a new world. Let there be justice for all. Let there be peace for all. Let there be work, bread, water and salt for all. Let each know that for each the body, the mind and the soul have been freed to fulfil themselves*' (South African Government Information 1994). This vision towards a healed and healthy nation has now been further developed in the vision from the National Development Plan 2012–2030 (www.npconline.co.za). Based on this vision, Njabulo Ndebele and Antjie Krog poetically verbalised our dream to become a positive and healthy nation by 2030 as follows: '*We feel loved, respected and cared for at home, in the community and the public institutions we have created; we feel understood, we feel trustful, we feel trusted, we feel accommodative, we feel accommodated, we feel informed, we feel healthy, we feel safe, we feel resourceful and inventive, we learn together, we talk to each other, we share our work, we play, we worship, we ponder and laugh, we are energised by sharing our resourcefulness, we are resilient*'. They further visualise, '*Now, in 2030, our story keeps growing as if spring is always with us. Once we uttered the dream of a rainbow. Now we see it, living it. It does not curve over the sky. It is refracted in each one of us at home, in the community, in the city, and across the land, in an abundance of colour*' (Ndebele and Krog 2012, p. 31). Thus, we see a positive nation as one in which a we-ness is experienced and expressed in all domains of life while vibrantly reflecting our colourful diversity in the process of moving forward. This is what Krog (2008) indicated as 'interconnectedness-towards-wholeness' which is not an end-state, but '*a process of becoming in which everybody and everything is moving towards its fullest self, building itself; one can only reach that fullest self though, through and with others*' (Krog 2008, p. 355).

Positive psychology, and a strengths perspective, can greatly contribute to a deeper understanding of what well-being or resilience in a group or nation means and how it can be facilitated in scientifically informed and sustainable ways with appreciation of cultural diversities (cf. Wissing 2013). Interpretation of the TRC processes through the lens of positive psychology and how these processes contributed to positive nation building forward our understanding of how the negative and the positive can be intrinsically linked and thereby then also contributes to the development in positive psychology as a science.

References

Alais, L. (2007). Forgiving without forgetting: Forgiveness and the TRC. *SA Publiekreg/Public Law, 22*(1), 255–263.

Aldwin, C. M. (1994). *Stress, coping and development: An integrative perspective.* New York: Guilford Press.

Antonovsky, A. (1987). *Unravelling the mystery of health: How people manage stress and stay well.* San Francisco: Jossey-Bass.

Baumeister, R. F. (1991). *Meanings of life.* New York: Guilford Press.

Blomfield, O. H. (1985). Parasitism, projective identification and the Faustian Bargain. *International Review of Psycho-Analysis, 12,* 299–310.

Boraine, A. (1996). *Alternative and adjuncts to criminal prosecutions.* Paper delivered at the conference on, Justice in cataclysm: Criminal tribunals in the wake of mass violence, Brussels, Belgium. http://www.truth.org.za

Borer, A. T. (2003). A taxonomy of victims and perpetrators: Human rights and reconciliation in South Africa. *Human Rights Quarterly, 25*(4), 1088–1116.

Brand, G. (2002). *Speaking of a fabulous ghost: In search of theological criteria, with special reference to the debate on salvation in African Christian theology* (Contributions to philosophical theology, Vol. 7). Frankfurt am Main: Peter Lang.

Brown, K. W., & Ryan, R. M. (2003). The benefits of being present: Mindfulness and its role in psychological well-being. *Journal of Personality and Social Psychology, 84,* 822–848.

Chapman, A. R., & van der Merwe, H. (Eds.). (2008). *Truth and reconciliation in South Africa: Did the TRC deliver?* Philadelphia: Penn Press.

Chenyang, L. (2008). The philosophy of harmony in classical Confucianism. *Philosophy Compass, 3*(3), 423–435.

Emmons, R. A. (2003). Personal goals, life meaning, and virtue: Wellsprings of a positive life. In C. L. Keyes & J. Haidt (Eds.), *Flourishing positive psychology and the life well-lived* (pp. 105–128). Washington, DC: American Psychological Association.

Emmons, R. A. (2007). *Thanks! How the new science of gratitude can make you happier.* Boston: Houghton-Mifflin.

Emmons, R. A., & McCullough, M. E. (Eds.). (2004). *The psychology of gratitude.* New York: Oxford University Press.

Fredrickson, B. L. (2001). The role of positive emotions in positive psychology: The broaden-and-build theory of positive emotions. *American Psychologist, 56*(3), 218–226.

Fredrickson, B. L. (2009). *Positivity.* New York: Random House.

Gibson, J. L. (2002). Truth, justice, and reconciliation: Judging the fairness of amnesty in South Africa. *American Journal of Political Science, 46*(3), 540–556.

Gobodo-Madikizela, P. (2002). Remorse, forgiveness and rehumanization: Stories from South Africa. *Journal of Humanistic Psychology, 42,* 7–42.

Gobodo-Madikizela, P. (2003). *A human being died that night: A South African story of forgiveness.* Boston: Houghton Mifflin.

Gobodo-Madikizela, P. (2008). Trauma, forgiveness and the witnessing dance: Making public spaces intimate. *The Journal of Analytical Psychology, 53,* 169–188.

Government Communications (GCIS). (2003, April 27). Truth and Reconciliation Commission (TRC): Build a people's contract for South Africa. *Sunday Times*, 8.

Gyekye, K. (1987). *An essay on African philosophical thought: The akan conceptual scheme.* Cambridge: Cambridge University Press.

Gyekye, K. (1997). *Tradition and modernity: Philosophical reflections on the African experience.* Oxford: Oxford University Press.

Hay, M. (1999). Grappling with the past: The Truth and Reconciliation Commission of South Africa. *African Journal on Conflict Resolution, 1*(1), 29–51.

Kagee, A. (2006). The relationship between statement giving at the South African Truth and Reconciliation Commission and psychological distress among former political detainees. *South African Journal of Psychology, 36*(1), 10–24.

Kashdan, T. (2010, August 23). *Why are we afraid of having regrets?* Retrieved from http://www.huffingtonpost.com/todd-kashdan/why-you-should-admit-havi_b_687439.html

Keyes, C. L. M. (1998). Social well-being. *Social Psychology Quarterly, 61*, 121–140.

Keyes, C. L. M. (2007). Promoting and protecting mental health as flourishing: A complementary strategy for improving national mental health. *American Psychologist, 62*(2), 95–108.

Kinman, C. (2010, September). *The nation as rhizome.* Presentation at the First Portuguese conference on positive psychology: Positive nations, September 29–30, 2010.

Krog, A. (1998). *Country of my skull.* Johannesburg: Random House.

Krog, A. (2008). This thing called reconciliation: Forgiveness as part of an interconnectedness-towards-wholeness. *South African Journal of Philosophy, 27*(4), 353–366.

Mamdani, M. (2002). 'Amnesty or impunity? A preliminary critique of the report of the Truth and Reconciliation Commission of South Africa (TRC). *Diacritics, 32*, 33–59.

Markel, D. (1999, Summer). The justice of amnesty? Towards a theory of retributivism in recovering states. *University of Toronto Law Journal, 49*(3), 389–445. doi:10.2139/ssrn.411783.

Markel, D. (2001). Are shaming punishments beautifully retributive? Retributivism and the implications for the alternative sanctions debate. *VanDerBilt Law Review, 54*(6), 2157–2242.

McCullough, M., Pargament, K., & Thoresen, C. (Eds.). (2000). *Forgiveness: Theory, research and practice.* New York: Guilford Press.

Méndez, J. E. (2005, April 1). *How to take forward a transitional justice and human security Agenda: Policy implications for the International Community*, Cape Town.

Ndebele, N., & Krog, A. (2012, August 9). The vision for SA in 2030. *City Press*, 31.

Peterson, C., & Seligman, M. E. P. (2004). *Character strengths and virtues: A handbook and classification.* New York: American Psychological Association/Oxford University Press.

Seligman, M. E. P., Reivich, K., Jaycox, L., & Gillham, J. (1995). *The optimistic child.* New York: Houghton Mifflia.

Setiloane, G. M. (1976). *The image of God among the Sotho-Tswana.* Rotterdam: A.A. Balkema.

Skaar, E. (1999). Truth commissions, trials—Or nothing? Policy options in democratic transitions. *Third World Quarterly, 20*, 1109–1128.

Snyder, C. R. (Ed.). (2000). *Handbook of hope: Theory, measures, and applications.* San Diego: Academic.

South African Government Information. (1994, May 10). *Statement of the president of the African National Congress, Nelson Mandela, at his inauguration as president of the democratic republic of South Africa*, Union Buildings, Pretoria. Retrieved from the internet http://www.info.gov.za/speeches/1994/990319514p1006.htm

South African Truth and Reconciliation Commission (SATRC). (1998). *Truth and Reconciliation Commission of South Africa report.* Cape Town: Author.

Soyinka, W. (1976). *Myth, literature and the African world.* Cambridge: Cambridge University Press.

Statman, J. M. (2000). Performing the truth: The social-psychological context of TRC narratives. *South African Journal of Psychology, 30*(1), 23–32.

Stein, D. J., Seedat, S., Kaminer, D., Moomal, H., Herman, A., Sonnega, J., & Williams, D. R. (2008). The impact of the Truth and Reconciliation Commission on psychological distress and forgiveness in South Africa. *Social Psychiatry and Psychiatric Epidemiology, 43*, 426–468.

Stevens, G. (2005). Truth, confessions and reparations: Lessons from the South African Truth and Reconciliation Commission. *African Safety Promotion: A Journal of Injury and Violence Prevention, 3*(1), 23–39. Retrieved from http://www.aspj.co.za/index.php/ASPJ/article/viewFile/75/68.

Van Binsbergen, W. (2001). Ubuntu and the globalization of Southern African thought and society. *Quest: An African Journal of Philosophy, 15*(1–2), 53–89.

Van der Merwe, E. J., Venter, C. A., & Temane, Q. M. (2009). Untold stories of a group of black South Africans about the apartheid era. *Journal of Psychology in Africa, 19*(3), 395–400.

Wissing, M. P. (2013). A framework for future research and practice. In M. P. Wissing (Ed.), *Well-being research in South Africa*. Volume in series Cross-cultural advancements in Positive Psychology with Antonella Delle Fave as editor in chief. Dordrecht: Springer.

Wissing, M. P., & Temane, Q. M. (2008). The structure of psychological well-being in cultural context: Towards a hierarchical model of psychological health. *Journal of Psychology in Africa, 18*(1), 45–56.

Wong, P. T. P. (2010). Meaning therapy: An integrative and positive existential psychotherapy. *Journal of Contemporary Psychotherapy, 40*, 85–94.

Part IV
Agency: From Passive to Active

Chapter 10
Gross National Happiness: A Case Example of a Himalayan Kingdom's Attempt to Build a Positive Nation

George W. Burns

10.1 Introduction

What is a 'positive nation?' Is national positivity the responsibility of the government, or the people, or both? And if the latter, what should be the balance of responsibility between both? Does a positive political philosophy actually convert into greater levels of happiness for the individual? In other words, do efforts to create happy, Positive Nations work?

This chapter examines the case example of the tiny Himalayan of Bhutan that has, for the past 40 years, initiated, applied and measured a concept based on the fourth king's statement that 'Gross National Happiness is more important than Gross National Product'. Considering it is the responsibility of government to provide a programme of development that ensures an environment for individual happiness – rather than just balancing the budget – Bhutan has defined four core 'pillars' of happiness and is constantly measuring these across nine domains in all provinces within the country.

What does this little-heard-of kingdom have to offer the world? Does its social experiment in building a positive nation offer replicable examples for other countries or communities? These are some of the questions addressed in this chapter.

Do we want our development – individually, nationally and globally – to be based primarily on a measure of greatest wealth or on measures of greatest happiness? How do we want such policies for happiness to look in our own country as well as

Over the last decade the author has visited Bhutan 12 times, working as a volunteer clinical psychologist and leading colleagues on study tours during which they explore the concept and practice of Gross National Happiness. At the invitation of the Prime Minister of Bhutan, he has participated in a High Level United Nations Meeting looking at shifting the world's developmental paradigm solely from economics to a more happiness-based model. He is the author of 7 books, including *Happiness Healing Enhancement*.

G.W. Burns (✉)
Adjunct Professor of Psychology, Cairnmillar Institute, Melbourne, Australia

Milton H. Erickson Institute of Western Australia, PO Box 289, Darlington, WA 6070, Australia

H. Águeda Marujo and L.M. Neto (eds.), *Positive Nations and Communities*, Cross-Cultural   173
Advancements in Positive Psychology 6, DOI 10.1007/978-94-007-6869-7_10,
© Springer Science+Business Media Dordrecht 2014

in the world? What are the values and evidence on which they can be based? How can we develop indicators to measure our progress? How can we provide feedback to policymakers? How can we establish the sort of institutions and tools necessary to implement the policies? In this chapter I want to raise such questions. These are the sort of questions that I think we should all be asking as individuals and as citizens of the world. We may not, as individuals or nations, yet have the answers, but one country has been experimenting with a political philosophy based on the happiness of its citizens for several decades. Here I want to offer the tiny Himalayan kingdom of Bhutan as an illustrative case example of *one* way to build a positive nation, and to do so, let me begin by quoting one of its citizens.

'I believe it is not the responsibility of the state to make every one of its citizens happy. The pursuit of happiness is not only personal but subjective. However, the state shoulders the responsibility of creating a healthy atmosphere to pursue happiness'. These words of local Bhutanese author, businessman and tourist operator, Tshering Tashi, expressed in personal correspondence, (a) highlight an important differentiation in the responsibility for happiness, (b) raise questions about a state's involvement in individual happiness and (c) reflect a long-held political philosophy from Bhutan, the land of Gross National Happiness. They also make assumptions about the roles and responsibilities of the state in regard to its people.

First, Tshering Tashi's comments emphasise that my happiness as an individual is my responsibility. I cannot rely or depend on other people, circumstances, communities or state to *make* me happy. My happiness falls in my ball court…and is ultimately my choice. It is a myth to think that other people or circumstances *make* us happy. This is something we have known from both ancient Greek philosophers who elicited it so clearly and modern-day researchers in the field of positive psychology who are affirming it from a basis of evidence (Burns 2010a). It is not what happens to us but how we *react* to what happens that determines our happiness or unhappiness. And we might question whether the right for individuals to have that reaction can or should be in the control of a big-brother state.

Second, Tshering Tashi's words raise the question of whether the state should be a stakeholder in its citizen's happiness or not…and, if so, to what extent? After all, what is a 'positive nation?' Surely, the assessment of what is positive and what is not is a very subjective matter. Who judges whether it is positive or not? Is national positivity the responsibility of the government, the people, both or neither?

History provides us with, unfortunately, far too many examples of how national leaders, governments and even a significant percentage of its people have considered it a positive national move to engage in ethnic cleansing, colonise another people's homeland, persecute adherents of different religions or stomp out an axis of evil. This raises important questions not only about what a positive nation is but also who is to define or judge what is a positive nation and what is not? Is a nation acting positively if it engages in activities that support the welfare of the majority of its citizens, even if that infringes on the rights of the minority?

Let us take a hypothetical example of a large nation that is running out of oil reserves. The lack of fuel could drive the country's economy to a standstill. Factories could no longer operate to provide necessary goods. People could not drive cars or get to work. The absence of fuel for heating and cooling would raise levels of discomfort and dissatisfaction. People would complain, perhaps engage in protests and riots. It may be seen as positive for a nation to guarantee those fuel reserves for its people but would it be seen as a positive nation if it invaded, overran or colonised another, weaker nation to do so? For the government and people of the fuel-starved nation it may well seem positive while the government and people of the invaded, fuel-rich country may have an entirely different perspective.

So what is a positive nation? Rather than provide a definition of a positive nation or community (which has already been offered elsewhere in this book), I want to offer a case example of a country that has been building a political philosophy of happiness for several centuries and has been expounding, measuring and operationalising the concept of Gross National Happiness (GNH) for the last four decades. When I speak about Bhutan, a common response from people is, 'Isn't that the country where everyone is happy?' or 'Isn't that the happiest nation in the world?' Are such expectations positive for the people of a country with a goal of happiness? Does it create an expectation that if I am a citizen of a country committed to GNH, I *must* be happy? I can imagine people thinking, *if I am not happy, then surely something is wrong with me*. Could such expectations of national happiness actually lead to people experiencing feelings of hopelessness, helplessness and, in the worst case scenarios, depression?

Third, in his personal correspondence, Tshering Tashi reflected a long-held and long-applied political view from his home in the tiny, landlocked Himalayan kingdom of Bhutan. In this chapter, I present the case example of this unique nation that has, for the past 40 years, initiated, applied and measured a concept based on the fourth king's statement that 'Gross National Happiness is more important than Gross National Product'. Considering it is the responsibility of government to provide a programme of development that ensures an environment for individual happiness – rather than just balancing the budget – Bhutan has defined four core 'pillars' of happiness and is constantly measuring these across nine domains in all districts within the country.

King Jigme Singye Wangchuck's seemingly simple play on words in juxtaposing Gross National Happiness and Gross National Product not only won international interest but has crystallised the basis for the country's political philosophy. It has been written into Bhutan's democratic constitution, is measured by a series of established indicators across all provinces, and has attracted the interest of multidisciplinary scientists in fields as seemingly diverse as economics, political science, religion and psychology.

10.2   What Is Gross National Happiness?

The principle of GNH describes development as a continuous process towards a balance between material and non-material needs of individuals and society. The country's philosophy of development, while recognising the importance of economic growth as essential to support and nurture the spiritual and social needs of the community, is not an end in itself but one among many means of achieving holistic development.

It is fitting here to point out the term 'happiness' as Bhutan uses it in Gross National Happiness differs in several ways from its usage in western literature where it commonly refers to a fleeting, heightened, pleasurable emotion (Ura et al. 2012). Positive psychology has largely defined happiness in line with the definitions of the ancient Greek philosophers, talking of temporary pleasure as 'common happiness' and the more sustained state of well-being as 'eudaemonia' or the big picture state of individual well-being. Positive psychologist Martin Seligman presents this in the anagram, PERMA, as the initials for the five essential elements that he claims should place us in a state of lasting well-being (Seligman 2011). These are (1) positive emotions (P) such as peace, gratitude, satisfaction, pleasure, inspiration, hope, curiosity or love; (2) engagement (E) or total, focussed absorption in a situation, task or project; (3) positive, meaningful relationships (R); (4) meaning (M) such as serving a cause bigger than ourselves; and (5) accomplishment or achievement (A) such as mastering a skill, achieving a valuable goal or winning a competitive event. While this is broader in its concept than the fleeting, pleasurable emotions referred to by Ura et al. (2012), Seligman's concept of happiness is still a primarily individual experience or pursuit, even though he has recently proposed the same model as a goal of international policy (Seligman 2012).

By comparison, happiness as perceived in GNH is both more expansive and deeper. It is more systemic than individualistic. First, the concept of happiness incorporated in GNH is seen as multidimensional – as will become apparent when we discuss the domains and indicators of GNH below. Though psychological or subjective well-being is included as one important domain, it is just one of nine and does not dominate to the exclusion of other domains. Second, happiness is seen as other regarding more than solely self-regarding. The Prime Minister of Bhutan has said, 'We know that true abiding happiness cannot exist while others suffer, and comes from serving others, living in harmony with nature, and realising our innate wisdom and the true and brilliant nature of our minds' (Ura et al. 2012, p. 110). Third, the Prime Minister refers to happiness as living in harmony with nature (Thinley 2012a, b), a variable neglected in most western notions of happiness but a variable that is ultimately logical. We cannot go on depleting our environment and expect that will contribute to our happiness (Burns 1998, 2005, 2009; Thinley 2012b). Finally GNH refers to even bigger picture dimensions such as happiness-based economics, happiness-based politics, social capital, human capital and, as mentioned, natural capital.

Gross National Happiness is based on the ideology that the pursuit of happiness is found in all people and is the strongest force of desires once basic needs such as food, shelter, security and health are satisfied. Included in the concept of GNH, and characteristic of Bhutan's Buddhist heritage, is a 'middle path' approach in which spiritual and cultural pursuits are balanced with material pursuits. Bhutan's concept of happiness thus follows a more systemic, rather than individualistic, concept. Happiness is perceived as being grounded in the systems of which individuals are a part: our relationships with other people, with other living beings, with the natural environment, with our culture and with the spiritual world.

At its core GNH holds the belief that development should promote happiness as its primary value. Equal importance must be placed on socio-economic development, along with the spiritual, cultural and emotional needs of the people. Economic growth, far from being the dominating force in development, is seen as just one aspect of the multi-armed developmental programme that aims to improve the social requirements of society and not just the financial balance sheet. Thus, GNH has become the philosophical foundation for the policies, processes and implementation of development in Bhutan (Burns 2010b).

A major political change occurred in 2008 when Bhutan became the world's newest democracy. It came about peacefully – interestingly, not from the will of the people but from the persuasion and personal efforts of the fourth king. In his first address to the United Nations, the newly elected Prime Minister of Bhutan Jigmi Y. Thinley said, 'Gross National Happiness is based on the belief that happiness is the single most important goal and purpose in life for every individual and that the end of development must be the promotion and enhancement of happiness. It must, therefore, we believe, be the responsibility of the State to create an enabling environment within which its citizens can pursue happiness. The concept emphasises a balanced life – matching material needs of the body with the spiritual, psychological and emotional needs of the mind. To this end the Royal Government of Bhutan has structured its development programs on four broad themes or "pillars" that constitute a paradigm of holistic and sustainable development' (Thinley 2008).

10.3   What Are the Pillars of GNH?

For the last 40 years, Bhutan's monarchy and government leaders have been exploring and developing the concept of GNH and its applications in their forward movement as a nation. Initially this led to breaking the definition down into the four pillars of GNH referred to by Prime Minister Tinley. They are:

10.3.1   Sustainable and Equitable Socio-economic Development

Economic growth is acknowledged as an integral part of development but is not seen as either the sole measure or the whole picture. Development needs to be both sustainable and equitable for the whole community. Putting this into practice, Bhutan commits over 30 % of its national budget to providing free health and education services to all citizens.

10.3.2 Environmental Conservation

It is a common belief in Bhutan that irresponsible activities in nature will lead to negative and therefore unhappy outcomes such as seen in neighbouring countries like Nepal where the denuding of forests on the slopes of the Himalaya has led to landslides that have destroyed villages and taken lives. The environmental benefits that have derived from this pillar of GNH include the listing of Bhutan as a world biodiversity hotspot, increased preservation policies and the constitutional protection of the environment. Bhutan's democratic constitution, adopted on 18 July 2008, states: 'The Government shall ensure that, in order to conserve the country's natural resources and to prevent degradation of the ecosystem, a minimum of 60 % of Bhutan's total land shall be maintained under forest cover for all time' (The Constitution of the Kingdom of Bhutan 2008, p. 12).

10.3.3 Promotion of Culture

With globalisation comes the risk of losing diverse cultural heritages. Believing that a decline in traditional heritage and culture will lead to a loss of long-held values and, in turn, a general dissatisfaction of society, Bhutan seeks to guard and maintain its culture as a high priority for the maintenance of happiness. In schools all children are taught Bhutanese cultural values and language; they do a daily mindfulness practice and are educated in the principles of Gross National Happiness – side by side with science, mathematics and English language.

10.3.4 Good Governance

The preceding pillars for promoting happiness and well-being cannot happen without good governance. To this end, the fourth king steered his people towards democracy by gradually withdrawing from the executive function of government in 1998, introducing universal voting rights in 2002 and overseeing the establishment of an elected democratic government in 2008. The pillars of GNH are written into the constitution as a basis for continuing good governance.

10.4 How Did GNH Originated?

Approaches to building a positive nation do not generally emerge from a political void. They have a history, a cultural context, a time of assessment, a period of contemplation and a process of development. To understand what Gross National

Happiness is, how it developed and how is it applied, it may therefore help to understand a little about the nation where it emerged and a little of its recent history. Bhutan follows religious, cultural and linguistic traditions similar to Tibet. Along with its architecture, language and Buddhist beliefs, Bhutan inherited a concept of the importance of happiness as a goal of existence for both self and others that dates back to the Buddha, two and a half millennia ago (Wangmo and Valk 2012).

By comparison to its populous northern and southern neighbours, China and India, Bhutan has a humble population of around 750,000 and territory that extends just 190 miles (300 km) from east to west and 95 miles (150 km) from north to south. Contours on the national map rise from a mere 330 ft (100 m) on the Indian plains to 24,800 ft (7,540 m) on the northern border with China. Isolated valleys, separated by high mountain passes, have resulted in Bhutan being one of the most culturally and linguistically diverse countries on the planet. Both its economy and culture have been based on agricultural subsistence from time immemorial with a more recent shift towards consumerism, particularly in the rapidly growing cities. Wedged between the two most populous nations in the world and facing rapid exposure to the outside world, Bhutan has had to develop its own also uniquely individual nationhood and wisely plan its pathway to socio-economic development.

The monarchy that governed Bhutan for just over a century began with the coronation of the first King on 17 December 1907. Under the third King, who was educated in India and England, Bhutan started to emerge from centuries of self-imposed isolation, opened itself to the outside world and began a process of planned development. This lasted barely a decade before the third King died prematurely at the age of 44 in 1972, leaving the throne to his 16-year-old son, Jigme Singye Wangchuck. King Jigme, the fourth king, adopted his father's programme of modernisation and economic self-reliance, emphasising education, health services, rural development and communication, as well as conservation of the natural environment. In this context, and with a keenness to preserve Bhutanese values from the influence of external factors, the king began to explore and speak about a specific Bhutanese path to development that would be consistent with Bhutanese values, culture, institutions and spiritual beliefs. Wanting to selectively choose from what had worked for the benefit of a population's well-being in developed countries and what had worked in the centuries' old traditions for the well-being of the Bhutanese, the king made his now-famed statement at his coronation in 1972: 'Gross National Happiness is more important than Gross National Product'.

This concept was nothing new for Bhutan. From the very time that the separate peoples of Bhutan were unified into the current nation, the Legal Code of 1729 declared that 'if the Government cannot create happiness for its people, there is no purpose for the Government to exist' (Ura et al. 2012, p. 109). Building on this long-standing concept, King Jigme's statement directly juxtaposed the concepts of GNH and Gross National Product (GNP) or Gross Domestic Product (GDP) as it is now more commonly known. Not only did it attract international attention, but it also challenged orthodox Western developmental theory that tends to see and measure development primarily in material, economic terms. Increasing material development as an end in itself, King Jigme foresaw, would come at a cost to the other values dear to his people – and it was these values that could and did make his country a positive nation. Material development, he proposed, was *not* an end in itself but was *one* means to enhance the overall well-being of his people and his nation. Gross National Happiness is therefore grounded in the premise that the principal goal of society should be the attainment of material progress hand in glove with psychological, environmental, cultural and spiritual well-being.

10.5   How Is a Positive Nation's Progress Measured?

If we are to develop Positive Nations with the ultimate goal of positive citizens, the next question becomes how can we measure if this new system is working to achieve that? Here Bhutan can continue its role as a case study given that it is perhaps the first country in the world to have already explored this. In 1999, the Centre for Bhutan Studies was established as a research institute that is at the forefront of investigating GNH at both theoretical and applied levels. The Centre's mission is to explore three main questions: How do you define GNH, how do you measure GNH and how do you operationalise GNH? (http://www.bhutanstudies.org.bt)

By comparison, measuring progress in GDP is a relatively simple process: if the economic balance sheet is in the blue, progress is assessed to be happening. Much the same as your household budget, if your income exceeds your expenses, all is well but if expenses exceed your income, you are in trouble. Hopefully, most families are aware, however, that their happiness and well-being are related to more than just the balance of their household budget.

What are those other factors for a nation and how do you assess them? In Bhutan, the Centre for Bhutan Studies has defined nine domains that articulate the core pillars of GNH more fully and form the basis of the GNH Index. These domains are measured by 33 indicators: four indicators for each domain except time use (2) and living standards (3). They were initially pilot tested in a 2006 survey with 350 respondents to assess the questionnaires, help researchers to understand the potential problems of a full survey and examine the actual data collected. This was followed by a nationally representative GNH survey in December 2007 that covered 12 of the country's 20 districts (dzongkhags), spanned both rural and urban areas and had a sample size of 950. The questionnaires included some 750 variables that took about 5–6 hours to complete.

Plans are to continue to administer the GNH Index at regular intervals so as to assess the citizens' levels of happiness, provide feedback to the government on its performance and plan future policies and interventions. In line with this a second survey in 2010 sampled 7,142 people across all of the country's 20 dzongkhags with a questionnaire that took an average 3 hours to complete (Ura and Penjore 2009; Ura et al. 2012; http://www.grossnationalhappiness.com/index/). Efforts were made to ensure that the survey was nationally representative, representative at a district level and representative of the rural-urban balance.

The nine domains surveyed in Bhutan's GNH Index include:

- Psychological well-being
- Health
- Time use
- Education
- Cultural diversity and resilience
- Good governance
- Community vitality
- Ecological diversity and resilience
- Living standards

While neither space nor content relevance permit me to provide a full explanation of each domain and its specific indicators – along with the results of the 2010 survey – this information can be found at http://www.grossnationalhappiness.com/index/ or in Ura et al. (2012).

These domains and indicators serve as a means for a country to objectively measure progress towards positive national development. They provide information on which policymakers, businesses, various agencies and the population can make informed decisions about continuing social and political development. Indicators can highlight areas of progress, areas that may need attention, programmes that are effective or not and efforts that need to be expanded or abandoned.

Speaking of Bhutan's indicators, Coleman says, 'Good evidence is essential for informed decision-making. Without such measures, policymaking would be blind, and have no understanding where the greatest needs are, and which population groups need to be targeted with which programs. They can also send early warning signals to policymakers if key indicators begin to trend downward, and thus allow and encourage timely remedial action' (Coleman 2009, p. 15).

10.6   How Do You Keep Accounts of Happiness?

'We will always need these indicators', the Prime Minister, Jigmi Thinley, has stated, 'for basic information about our country – and particularly as the important policy screening tool they have become. But they are not enough. Indicators and accounts are two entirely different, though fully complementary, sets of measures. Indicators assess trends over time. Accounts assess value – what something is worth' (Thinley 2012a).

Why introduce a set of National Accounts that assess the value of natural, human and social capital rather than stay with the dollar-based GDP? Again the idea was not entirely new as it had already been recommended by the Stiglitz Commission that was appointed by French President Nicolas Sarkozy (Stiglitz et al. 2009; Isensen 2009). Bhutan was simply the first, and at the time of writing, so far the only country in the world to put it into practise.

Coleman has claimed that GDP is not an indicator of national well-being but simply an accounting system (Coleman 2009, p. 17). Surprisingly, this view has found support among economists who, given their background and training, might be expected to show strong preferences for economic indicators. UK economist Richard Layard and American Nobel Prize-winning economist Joseph Stiglitz take stances similar to that long held by the Bhutanese government, asserting that happiness should be the goal of a country's political philosophy and that progress towards it should be studied and measured with the same level of scrutiny as GDP. The primarily economic model of GDP, Layard argues, is far too limited and restricted in its approach (Layard 2005), while Stiglitz has described it as an antiquated standard open to the criticism of being an overly narrow indicator (Stiglitz et al. 2009; Isensen 2009).

Bhutan's Prime Minister, along with these and other leading economists, has argued that there is a conventional, almost universally held, but false belief that the more GDP grows the better off, more prosperous, and the happier we will be. But is this so? 'If we were to cut down all our forests in Bhutan', he has said, 'GDP would mushroom, because GDP only counts the timber value of our forests once they are cut down and sold at market. GDP…entirely ignores the value of our standing forests' (Thinley 2012a). Yet these forests, which the Constitution wisely preserves, hold immense value by reducing the risk of landslides that could wipe out whole villages, providing watersheds, biodiversity and sacred sites, protecting wildlife, securing good, clean water sources, offsetting carbon from the atmosphere and indeed much more. Such values are invisible in GDP and thus account for much of the degradation and depletion of our natural wealth worldwide. Analogously, the Prime Minister described it as being like a factory owner who sold off all his machinery and counted it as profit, only then to discover that he had nothing to produce the next year.

To offer another example, take the production of cigarettes, alcohol and illegal drugs. They provide employment to workers and profits to manufacturers and so, in GDP terms, contribute to economic growth, making us 'better off'. The health consequences of using such substances means the community needs to build hospitals (which helps the construction industry to grow), train doctors and nurses (which helps universities to grow), employ doctors and nurses and manufacture pharmaceuticals and hospital equipment (which contributes to peripheral employment). These income earners then spend money on goods and services which further helps GDP to grow. Substances like cigarettes, alcohol and illegal drugs and their huge health consequences are therefore seen as a positive in an accounting system that values no more than economic progress. Similarly, the more crime, the more war, the more pollution we have, the more the economy will grow because we have to spend on prisons and police, weapons and soldiers, and pollution clean-ups.

Consequently, GDP accounting methods can send highly misleading messages to policymakers and, therefore, can be counterproductive to taking timely action about many of the issues our world currently faces with climate change, environmental degradation, disease prevention and other important preventative actions. For these reasons, Bhutan has become the world leader in moving towards creating a balanced GNH accounting system for the country. Its first step in this direction was to measure the economic value of its natural capital of which nearly 94 % was provided by its forests. Because Bhutan's forests help store carbon, regulate the climate, protect watersheds and provide benefits to peoples and nations outside of its borders – indeed, a total of 53 % of the value is accrued beyond Bhutan – it is performing a huge service to the world. The value accredited to its per annum ecosystem capital amounted to 4.4 times the country's total GDP.

Social capital was assessed by putting a value on voluntary work that Bhutan's citizens generously provided in activities such as assisting others, fighting fires, cleaning up litter, repairing temples or helping the sick, elderly and disabled. Through such voluntary acts of caring and compassion, people are both living the GNH life and assisting the country's economy. GDP does not take voluntary work into account, but if the Bhutanese people had been paid for the generosity of their time, it would add up to about 6.5 million US dollars per year.

In the area of human capital, Bhutan faced a deficit in the health-care costs for alcohol abuse, unlike in a GDP account where alcohol use could be seen as contributing to economic growth.

Some may ask, 'But isn't putting the value of natural, social and human capital in dollar terms just falling back into the GDP model that GNH wants to escape? Shouldn't things like natural capital be appreciated for their intrinsic rather than monetary value?' While this would be ideal, unfortunately not everything in life – or account systems – is ideal. Ideas and new models need to develop, step by step. Placing a monetary value on resources allows for comparisons to be made and may help people see value where it was not appreciated before. If people and policymakers can attach a value to natural, social, human and cultural capital, they are, simply, more likely to value them. Seeing the immense value in its forests allows Bhutan to view preserving, protecting and planting more trees as a capital investment rather than as a non-returnable expense. Seeing deficits in human capital accounts, such as with alcoholism, allows Bhutan to view expenditure on preventative strategies as an investment in human capital. In the words of the Prime Minister, 'The new accounts will point accurately to our hidden strengths (like our rich natural and cultural heritage), on which we need to build rather than taking them for granted, and they will identify weaknesses and investment requirements in our national wealth that are overlooked in conventional market measures' (Thinley 2012a).

10.7   How Is GNH Applied?

Knowing how well a nation is doing on the indicators and how you value that is one thing. Putting that knowledge into practice can be another. To this end, Bhutan has a long-established Planning Commission charged with overseeing the country's development in accord with the principles of GNH. On 18 January 2007, the Royal Government announced the establishment of the GNH Commission to revamp and rename the former Planning Commission (www.bbs.com. bt/GNH%20Commission%20formed.html). All development projects, including funding, have to be processed through by the GNH Commission to ensure they pass the standards of the pillars, domains and indicators for national happiness and well-being.

Given that the Centre for Bhutan Studies was charged with providing feedback on issues under consideration by the GNH Commission, the Centre has sought to operationalise this process by developing what they call GNH Tools. These tools are designed to systematically assess impacts of any policy and project on GNH, thereby allowing the Commission and policymakers to select GNH enhancing policies and projects while rejecting projects and policies that adversely affect the key determinants of GNH. They cover all nine domains of GNH, are measured on a 4-point scale and are applied at both project levels and policy levels. Before policies or projects can go ahead, they have to be assessed to see if they are in accord with Bhutan's positive nation policy of GNH. Details of these tools can be found at http://www.grossnationalhappiness.com/gnh-policy-and-project-screening-tools/.

One historic example of this is in the potentially lucrative area of mountaineering that makes a significant contribution to the national coffers of neighbouring Nepal. The fee for a team climbing Mt Everest in 2007 was USD50,000, and that is just one of the 325 peaks available to climbers. Not surprisingly, mountaineering has become Nepal's highest per capita source of income due to the fact that each mountaineer spends 27 times more than an ordinary tourist (Dhakal 2009). If Bhutan, like Nepal, assessed mountaineering from a solely GDP approach, it would seem like a logical financial decision for a relatively poor country. One alpine club alone has offered the Bhutan government one million US dollars for the opportunity to climb the world's highest unclimbed peak of Gangkar Puensum (Tashi 2009).

Poverty levels in Bhutan, especially in rural areas, are high. On the United Nation's Human Development Index (HDI) – a quantified score that is calculated by averaging three indicators of income, educational attainment and life expectancy – Bhutan is rated 130 on a list of 160 countries (Carpenter and Carpenter 2002). Mountaineering could provide an instant and continuing source of income. So why then is climbing of the major peaks banned?

Previously, it had not been banned. Previously, several of Bhutan's important peaks had been climbed but the Bhutanese people believe their mountains are sacred. For centuries they have provided retreat sites for revered ascetics and saints. They are places for religious pilgrimages. They have served as a natural barrier to deter invaders. They are the place for sky burials and the abode of local protector deities. They are, in sum, holy and sacred (Tashi 2009).

Because of these associations with their mountains, the people approached the king with their concerns about mountaineering. The National Assembly assessed their concerns from the perspective of the four GNH pillars, examining the economic factors as well as the cultural and religious sentiments of the people, the preservation of the regional environment, the potential costs of ecological imbalances resulting from the sport and the need to provide good governance to the people. Deeming that the noneconomic pillars of GNH outweighed the potential monetary income from mountaineering, the National Assembly placed a total ban on mountaineering that remains to this day.

10.8   Does GNH Actually Enhance Citizen's Happiness?

The ultimate questions we need to ask, of course, are *'Does GNH work?' 'Have applications, such as the banning of mountaineering, enhanced the happiness of Bhutan's citizens?' 'Is it a workable basis for defining a positive nation?'*

In 2005, the government of Bhutan conducted a nationwide census to measure the country's level of happiness (Population and Housing Census of Bhutan 2005). Efforts were made to ensure that the census followed prescribed UN procedures and standards so that the outcomes would have international conformity and thus be meaningful and acceptable at an international level. It was a universal census, covering the whole country and all citizens in a particular specified time period. The results revealed that a little under half of the population (45.2 %) reported being very happy with just over half (51.6 %) claiming to be happy. With almost 97 % of the country's citizens purporting to be happy and a mere 3.2 % describing themselves as not being happy, this initially seems like a strong endorsement for a nation to adopt and implement a policy of Gross National Happiness.

It is one thing to have an internal report where the people are not only familiar with GNH but are also taught it in school. Caution should be taken in interpreting these results for a couple of reasons. First, there could be an expectancy that people should respond on the happy side given their government's strong emphasis on GNH, and second, assessment of life satisfaction was undertaken solely on a three-point scale.

So how do Bhutan's happiness levels stand up when compared to other nations? The answer to that basically depends on the measurement used and what it measures. In 2006, the London-based New Economics Foundation reported the results of the global *Happy Planet Index* (Marks et al. 2006). This index measures the extent to which countries deliver long happy and sustainable lives for the people that live in them. To do this it assesses data on national life expectancy, experienced well-being and the country's ecological footprint. Countries are then rated on how many long and happy lives they produced per unit of environmental input.

Bhutan rated highest on the index for its subregion of South Asia, was within the top 10 % of nations worldwide for its level of life satisfaction and ranked number 13 out of the 178 nations included. By the time of the second Happy Planet Report in 2009, it still topped the ladder for its region of South Asia and was ranked 17th of the 143 nations included (Abdallah et al. 2009). While many economically stronger countries had higher life expectancy and life satisfaction, they had a much larger environmental footprint that had them sliding further down the scale. What helped Bhutan maintain such a high ranking was one of the four pillars of GNH – the conservation of the environment.

10.9   Is Bhutan's Case Example Applicable Internationally?

Does Bhutan's experiment with creating a positive nation through GNH have applicability for the rest of the world? In an article entitled *The Causes of Happiness and Misery*, Layard et al. (2012) discuss some 30 years of research defining the numerous key 'external' and 'personal' determinants of happiness. They conclude by saying, 'We have shown above all that happiness depends on a huge range of influences, many of which can be influenced by government policy' (Layard et al. 2012, p. 79). Given that government can play a role in facilitating citizens' happiness, the next questions raised are 'Do we want governments to be more involved in happiness rather than in just keeping a balance on the nation's accounts?' 'Do citizens want the state to be responsible for creating and enabling an environment in which they can pursue happiness?' Some researchers, such as Marks, claim that there is indeed 'considerable support among the public for governments to use broader measures of progress' (2009, p. 103). In support of this, data from a UK poll found that 81 % of people endorsed the idea that a government's prime objective should be 'greatest happiness' rather than the 'greatest wealth'. Only 13 % of respondents thought that government should not be involved in the matter of happiness (BBC 2006).

Bhutan's approach to building a positive nation is not one of a simplistic, idealised philosophy from a country that can easily afford to buck the pressures of larger GDP-based economies. Instead its wise leaders in the kings and the first Prime Minister have created a sound, practical and scientific approach for establishing a political environment conducive to the pursuit of happiness. The political experiment of the last four decades, with much longer term antecedents, has been measured carefully with two surveys to assess its progress. There are institutions, established procedures and feedback systems in place for the continuing movement towards the country's GNH goals – and these will remain in place to continue monitoring progress.

These steps may seem like a tiny stone that Bhutan has dropped into the world pool of development and sustainability, but its actions have created ripples that are spreading well beyond its own borders. The concept of GNH has appeal to a world that is seeing the negative effects of the GDP model in unaccountably depleting the environment, creating growing schisms between the rich and poor, leaving at least one billion of the world's people without sufficient food to eat each day, facing escalating rates of depression and cycling on a treadmill of consumerism.

Other nations have, metaphorically, picked up the torch, carried it into new areas and are exploring alternate paradigms to building more Positive Nations. As already mentioned, France's President Nicolas Sarkozy drew a group of leading economists into a think tank to re-examine the validity of continuing with GDP as a sole or primary measure of a nation's well-being. In a ground-breaking initiative in September 2009, Sarkozy raised the idea of a GNH-type model of development at the G20 meeting in Pittsburgh, USA.

In 2010, the conservative government in Britain introduced a happiness index to measure and track the nation's well-being. This project was designed to inform civil servants (a) about what makes people happy and (b) use that information for incorporating happiness in the formulation of public policy. Early results from the study have highlighted citizens' desire for government to assist in reducing loneliness, improving work-family balance, enhancing public spaces, strengthening relationships and staunching a growing culture of consumerism (http://www.thesolutionsjournal.com/node/1111).

Gradually passing from nation to nation, our metaphoric torch now appears to have reached its Mt Olympus of the United Nations. Inspired by Bhutan's development philosophy of GNH, a 2011 UN Resolution to pursue the elaboration of additional measures that better capture the importance of the pursuit of happiness and well-being in development with a view to guiding their public policies was endorsed by all 193 member nations of the United Nations.

Following on from this, on 2 April 2012, the Royal Government of Bhutan convened a High-Level Meeting on 'Happiness and Well-Being: Defining A New Economic Paradigm' at the UN headquarters in New York City, taking a major step towards a sustainable, holistic, inclusive and equitable new economic development paradigm for the global community. Some months before I was surprised to find in my Inbox an email from the Prime Minister of Bhutan inviting me, given my 'profound contribution to the psychology of well-being', to join 700 other invited political and government leaders, scholars, economists, philosophers, scientists, media, civil society, UN officials, entrepreneurs and spiritual leaders from the world's major faiths at this high-level meeting. Following the initial day, 200 of us remained to continue the intensive discussions for another 2 days.

The meeting focused on a new economic paradigm that will ensure a fully sustainable balance among natural, social, cultural, human and built capital assets. It concluded that the paradigm should be based on four fundamental tenets:

- Happiness and well-being
- Ecological sustainability
- Fair distribution of wealth and resources
- Efficient use of resources

For me, the meeting was highly inspirational in that world leaders from various disciplines had all come together with a consensus of opinion that our current economic-based model of development was not offering the planet or its people the best service. All agreed that we need a better model to better serve equality, happiness and quality of life for all people. This involves a huge paradigm shift from the current model – that many people, corporations and governments are heavily invested in – to one that at this stage is little more than a political ideal. I do not think anyone left the meeting deluded about how long and difficult the road to achieving this new paradigm is likely to be. Nonetheless, I found myself, along with others, leaving with a sense of hope for the future of our planet. Ideas are the precursors to action and that in itself is enough to inspire hope.

10.10 What Hope Does GNH Offer for Building More Positive Nations?

Based on its philosophy of GNH, Bhutan has pioneered an innovatively different approach for broadening the overly narrow approach of GDP and creating a more equitable and holistic model for socio-economic development. It is not just a quaint idea from a somewhat mystical kingdom in the Himalaya but a social, political and economic approach to development that has been tried, tested and developed over the last four decades. It has four established pillars on which this philosophy is based. It has defined nine domains that have been rigorously studied throughout the country and closely analysed. It has created tools for assessing whether policies and projects meet the criteria of GNH and established a National Accounts system that includes natural, social and human capital as well as financial and built capital. The indicators provide feedback to the public and politicians about what programs are facilitating development towards happiness and what might need to be modified. Institutions such as the GNH Commission and the Centre for Bhutan Studies provide the vehicles for putting policies and projects into GNH-based practice. Instruments like the GNH Tools contribute systematic means for operationalising the whole concept, and the broader-based accounts system is a way of assessing the value of those measures.

In this chapter, I have sought to present Bhutan as an illustrative case example of *one* way of building a positive nation. I have also been asked to give my own personal observations as someone who has visited Bhutan in various capacities (from a study tour leader to a conference presenter to a volunteer clinical psychologist) some 12 times over the last decade. During those visits I have been honoured to lunch with the King, meet with the Prime Minister and meet and dine with several other government ministers. I have been honoured to meet with many professional people especially in the health field, have had business dealings with people in tourism and have worked alongside guides and drivers. I have also been honoured to sleep with rural families on the floors of their farmhouses, trek with traders plying their trade across the treacherous Himalaya and been privileged to hear personal life stories in a way that one could only hear in the confidence of a psychologist-client relationship. I initially travelled in Bhutan as a tourist and, more recently, have lived there for extended periods in a small apartment adjacent to one of the economically poorest areas in the capital city. In other words, my contacts have allowed me to meet with the wide variety and diversity of people across the socio-economic range.

Based on this, what has my experience shown? Has Bhutan got it perfectly right? Is all happy in the land of happiness? Most of us would probably like to dream of a Shangri-La, as Bhutan has often been called. It would be nice to think that there is a land of ultimate happiness tucked away in some hidden place where people are free of worries, stress or problems; where governments are benevolent to all; and life is ultimately idyllic. Perhaps this is why the fictional place, Shangri-La, created by James Hilton in his novel *Lost Horizon* has crept into our everyday language and consciousness.

Though it often bears the label, Bhutan is not that fantasy. Its policy of GNH does not make it immune from the problems faced by all developing countries any more than a medical practitioner is immune from contracting the same diseases as his patients. Neither does Bhutan's policy make its people free of all the frailties, foibles and fears that make up the human condition. Its people are people and, like people everywhere, are subject to the stresses, sorrows and sadness of life. Bhutan also has extremely poor rural communities and is, consequently, facing major issues of an urban migration to the capital city. With this comes a breakdown of community and extended family networks as people take up residence in city apartments that house no more than a nuclear family. In addition, the community has long faced a significant alcohol problem, and this is joined by a relatively new issue of growing youth drug dependency. These are all problems that those in office, along with the general public and the media, are aware of. In fact it seems to me that the country is currently walking a tightrope strung between two skyscrapers of traditional values and rapid modern development. How well it keeps its balance and manages to bridge that gap is yet to be seen.

Despite these challenges, the majority of people that I have spoken with – from the son of the king who coined the term Gross National Happiness through professional people with whom I have worked to people I have met on the street – endorse the GNH policy. This is evidenced in the fact that the political party with the strongest GNH basis was overwhelmingly elected by the majority of people. While occasionally one sees a press article asking *Why is the Prime Minister taking GNH to the United Nation's when we have our own problems at home?*, the majority of people seem to support the idea – expressed by Tshering Tashi at the beginning of this chapter – that the state shoulders the responsibility of creating a healthy atmosphere in which individuals can pursue their own happiness.

To further the analogy of the medical practitioner, while a doctor may not be immune to common diseases, what he does have is knowledge about the cause, prevention and treatment of the illness. While Bhutan faces many challenges, what it does have is a clear vision for how it wants to see its future, established pathways to follow and a strong motivation to make it work. It may not have it perfectly right but it is pioneering a path towards creating a happy state and happy citizens.

Given this, can Bhutan's GNH model serve as a template of social policy for other cultures, societies and nations? To answer this, let us bear in mind that Bhutan's people are closely united under their monarchy and consolidated with a stable government overwhelmingly elected by more than 90 % of voters. It is a relatively, but not solely, monocultural, monoracial country with a small population. In these ways it differs from more populous, multiracial, multicultural nations such as the USA, the UK and Australia. Though Bhutan offers a good, well-established and well-investigated model, it could be expected that social and political policies based on the enhancement of happiness might look different in different countries. For example, the nine domains defined by Bhutan (and described earlier in this chapter) are different from the eight psychological and social indicators based in Western research as described by positive psychology researchers Ed and Carol Diener (2010). Here, I think it is important not to get caught up in the potential differences but rather to look at the underlying principles and processes for creating more Positive Nations.

Bhutan's Gross National Happiness is not only coming to the awareness of the world's politicians and policymakers but also seems to be emerging as a basis to shift political and social philosophy from wealth to well-being. As nations of the world begin to explore whether GDP should or will remain an adequate measure of their current and future well-being and the well-being of the whole planet, can we hope that Gross National Happiness will provide an inspirational, well-investigated and applied example of a way to build a world of many more positive, happy nations?

If a nation facilitates the opportunities for individual happiness, we know that the resultant happy citizens will in turn contribute much to the social fabric of society and its effective functioning as well as be less of a drain on its resources. It is therefore in the interests of countries and communities to (a) examine the research on what facilitates happiness, (b) provide a context in which these factors can develop, (c) measure the progress of these policies and (d) examine the feedback for continued individual and national well-being. Not only will individual citizens be healthier, happier and more productive, but so will the community and the world as a whole (Burns 2012). Simply put, while the pursuit of happiness is both personal and subjective, and ultimately an individual responsibility, if any nation wants its citizens to be functioning optimally and contributing to the well-being of society, then it needs to create an environment in which individuals can pursue their goal of happiness.

In the words of Bhutan's Prime Minister, 'The time has come for a global effort to build a new economic system no longer based on the dangerous illusions that irresponsible growth is possible on our finite planet and that endless material gain promotes wellbeing. Instead, it will be a system that promotes harmony and respect for nature and each other, that respects our ancient wisdom traditions and protects our most vulnerable people as our own family, and that gives us time to live and enjoy our lives and to appreciate rather than destroy our world' (Thinley 2012b, p. 64).

References

Abdallah, S., Thompson, S., Michaelson, J., Marks, N., & Steuer, N. (2009). *The Happy Planet Index 2.0.* http://www.happyplanetindex.org/public-data/files/happy-planet-index-2-0.pdf. Accessed 10 Apr 2012.

BBC. (2006). *Britain's happiness in decline.* http://news.bbc.co.uk/2/hi/programmes/happiness_formula/4771908.stm. Accessed 5 Dec 2009.

Burns, G. W. (1998). *Nature-guided therapy: Brief integrative strategies for health and wellbeing.* Philadelphia: Brunner/Mazel.

Burns, G. W. (2005). Naturally happy, naturally healthy: The role of the natural environment in well-being. In F. A. Huppert, N. Baylis, & B. Keverne (Eds.), *The science of well-being* (pp. 405–431). Oxford: Oxford University Press.

Burns, G. W. (2009). Can we have both psychological and ecological well-being? In K. Ura & D. Penjore (Eds.), *Gross National Happiness: Practice and measurement* (pp. 127–148). Thimphu: Centre for Bhutan Studies.

Burns, G. W. (Ed.). (2010a). *Happiness, healing, enhancement: Your casebook collection for using positive psychotherapy.* Hoboken: Wiley.

Burns, G. W. (2010b). Gross National Happiness: A gift from Bhutan to the world. In R. Biswas-Deiner (Ed.), *Positive psychology as a mechanism for social change* (pp. 73–88). New York: Springer.

Burns, G. W. (2012). Happiness and psychological well-being: Building human capital to benefit individuals and society. *Solutions, 3*(3), 80–82.

Carpenter, R., & Carpenter, B. (2002). *The blessings of Bhutan*. Honolulu: University of Hawaii Press.

Coleman, R. (2009). Measuring progress towards Gross National Happiness: From GNH indicators to GNH national accounts. In K. Ura & D. Penjore (Eds.), *Gross National Happiness: Practice and measurement* (pp. 15–48). Thimphu: Centre for Bhutan Studies.

Dhakal, D. P. (2009). *Mountain tourism and mountaineers*. http://news.visitingnepal.com/archives/129. Accessed 17 Aug 2009.

Diener, E., & Diener, C. (2010). Monitoring psychosocial prosperity for social change. In R. Biswas-Deiner (Ed.). *Positive psychology as a mechanism for social change* (pp. 53–72). New York: Springer.

Isensen, N. (2009). *Sarkozy calls for a new international prosperity barometer*. http://www.dw-world.de/dw/article/0,,4692507,00.html. Accessed 16 June 2012.

Layard, R. (2005). *Happiness: Lessons from a new science*. London: Allen Lane.

Layard, R., Clark, A., & Senik, C. (2012). The causes of happiness and misery. In J. Helliwell, R. Layard, & J. Sachs (Eds.), *World happiness report* (pp. 58–89). New York: The Earth Institute, Columbia University.

Marks, N. (2009). Creating national accounts of well-being: A parallel process to GNH. In K. Ura & D. Penjore (Eds.), *Gross National Happiness: Practice and measurement* (pp. 102–123). Thimphu: Centre for Bhutan Studies.

Marks, N., Abdullah, S., Simms, A., & Thompson, S. (2006). *The Happy Planet Index*. http://www.happyplanetindex.org/public-data/files/happy-planet-index-first-global.pdf. Accessed 10 Apr 2012.

Population and Housing Census of Bhutan. (2005). http://www.bhutancensus.gov.bt/census_results_7.htm. Accessed 16 June 2012.

Seligman, M. E. P. (2011). *Flourish: A visionary new understanding of happiness and well-being*. New York: Free Press.

Seligman, M. (2012). Flourishing as a goal of international policy. *Solutions, 3*(3), 66–67.

Stiglitz, J. E., Sen, A., & Fitoussi, J. P. (2009). *Report by the commission on the measurement of economic performance and social progress*. http://www.stiglitz-senfitoussi.fr/documents/rapport_anglais

Tashi, T. (2009). The tallest virgin mountain in the world. In T. Fisher & T. Tashi (Eds.), *From Jesuits to Jetsetters: Bold Bhutan beckons: Inhaling gross national happiness* (pp. 114–125). Brisbane: CopyRight Publishing.

The Constitution of the Kingdom of Bhutan. (2008). http://www.constitution.bt. Accessed 16 June 2012.

Thinley, L. J. (2008, September 26). A statement to the 63rd session of the General Assembly of the United Nations, New York.

Thinley, J. Y. (2012a, February 26). Remarks of the Honourable Prime Minister at the press conference releasing the first natural, social, and human capital results of Bhutan's new National Accounts, Prime Minister's Office, Thimphu.

Thinley, L. J. (2012b). Sustainability and happiness: A development philosophy for Bhutan and the world. *Solutions, 3*(3), 64–65.

Ura, K., & Penjore, D. (Eds.). (2009). *Gross National Happiness: Practice and measurement*. Thimphu: Centre for Bhutan Studies.

Ura, K., Alkire, S., & Zangmo, T. (2012). Gross National Happiness and the GNH index. In J. Helliwell, R. Layard, & J. Sachs (Eds.), *World happiness report* (pp. 108–147). New York: The Earth Institute, Columbia University.

Wangmo, T., & Valk, J. (2012). Under the influence of Buddhism: The psychological wellbeing indicators of GNH. *Journal of Bhutan Studies, 26*, 53–81.

Chapter 11
The Revolution of Happiness and Happiness in Revolutions: The Case of the First Portuguese Republic

Miguel Pereira Lopes, Patrícia Jardim Da Palma, and Telmo Ferreira Alves

> *We hold these truths to be self-evident, that all men are created*
> *equal, that they are endowed by their Creator with certain*
> *unalienable Rights, that among these are Life, Liberty*
> *and the pursuit of Happiness.*
>
> Declaration of the United States of America, July 4, 1776

11.1 Introduction

Research on well-being and happiness is one of the most extraordinary and revolutionary advancements in economic and social theory. The present chapter aims to discuss three essential issues: (1) How did research on happiness revolutionized economic theory and the way we see our world? (2) Is people's happiness related to their will to support a sociopolitical revolution? If yes, in what way? (3) How can nations increase their citizens' happiness at a macro-level? After outlining an answer to each of these questions, a brief discussion will be made about some of the events that took place when the First Portuguese Republic was established at the beginning of the twentieth century.

Studies about well-being and happiness are one of the most extraordinary and revolutionary advancements in today's economic theory (Frey 2008). Along with a tradition that is already making its name in Economic Psychology, a variety of happiness studies and empirical results have found their space by questioning traditional

M.P. Lopes (✉) • P.J. Da Palma • T.F. Alves
School of Social and Political Sciences, ISCSP, CAPP – Center for Public Policy and Administration, Technical University of Lisbon, Lisbon P-1349055, Portugal
e-mail: mplopes@iscsp.utl.pt; ppalma@iscsp.utl.pt; telmo.ferreira.alves@gmail.com

H. Águeda Marujo and L.M. Neto (eds.), *Positive Nations and Communities*, Cross-Cultural Advancements in Positive Psychology 6, DOI 10.1007/978-94-007-6869-7_11, © Springer Science+Business Media Dordrecht 2014

economic theory assumptions, such as the agent rationality, the possibility of altruistic behavior, or even the assumption that money always brings a state of greater happiness and well-being.

Taking all of these developments into consideration, knowledge and research models of the so-called Economics of Happiness may be used as ways to understand social and political revolutions. Among other central questions, studying happiness may be necessary to understand if our satisfaction with life and the emergence of revolutionary acts are linked in any way.

In Portugal, the timeliness of such a research question couldn't be better. Both the Centennial Commemorations of the First Portuguese Republic and the current socioeconomic situation of Portugal call for the benefits of achieving a better understanding of the causes, consequences, and processes that link revolutionary acts to the state of well-being/ill-being of populations. This pioneering reflection is the pith of our text.

Our subject matter develops on the basis of three fundamental questions: (1) How research about happiness is revolutionizing economic theory and the way we see our world? (2) Is people's happiness related to their will to support a sociopolitical revolution? If yes, in what way? (3) How can nations increase their citizens' happiness at a macro-level?

After outlining an answer to each of these questions, a brief discussion will be made on some of the events that took place when the First Portuguese Republic was established at the beginning of the twentieth century.

11.2 The Revolution of Happiness

As previously mentioned, we start our analysis by outlining an answer to "how research about happiness is revolutionizing economic theory and the way we see our world." Frey and colleagues (Frey and Benz 2008; Frey and Stutzer 2002), for example, have been trying to answer this question by framing it in vast economic literature that questions economic traditional models. These models defend the rationality of actors and their exclusive self-interested behavior and are based on the idea that human beings are only guided by material and financial motives.

Psychological research has demonstrated over the last few decades that human rationality is largely limited and biased in several situations. Examples of such biases were described by several authors, such as Kahneman and Tversky (1979) who won the Economic Sciences Nobel by showing that people do not follow formal logical rules when rationalizing over things, namely, when they try to reason about finances or economy. Among some of these "mistakes" or biases, we find the conjunction fallacy, the base-rate neglect, and the sample size neglect. Despite not entering into too much detail, we would like to state that today there is a clear refutation of the agents' rationality presumption, something that is contributing to a better conceptualization of the economic science.

Another basic assumption of the classic economic perspective is the idea that the sum of choices would redound in a freer, more efficient and effective economic system if all individuals acted in an exclusively self-interested way. This assumption has been refuted by several studies in Psychology and Economics that show evidence of how people are capable of altruistic behavior, at least to a certain point (e.g., Fehr and Gächter 2000). And these include behaviors in the economic and financial domains. Bewley (1999), for example, during the 1990s questioned why human resource managers, even in the middle of a recession, did not reduce managers' salaries, as predicted by the economic theory at the time. Their answers stressed how unfair it was to have companies paying above the average price in the market.

A recent ingenious test performed by the Swiss economist Bruno Frey and his colleagues (Frey et al. 2010) shows that human beings are capable of displaying altruistic behavior, even in life-or-death situations. In their study, Frey and colleagues compared the probabilities of surviving with the effective survival of different groups of people in the sinking of the Titanic. If exclusively self-interested behavior theories were to be correct, a huge number of men should have survived, in comparison to women, given that men are physically stronger and sturdier. The same should have happened with adults, in comparison to children. However, a careful analysis of the survival ratios showed that this was not the case. Actually the opposite was registered, probably due to the psychological activation of the norm that one must protect the weaker first in life-or-death situations. So there is not much room for any doubt. At least under certain conditions, human beings are capable of behaving altruistically, which totally contradicts the classical assumption of universal self-interest.

But the main issue has to do with the idea that happiness studies' contribute to a better and wider understanding of economic behavior.

To illustrate the impact of the happiness studies in the economic theory, we will focus on two impressive studies. Both of these studies try to reveal how limited the traditional macroeconomics parameters are in analyzing people and societies and how restrictive and insufficient is the notion of the *utility* of people's decisions.

In this new framing, some authors have proposed the need to evaluate and monitor the countries' "gross domestic happiness" (GDH), along with the known "gross domestic product" (GDP). Research has already shown how GDP is often positively influenced by negative aspects of society, such as terrorist activities or road accidents. These activities stimulate economic transactions in a country, as terrorists have to move money in so that they may carry out their missions, but hardly anyone will judge them as positive contributors to happiness and well-being. On the other hand, though many events contribute to human happiness, they are not taken into consideration nor add value to GDP. For instance, when a person helps another by giving her something, it contributes to reduce the acquirement and consumption of goods, hence penalizing GDP. Notwithstanding, generosity and social support are among the relations that most contribute to our happiness and well-being, thus increasing a nation's GDH. These examples reveal the importance of happiness studies on rethinking classical economic models.

It is well known that inflation, alongside with unemployment, has a negative impact on citizens' perceived well-being (inflation and unemployment cumulating effect form what economists call the "misery index"). Classic economic models tend to assume an inverse relationship between inflation and unemployment (the so-called Phillips curve) and give the same weight and importance to both these factors. However, latest research has showed that the perceived negative impact of inflation and unemployment are different. When the time comes for us to choose between inflation and unemployment, we therefore must not consider them as having the same weight.

For instance, a study of Di Tella and colleagues (2001) showed that unemployment has a much greater negative impact on people's well-being than inflation. Specifically, the rise of 1 % in unemployment produces the same reduction in satisfaction and well-being that would be produced by an increase of 1.7 % in inflation! The conclusion is simple: people become unhappier with unemployment rising than with inflation rising equivalently, even though from a financial point of view, the balance remains the same.

Such understanding is only possible by carrying out measurements of people's happiness and well-being. Without the happiness approach used in this first example, perhaps economic models would still draw on inflation and unemployment as having the same weight, therefore biasing or misleading politicians and economists in their decisions.

Another recent example of the major importance that happiness studies have on economic behavior analysis comes from research on terrorism. It's not easy to quantify the social costs of terrorism, but when well-being and satisfaction with life indexes reported by citizens are monitored, such impacts are determinable. That's precisely what Frey et al. (2009) made in their study about terrorism and happiness, based on incidents and fatalities caused by terrorist attacks between 1972 and 2002 in France and the British Isles. The results found by these researchers showed that the frequency and intensity of terrorist acts negatively predicted the satisfaction with the life of citizens in general, even in people who did not live at the locations where the attacks occurred.

These studies demonstrate that particular events (e.g., terrorism) may be analyzed in terms of their impact over well-being in general (and not only on those who are direct targets of such actions). This would not be possible if the citizens' levels of happiness and satisfaction with life were not measured. In addition, these studies relaunch a positive debate on nations' investment on public goods, whether in terms of security, health, education, and others.

Considering these new avenues of research on happiness on the one hand and the possibility of monitoring life satisfaction across countries on the other, we turn our attention to the central aspect of this chapter, which is to understand in what way people's happiness is related to their "revolutionary" tendencies.

11.3   (Un)Happiness in Revolutions

In this section we will try to respond to the second question asked at the beginning of this chapter: Is people's happiness related to their will to support a sociopolitical revolution? If yes, in what way?

Research on happiness has not revealed a clear answer to this specific question yet. However, research concerning the causes and consequences of a revolutionary attitude provide the lens to analyze this question. In addition, available international data makes it possible to compare attitudes and happiness among nations and within nations over time, thus allowing exploratory analyses that will be presented later on en route for sketching a response to this section's question.

Taking the MacCulloch and Pezzini (2007) study on economic development, unemployment, and what they refer to as "taste for revolt" or revolutionary attitude as a starting point, the authors analyzed a sample of 107,985 individuals from 61 nations that were inquired between 1981 and 1997 by the *World Values Survey*[1] international panel. Here is an example of one of the questions asked: "*On this card are three basic kinds of attitudes vis-à-vis the society in which we live in. Please choose the one which best describes your own opinion (one answer only).*" To give an answer, respondents were forced to choose one position among three: (1) "*The entire way our society is organized must be radically changed by revolutionary action.*" (2) "*Our society must be gradually improved by reforms.*" (3) "*Our present society must be courageously defended against all subversive forces.*" Depending on respondents' choices, they could be labeled as "revolutionaries," "reformists," or "conservatives."

The results obtained by MacCulloch and Pezzini (2007) showed that 9.8 % of this worldwide sample agreed with the first statement, hence manifesting a noteworthy "taste for revolt." But this revolutionary attitude was not only translating the expression of the respondents' attitude. Quite the opposite, data also showed that "revolutionary" individuals were more likely to join boycotts and nonofficial strikes, as well as occupy factories and working posts. Putting it in another way, these people's preference for revolt wasn't only just "small talk." They could actually act rebelliously as soon as the opportunity came up.

Therefore, these studies make it possible to identify the "revolutionary propensity" levels of a given population, and along with these, the consequences of this revolutionary attitude become evident as well. Given this chapter's focus, we may now ask how such a revolutionary attitude is related to the levels of happiness and satisfaction with life that people report. As there is no validated answer to this question, we took the initiative of exploring it by using the same database, which is also used in several international comparison studies on happiness and well-being. Our benefit of using the *World Values Survey* database lies in the access to each respondent's answers, concerning both their revolutionary attitude and happiness levels. The descriptive graphic results collected in 2000 comparing four countries with distinct cultures – the United States, Venezuela, Japan, and Canada – are illustrated in Fig. 11.1.

As we can see, even considering how distinctive these countries are concerning their historical-cultural background, the association pattern of lower happiness levels with higher revolutionary attitudes is striking. Indeed, the "revolutionaries" is the sole group where unhappiness levels are higher than happiness levels. This

---

[1]http://www.worldvaluessurvey.org

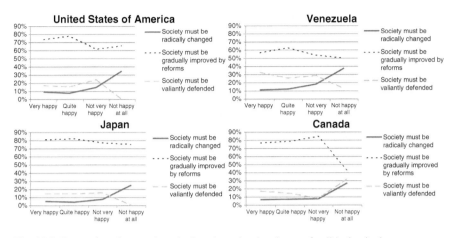

Fig. 11.1 Proportion of respondents by happiness level and type of political attitude

means that lower happiness levels go "hand in hand" with greater revolutionary propensity. Despite being intuitive data, it has not been validated yet.

Given the correlational nature of these data, we must stress that no conclusion can be attained concerning the causality of the relationship between "revolutionary attitude" and "happiness" variables. In accordance to the results, it is possible to consider that lower happiness is one of the bedrock layers forming the revolutionary attitude. But it's also plausible that "revolutionary" individuals evaluate their life as being less happy. As such, we cannot infer a causal relationship between both variables. But one thing remains clear: both states coexist and, eventually, reinforce each other interactively.

The implications of this association between revolutionary attitude and lower levels of happiness are also a hot topic. One thing seems to be true: avoiding revolutionary actions must not be necessarily a public and political priority. When considering the earlier-cited Declaration of Independence of the United States, which claims that all human action must be guided by the "search of happiness," a fundamental question arises: If we have to rebel ourselves when low happiness levels are present, then where should we place our focus?

11.4   How Can Nations Increase People's Happiness?

Given the above-described evidence, highlighting the importance of happiness to people, we now look upon the third and last question proposed in the chapter, i.e., "How can nations increase their citizens' happiness at a macro-level?" Avoiding an ideological appreciation, we will try to describe scientific research comparing political systems and the role of both democracy and public participation in promoting people's happiness.

The old dichotomy between "utilitarianism" and "egalitarianism" has been used to approach this essential question of promoting happiness at macro-societal level (Veenhoven and Kalmijn 2005). Utilitarians contend that promoting social and economical welfare must follow the logic of "the greater good for the greater number," thereby propping up healthy competition among individuals, which in the end will be better for everyone, even for those who stayed at the rear. Egalitarians, on the other hand, argue that the quality of life of a society depends on the degree of equality that exists between citizens, defending the view that it is the role of the state to intervene and limit the effects of the economic markets. Whereas utilitarianism apologists support the idea that an egalitarian state adds little motivation and stimulation to initiative, egalitarians claim that a state based on unregulated competition promotes a generalized feeling of insecurity among citizens, which becomes counterproductive.

Frey et al. (2008) recently embarked on research where they explored this tension between utilitarianism and egalitarianism by analyzing the objective performance of players from the *Bundesliga*. If utilitarianism apologists are right, then inequality between the football players' income of members of the same team would be a stimulus and motivation for all team players, especially for those who earn less, since they will feel more motivated to improve their performance. In contrast, if teams with more egalitarian income distributions enjoy superior performance, this is a strong argument for supporting the egalitarianism proponents. However, there might be a level of inequality (note that it is the "inequality" that is the subject matter and not "unjustice"!) from which performance differences become unmotivated to all. While some individuals earn much more than others, there are some who have stopped believing that they could someday change their situation.

Based on the objective performance measures of each football player (retrieved from specialized magazines throughout the season), on the one hand, and the players' income estimates of the several *Bundesliga* teams, on the other, Frey et al. (2008) found enough proof to infer that a certain level of equality is necessary to improve not only the citizens' well-being but also their performance. In another way, football teammates who shared higher levels of equal income salary had, on average, superior performance when compared to those belonging to teams with greater salary inequality. Furthermore, this happened because those players who perceived themselves as being on the bottom of the curve (i.e., as earning less) decreased their performance, while the others kept it. On the whole, the average performance of players from these teams was therefore worse than those from teams with less salary inequality. Nevertheless, we cannot consider this type of research as a final and unequivocal test to the old problematic opposing utilitarians and egalitarians. Evidence, however, seems to support the idea that equality promotes the performance of everyone, at least to a certain extent, and, consequently, the performance of the collective.

In addition, other studies conducted at a macro-societal level seem to corroborate Frey and colleagues' findings. Radcliff (2001), for instance, used the 1990 collection data from *World Values Survey* to analyze the political determinants to peoples' satisfaction with life. He based his research on a simple question: Do citizens' levels of satisfaction with life differ in a systematic fashion according to the type of political regime in which they live in? Or in another way, is satisfaction with life greater in countries with socialist, liberal, or conservative dominance?

To categorize the type of political system prevailing in each country, Radcliff considered the indicators previously used by Esping-Anderson, which include the ease to access to social benefits, such as health-care, unemployment benefit, and pension programs. In a simpler way, there is a minimum universal protection for all citizens. Attention must be given to the term "socialist" used in the study, as it actually refers to a social-democratic model, which is quite different from the "statist socialism" (the latter will more properly be included in the "left wing conservatives" group, according to Esping-Anderson's logic).

Radcliff's (2001) results heightened how socialist/social-democratic predominance in a country influences people's satisfaction with life positively and significantly. In contrast, liberal policies have a negative impact on the satisfaction with life reported by people. Although predominantly conservative politics tend to negatively influence satisfaction with life, such influence is not significant as it shows neutrality toward their influence over citizens' satisfaction. In addition, tracing the linear correlation between the satisfaction with life and the left wing parties' dominance (categorized according to the criteria described above), we unequivocally see that countries with left wing political predominance are the ones where citizens report higher levels of happiness.

It is true that Radcliff's (2001) study and others with similar conclusions are not beyond conceptual and methodological criticism. Specifically, one criticism is the fact that only very developed nations are included in the sample, such as Japan, France, the United Kingdom, the United States, Germany, Canada, Finland, Denmark, Norway, and Sweden. And we must not put aside that these left wing governments might be consuming resources hoarded during other governmental periods, therefore bringing happiness at the present moment, which was compensated by a lower happiness in the past that was associated by a cut in expenses. But the consistency of these studies make undeniable the fact that at least a minimum level of security and equality seems to be required for people to report higher levels of satisfaction with life and happiness in a given nation.

One possible explanation for this may rely on a neglect of research in this matter, regarding the distribution of happiness on a population. As is happening in other domains of analysis, the statistical average values tell us very little about a variable's distribution over a population, mainly when they are not accompanied by dispersion and inequality measurements. For example, two countries may have similar average means of well-being in their populations (e.g., South Africa and the United States) but highly asymmetric well-being levels. South Africa, for instance, has a much higher level of well-being distribution asymmetry than the United States, something that confirms other authors' studies (e.g., Ott 2005). Taking into account similar well-being and happiness averages, this might highlight that in one of these countries, well-being is actually concentrated in a privileged minority of the population, while in the other country that well-being is more evenly distributed throughout the population in general.

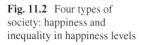

Fig. 11.2 Four types of society: happiness and inequality in happiness levels

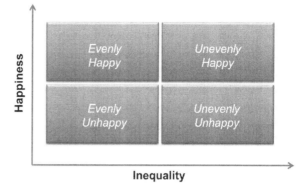

Inspired by this crucial distinction between a nation's average level of happiness and its more or less equalitarian distribution, we present in Fig. 11.2 a table with the possible relationships among these two factors.

As one can see in Fig. 11.2, it's possible to conceptualize the existence of nations where high average levels of happiness co-occur with low levels of inequality. We can call these *Evenly Happy* nations. Others, however, may also present high average levels of happiness but in co-occurrence with high inequality levels, something that makes these nations *Unevenly Happy*. This conceptualization can also be stretched to those nations with low average levels of happiness, in which the combination with low inequality among their population makes them *Evenly Unhappy*, but if inequality is high, such a nation is *Unevenly Unhappy*.

In order to validate this model and find out if each of the four nation types conceptualized correspond to real countries – relying on Ott's (2005) philosophy which considers the standard deviation of answers about happiness an acceptable indicator of the distribution's *inequality* degree of a population's feature – we use the latest *World Values Survey* data available of 2008. In Fig. 11.3, we can see how the collected data about people's happiness distributes across countries, in a way that perfectly fits many of them in each of the four types presented in Fig. 11.2.

However, though all sorts of examples are found for all four nation types, the sample's distribution looks relatively linear and negative. A detailed analysis of the correlation between happiness average and happiness level of inequality, both considered by their standard deviation indexes, shows a negative linear relation. Specifically, when we make a linear regression of the inequality levels over their respective country's averages, we find a considerable explained variance of 12.5 %. Such results show that countries with higher equality levels of happiness are also generally those with higher happiness averages (e.g., Canada, Sweden, or Norway), and vice-versa, which means that higher inequality levels go "hand in hand" with lower average levels of happiness in some countries, such as Iraq, Bulgaria, Zambia, and Ethiopia.

This finding has significant implications over the dichotomist opposition between utilitarianism and egalitarianism, which actually seems to be a false question. Still, those countries where average happiness is maximized in its totality (thesis

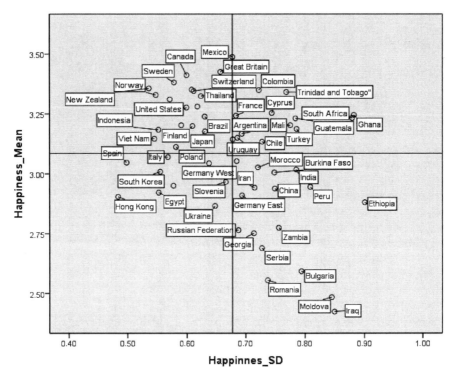

Fig. 11.3 Relationship between average happiness level (average) and inequality in happiness (standard deviation)

contended by the totalitarians) are also those where equality in happiness is higher (thesis contended by the egalitarians). As such, accordingly, equality and the maximization of "greater good for greater numbers," i.e., egalitarianism and utilitarianism, seem possible to reconcile rather than being philosophical opposites, though the mechanism through which this occurs is something yet to be studied in a more systematic fashion. The most likely thing is that both phenomena – the higher egalitarian distribution of happiness and higher happiness average – have in their genesis common institutional and sociopolitical factors. As we shall see next, the best explanation relies on the citizens' involvement and participation on political decisions.

In this way, in order to know how nations can increase their citizens' happiness at a macro-level, we will focus on one of the most researched leverages of happiness: the role of democracy and decentralized governance.

We highlight Frey and Stutzer's (2000) research about satisfaction levels with life in the Swiss cantons. These authors conducted 6,000 interviews, inquiring citizens from 26 Swiss cantons about their satisfaction with life. They also categorized each canton according to their degree of local autonomy and the rights of direct democratic participation, considering both the ease to begin a popular voting and the ease to promote a referendum as indicators (including the number of signatures and the time needed to kick off these processes). Frey and Stutzer's (2000) results clearly give evidence to the importance of the decentralized decision and political-administrative management but also of direct democratic participation in people's satisfaction with their lives. In cantons where local autonomy and direct democratic participation is higher, the reported satisfaction with life is also significantly higher.

Frey and Stutzer (2000) interpret these results by assigning it as "procedural utility." As a matter of fact, it seems that the more the will of voters is represented (which is indeed the basic assumption of representative democratic systems), the more their satisfaction with life, probably because politicians' decisions tend to be closer to the electors' preference, independently of any political decision. Hence, beyond translating the notion of the contingent utility defended by the classic economic models, the "procedural utility" label also postulates that there is also a utility that comes from the process through which choices are carried out.

In sum, research on happiness contributed to a better understanding of what we can do at a macro-level to promote the general well-being of citizens. As we've seen so far, these studies have shown that, among other things, (1) global happiness and equal distribution of happiness in nations are highly correlated, and for that reason the promotion of one does not necessarily oppose the promotion of the other; (2) there is no real tension involving the presumptions contended by utilitarians and the premises advocated by egalitarians; and (3) the causes explaining a high happiness average index are the same of those promoting an equality in happiness distribution in a given population, and some of those causes are local autonomy and direct democratic participation.

Based on the knowledge so far transmitted by happiness studies, we now take another step en route for our last section, where a generic but sustained analysis will be made over the events that occurred during the establishment of the First Portuguese Republic.

11.5   The Case of the First Portuguese Republic's

Keeping in mind what happiness research has told us, we will now turn our attention toward the way the changes in the happiness of Portuguese people can help understand the events which occurred, given the social-political shifts registered during and after the revolution and implementation of the First Republic.

As demonstrated in the previous sections, a growing wave of dissatisfaction may lead to rebellious actions, which can ultimately converge into a broader social and political revolution. In line with the historical facts mentioned by authorities in the subject (e.g., Teixeira 1987), a group of individuals were dissatisfied, both internally and externally (namely, the famous political question of the British Ultimatum), with the country's situation at the end of the Monarchy Regime, which was the root of the revolt. This unsatisfied group was the center of the subsequent revolutionary action that spread all over the country, although Lisbon and Porto were renowned as the main sites of clashes. Such events explain that dissatisfaction with life and the national situation may have ignited revolutionary attitudes as those mentioned by MacCulloch and Pezzini (2007).

But, the consequences born out from the political changes introduced by the leading figures of the new republican regime, in terms of happiness and well-being of citizens, are perhaps the most interesting feature to underscore this extrapolative comment about happiness in the First Portuguese Republic. Inspired by the illuminist canons of the French Revolution and the liberal roots bursting throughout Portugal at least since the 1640 Revolution (Braga 2010), ideologists of republican inclination defended and implemented measures aligned with the factors that predict high happiness and well-being levels, namely, the democratic participation and the decentralized and autonomous administrative regions, as well as the promotion of equality among all citizens, and religious freedom and civil rights, such as the right to divorce.

However, a central question crosses our mind immediately: if that's what happened, then why was the regime established by the First Republic so short lived? Why did it lead to the emergence of a totalitarian regime so shortly after? Why didn't the political actors of the First Republic manage to sustain the Portuguese's happiness and well-being to sufficient standards, enough to prevent the birth of the *Estado Novo* regime (the "New State"), in which an unequivocally fascist tendency generated less satisfaction with life in people? We will next comment on this last question, arguing that two main reasons might explain why the First Republic of Portugal collapsed so relatively quickly.

First, though republicans aimed to achieve a free society embedded in democratic principles, it seems true that, pragmatically, their plan never actually occurred. Quite the opposite in fact, as many historians refer (e.g., Valente 2009), this never came to happen. Though several interpretations of the events, occurred during that time, are still under dispute, republicans' actions were guided by openness to certain rights and freedoms but also by the persecution of other rights and freedoms, such as the persecution of Catholics. So, these early twentieth century republicans shared a narrow-minded vision regarding democratic rights, for a movement inspired by freedom ideals and public participation.

One clear example is the universal right to vote, of which universal suffrage never came into practice given that women weren't allowed to put a cross on the ballot paper. In order to maintain their power, republicans did not fulfill their ideal of a universal suffrage, given that they could suffer an electoral defeat against their monarchist opponents. In the same way, some argue that the censorship carried out on newspapers and the press masked the ideals of freedom and public participation.

To sum up, after the 1910 republican revolution, some democratic freedoms and rights were alienated or diminished, perhaps paradoxically. As a consequence, people's dissatisfaction lengthened until the establishment of Salazar's *Estado Novo*. Probably due to pragmatism, republican's actions were in the antipodes of the ideals defended by the Republic movement itself, thus placing the seed for the totalitarian rule that followed in 1928 and lasted until 1974.

The second reason that might explain the First Republic's collapse derives from recent research which we have been building on, in collaboration with other colleagues, in the domains of regional development and happiness and well-being. Among other relevant conclusions, we have found that the "tolerance" proclaimed by liberal ideals may possibly pose limitations to the creation of an effective economically and socially productive and sustainable society. In that research (Lopes et al. 2011) we studied how perceived tolerance in a given geographical area encourages economic development. We based our work on the "creative cities" research, a phenomenon popularized by Florida (2003), to whom the regional economic development based on knowledge and technology lies in the "creative capacity" of the people who work and live in a given region. According to Florida (2003), such creativity is, in turn, an outcome of the existing tolerance among the inhabitants and other actors of a region, who may impose, or not, obstacles to cultural integration of newcomers and diversified ideas. Hence, creative acts, which can lead to high economic value-added innovations, might be encouraged.

To test the linearity of Florida's (2003) proposals, we have compared several Portuguese municipalities. This research shows that "tolerance is not a sufficient element" to explain a region's economic development (Lopes et al. 2011). Specifically, we found that optimism had a moderating effect on the relationship between tolerance and economic development, as perceived by citizens. In other words, the economic performance perceived by residents was influenced by the cultural tolerance reported by the 3,757 respondents, but only for those citizens who were optimistic about their future. Regarding pessimists, who felt low well-being, we did not observe any effect of tolerance on reported economic performance.

A more straightforward interpretation of these results concerns the crucial role of well-being on the advantages of the diversity that is generated in tolerant contexts. But when quality of life and well-being levels are low, then tolerance (and eventually freedom and democratic participation) stops being so important to people. Perhaps this is another aspect that helps in explaining why freedom and democracy measures and policies, carried out by the early-twentieth-century republicans, didn't have a significant effect on happiness and satisfaction with life. Moreover, maybe this same result helps to explain why the *Estado Novo* regime and its iconic leader António Oliveira Salazar ascended to power in such a meteoric way. As put forward in our paper's discussion (Lopes et al. 2011), research suggested that leadership is indeed one of the main mechanisms for generating hope and optimism in times of crisis. Facing the discontentment and dissatisfaction of people during that time, Salazar's leadership might have found the best fertile soil to prosper, for the better and for the worst.

11.6   Conclusion

Relying on the most recent research in economics, sociology, and happiness psychology, we have tried to illustrate how people's well-being and quality of life influence their behavior and explain many decisions and collective events we live.

As such, it can be critical to understand our past and present life, as well as to project a future with higher levels of happiness and well-being for humans of all nations.

But we must be careful in order not to fall into the illusion that others take the initiative of doing it or that mankind runs "naturally" toward a global state of growing happiness. Not at all! Quite the contrary, it is on our hands to inspire others and to act on an interpersonal level en route to harnessing happiness potential to its fullest level. As we have seen throughout this chapter, we must not despise a macro-social and macroeconomic act, since we need to take action upon political and institutional factors, of which role is central to improving human happiness, such as public participation, direct democracy, and the existence of a state that guarantees every citizen's minimal safety and assures a minimum level of equality in happiness distribution throughout the nation.

With reference to the socioeconomic period we face today, this seems to be the time to act in that direction, transforming what might be seen as adversity into opportunity for positive action. Armed with all the required knowledge to promote the happiness of nations, we must assume the historical responsibility of accomplishing the purpose we are able to fulfill.

Acknowledgments *The authors thank the support given by the Public Administration and Policy Centre (CAAP) of the School of Political and Social Sciences of the* **Lisbon Tech University (ISCSP-UTL).**

References

Bewley, T. (1999). *Why wages don't fall during a recession*. Cambridge: Harvard University Press.
Braga, T. (2010). *História das ideias republicanas em Portugal* (2nd ed.). Lisboa: Veja.
Di Tella, R., MacCulloch, R. J., & Oswald, A. J. (2001). Preferences over inflation and unemployment: Evidence from surveys of happiness. *American Economic Review, 91*(1), 335–341.
Fehr, E., & Gächter, S. (2000). Fairness and retaliation: The economics of reciprocity. *Journal of Economic Perspectives, 14*(3), 159–181.
Florida, R. (2003). Cities and the creative class. *City & Community, 2*(1), 3–19.
Frey, B. S. (2008). *Happiness: A revolution in economics*. Cambridge: MIT Press.
Frey, B. S., & Benz, M. (2008). *Economics and psychology: Imperialism or inspiration?* Working paper presented at the 1st IESE conference on humanizing the firm and the management profession. Available at: http://ssrn.com/abstract=1295285
Frey, B. S., & Stutzer, A. (2000). Happiness, economics, and institutions. *The Economic Journal, 110*(446), 918–938.
Frey, B. S., & Stutzer, A. (2002). What can economists learn from happiness research? *Journal of Economic Literature, 40*(2), 402–435.
Frey, B. S., Schmidt, S. L., & Torgler, B. (2008). Relative income position, inequality and performance: An empirical panel analysis. In P. Andersson, P. Ayton, & C. Schmidt (Eds.), *Myths and facts about football: The economics and psychology of the world's greatest sport* (pp. 349–369). Newcastle: Cambridge Scholars Publishing.
Frey, B. S., Luechinger, S., & Stutzer, A. (2009). The life satisfaction approach to valuing public goods: The case of terrorism. *Public Choice, 138*, 317–345.
Frey, B. S., Savage, D. A., & Torgler, B. (2010). Noblesse oblige? Determinants of survival in a life-and-death situation. *Journal of Economic Behavior & Organization, 74*, 1–11.

Kahneman, D., & Tversky, A. (1979). Prospect theory: An analysis of decision under risk. *Econometrica, 47*(2), 263–291.

Lopes, M. P., Palma, P. J., & Cunha, M. P. (2011). Tolerance is not enough: The moderator role of optimism on perceptions of regional economic performance. *Social Indicators Research, 102*(2), 333–350.

MacCulloch, R., & Pezzini, S. (2007). Money, religion and revolution. *Economics of Governance, 8*, 1–16.

Ott, J. (2005). Level and inequality of happiness in nations: Does greater happiness of a greater number imply greater inequality in happiness? *Journal of Happiness Studies, 6*, 397–420.

Radcliff, B. (2001). Politics, markets, and life satisfaction: The political economy of human happiness. *American Political Science Review, 95*(4), 939–952.

Teixeira, N. S. (1987). Política externa e política interna no Portugal de 1890: o Ultimatum Inglês. *Análise Social, XXIII*(98), 687–719.

Valente, V. P. (2009). *Portugal: Ensaios de História e Política*. Lisboa: Alêtheia.

Veenhoven, R., & Kalmijn, W. (2005). Inequality-adjusted happiness in nations: Egalitarianism and utilitarianism married in a new index of societal performance. *Journal of Happiness Studies, 6*, 421–455.

Chapter 12
Positive Community Psychology and Positive Community Development: Research and Intervention as Transformative-Appreciative Actions

Luis Miguel Neto and Helena Águeda Marujo

12.1 Introduction

In this chapter we aim to address the issues related with the amplification of the relationship between Positive Psychology and Community Psychology and their future development. In that disciplinary future, we include a probable emergence of a subdiscipline under the title of Positive Community Psychology and Positive Community Development. However, we would like to start by considering, as a metaphor, the work of a Swiss engineer, Toni Rüttimann, known as "Toni el Suizo" (El Diario 2008). During the 1970s, after knowing about the isolation of several villages in Ecuador, following an earthquake, Toni decided to offer his engineering knowledge and started to build a bridge that enabled the local habitants to become in contact with the outside word. Once he watched the useful and positive consequences of his initiative, Toni started bridge building in at least three continents. In one of the videos made available to the public, Toni explains some of the strategies of bridge construction: All the participants are local habitants who later on enjoy the fruits of the common labor. The support and sponsorship of engineering products and manufacturing companies from abroad is also essential.

Referring to the bridge-building techniques of construction, Toni says "it should start from the two margins and finish in the connection more or less at the center of the river."

This bridge construction technique and its context of use will serve as an analogy for our endeavor of connecting the future development of Positive Psychology in close association with Community Psychology (CP). From the CP "margin," we will take into concern one of its main characteristic features: the consideration of values, particularly social justice, and the participants' well-being. This sharply contrasts

L.M. Neto (✉) • H. Águeda Marujo
School of Social and Political Sciences, ISCSP, CAPP – Center for Public Policy and
Administration, Technical University of Lisbon, Lisbon P-1349055, Portugal
e-mail: lneto@iscsp.utl.pt; hmarujo@iscsp.utl.pt

H. Águeda Marujo and L.M. Neto (eds.), *Positive Nations and Communities*, Cross-Cultural   209
Advancements in Positive Psychology 6, DOI 10.1007/978-94-007-6869-7_12,
© Springer Science+Business Media Dordrecht 2014

with mainstream Psychology. From the Positive Psychology "margin," we will contemplate issues related with research, particularly an "essential tension" present since the origin of the subdiscipline: to be challenged to do rigorous scientific research and simultaneously being useful in its individual and societal consequences. Both domains share a common intellectual tradition that is rooted in utilitarian seventeenth-century thinking of Jeremy Bentham and other Enlightenment thinkers.

Within the frame of the first "margin," we will stress the need of balancing the collective values, common in CP literature and practice, with the more individual values in Positive Psychology.

After that, we will envision the other "margin," meaning some of the issues related with research in Positive Psychology, particularly – paraphrasing Thomas Kuhn (1977) – in what concerns the "essential tension" between scientific-academic research and individual, cultural, and societal needs. We will conclude this section by connecting the two "margins," using some "materials" borrowed from different works and lines of research and thinking, chiefly by exploiting ideas taken from Donna Mertens' transformative research (Mertens 2009), issues related with the Economy of Happiness (Stiglitz et al. 2009) and Civil Economy and Economy of Communion (Bruni 2012). The final piece for connection has its origins from Paulo Freire's "conscientization" strategies in association with Marujo and Neto's (2011) transformative-appreciative action-research model that is based on Positive Psychology's techniques and is aimed to build empowerment strategies at the speech act level, in research and application.

12.2 Bridge Building from the "Margin of Values": Balancing Collective Values in Community Psychology with Positive Psychology's Individual Values and Strengths

> Poverty leads to an intolerable waste of talent (A. Sen 1999)

> (Values) imply a recognition of the sanctity of human life and the universal right to happiness and self actualization – coupled to the obligation to promote cosmopolitan solidarity and an attitude of respect (A. Giddens 1994, p. 25)
> We expect journal authors to give a detailed account of the statistics employed in their research but there is no demand to justify their values (I. Prilleltensky 2001, p. 747)

Some of the movement initiators like Martin Seligman, Mihaly Csikszentmihalyi, and Chris Peterson explicitly and implicitly used the term "values" almost as a flag or a symbol in major works like the *Values in Action* (VIA) and major titles like *The Life Worth Living*. Other authors also link their empirical research with values, although less directly. This is the case with the Massicampo and Baumeister's (2011) chapter *Finding Positive Value in Human Consciousness: Conscious Thought Serves Participation in Society and Culture*. This special focus on values is particularly significant since in the history of psychology the topic was not always welcome or even considered suitable for scientific study.

The frequent use of the term "values" in distinctive domains, and the different meanings and definitions implied in Psychology's subdisciplines, made its study elusive and marginal when compared with other topics such as personality and individual differences. Prentice (2000) justifies its sparse use in mainstream Psychology given that "theories and research in personality have not encompassed individual differences in views of what is desirable or good (…) Social Psychology, on the other hand, have devoted most of their energies to investigating those psychological states that can be produced or modified by changes in situational contingencies," and "values have not been well positioned to become a central concern of either personality or social psychologists" (Prentice 2000).

However, the above epigraphs point to the explicit use and centrality of values in current social thought. Different domains like Economy, Mathematics, or even Biology use the term with different definitions and meanings. Particularly in Economy, the concept inherits a legacy coming from the Enlightenment's thinkers, such as Adam Smith, Jeremy Bentham, and others. This is so because the concept of value is closely associated with utility, a central concept in Economy. Amartya Sen's and Anthony Giddens' epigraphs above are examples of the importance attributed to values making them some of the most "profound" quotations in all of current literature regarding social sciences. However, this line of thought and these authors are rarely quoted in Positive Psychology and CP, or even taken into consideration.

In this chapter we will try to relate the study of values made in Positive Psychology and CP with the generic understanding of values and life expressed in Sen's and Giddens' perspectives. Additionally, and following Geoffrey Nelson and Isaac Prilleltensky's idea, we will take into consideration the need for balancing values as a pivotal issue. If we assume that the ideals of the French Revolution – freedom, fraternity, and equality – helped to define modernity, the need to give them similar weight is of particular importance (Nelson and Prilleltensky 2005). Expanding the values' balance idea, we also consider the need to establish an equilibrium between the more individual values considered in Positive Psychology with the collective ones, which are part of CP intervention and research. Considering again Sen's perspective, it is worth reflecting his notion of capabilities, a derivation of the mentioned concept of utility and later expanded by Martha Nussbaum (Jayawickreme and Pawelski 2012). Later we will relate it with the study and practice of values considered in Positive Psychology and CP.

Sen defines capabilities in a way that gives large possibilities for positive and community psychologists to expand the common definitions and uses of values. He defines and contextualizes capabilities in the following manner:

> Each of these distinct type of rights and opportunities help to develop the general capability of a person. They may also serve to complement each other … Freedoms are not only the primary ends of development they are also among its principal means. In addition to acknowledging, foundationally, the evaluative importance of freedom, we also have to understand the remarkable empirical connection that links freedoms of different kinds with one another. Political freedoms (in the form of free speeches and elections) help to promote economical

security. Social opportunities, (in the form of education and health facilities) facilitate economic participation. Economic facilities (in the form for participation in trade and production) can help to generate personal abundance as well as public resources for social facilities. Freedoms of different kinds can strengthen one another. (Sen 1999, pp. 10–11)

12.3   The Study of Values Within Social and Mainstream Psychology

Before the questions related with values emerged in Positive Psychology, some basic research, especially in Social Psychology, pointed to its importance. This is particularly true in a very unique exemplar of research published by Adorno and colleagues (1950) on *The Authoritarian Personality*. Later on, Social Psychology explored the issues related with discrimination, race, gender, or age prejudices (North and Fiske 2012). All of these and other related researches were somewhat minimalist and based on "negative values" even when aimed at solving very important social issues, especially in North American society. This line of research framed in the Social Psychology tradition defined values in diverse ways. For instance, Prentice (2000) defined values as "beliefs pertaining to desirable states or modes of conduct that transcend specific situations, are organized into coherent systems and guide selection and evaluation of people, behaviors and events." The issue of the functions of beliefs was also addressed in Social Psychology literature: "They are presumed to regulate a person's adjustment to his or her social world. Other members of this family include attitudes, needs, traits, norms and interests, all of which overlap" (idem). However, even if the study of values in Social Psychology corresponds to an objective of dealing and offering solutions in socially relevant matters, some social psychologists consider that "values have been an important topic of theory and research in social sciences: By contrast, psychologists have devoted little research attention to values, especially relative to traits and attitudes" (ibidem). More generally, in terms of definition, Kekes (1993) defined values as "benefits that human beings provide to each other." The same author also gives the examples of love and esteem as "moral goods." To frame the concept of values in this kind of definition and equating them with "moral goods" is important when one tries to relate the development of Positive Psychology and CP with Economy, as we will do in the end of this chapter. Another important contributor, Schwartz (1994), defines values as a "guiding principle in the person's life or other social entity."

12.3.1   The Issue of Value Assessment

In *The Study of Values* (SOV), Gordon Allport et al. (1960) measured the relative prominence of six basic interests or motives in personality, namely, Theoretical, Economic, Aesthetic, Social, Political, and Religious. The respondents were expected to express preferences among pairs of sets of options that involve trade-offs along with these six basic values. They were asked questions like "Which of the following men do you think should be judge as contributing to the progress of mankind? (A) Aristotle (B) Abraham Lincoln." Respondents were supposed to distribute three points between the two options – reflecting theoretical and social values.

In 1973 Milton Rokeach wrote *The Nature of Human Values*, where he created the RVS, i.e., Rokeach Value System, in an easier way to administer the procedure. The RVS included 18 modes of conduct and 18 end-states of existence. The respondents were presented with 2 lists of 18 values each and asked to rank the items on each list "in order of importance to you, as a guiding principle in your life." One list contains terminal values, i.e., desired end-states of existence: comfortable life, exciting life, sense of accomplishment, a world at peace, a world of beauty, equality, family security, freedom, happiness, inner harmony, mature love, national security, pleasure, salvation, self-respect, social recognition, true friendship, and wisdom.

The other list contains instrumental values and desirable modes of conduct: ambitious, broad-minded, capable, cheerful, clean, courageous, forgiving, helpful, honest, imaginative, independent, intellectual, logical, loving, obedient, polite, responsible, and self-controlled.

Like the Gordon Allport's and team SOV's, Milton Rokeach and team RVS's meets acceptable standards of reliability and distinguishes sensibly between demographic groups. However, both research teams had to face the almost insurmountable issue of little consistency and predictability between expressed values and behavior. Posterior research somehow tried to solve this issue. For instance, S. Schwartz (2001) followed and adapted M. Rokeach's (1973) assessment of values and Inglehart followed Abraham Maslow's hierarchy of needs in his own taxonomy (Inglehart and Klingemann 2000).

All things considered, "when significant correlations between values and attitudes or values and behaviors have emerged, they have been weak, with values typically accounting for less than 5 % of the variance in attitudes and behaviors" (Prentice 2000). (See Tables 12.1 and 12.2 for a historical perspective on Social Psychology values research.)

12.3.2   The Authoritarian Personality Study and the Mandate to Change Toxic Values

It's worth noting the study Adorno et al. (1950) oversaw entitled *The Authoritarian Personality*, giving its sensitive nature and societal consequences. After World War II, the issues related with dictatorships and the psychological origin of abuse of power were particularly significant. Theodor Adorno, a German *émigré*, lead that remarkable research in which values where addressed both at the personal and societal levels.

Also as a part of the history of the study of values in Social Psychology, encouraging evidence has come from experimental studies labeled as "value self-confrontation." Pioneered also by Milton Rokeach (1968, 1973, 1979), value

Table 12.1 Values' content in Social Psychology research: a historical view adapted from Peterson (2006)

Allport et al. (1937)	Scott (1959)	M. Rokeach (1973)	Inglehart (1990) – after A. Maslow	Sissela Bok (1995)	S. Schwartz (1992)
1. Theoretical	1. Achievement	1. Comfortable life	1. Survival	1. Positive duties: caring and reciprocity	1. Achievement
2. Economic	2. Creativity	2. Exciting life	2. Self-expressive	2. Negative injunctions: violence, deceit, and betrayal	2. Benevolence and welfare of others
3. Aesthetic	3. Honesty	3. Sense of accomplishment		3. Fairness and procedural justice	3. Conformity
4. Political	4. Independence	4. Peace			4. Hedonism
5. Social	5. Intellectualism	5. Beauty			5. Power
6. Religious	6. Kindness	6. Equality			6. Security
	7. Loyalty	7. Family security			7. Self-direction
	8. Physical prowess	8. Freedom			8. Stimulation
	9. Religiousness	9. Happiness			9. Tradition
	10. Self-control	10. Inner harmony			10. Universalism
	11. Social skills	11. Mature love			
	12. Status	12. National security			
		13. Pleasure			
		14. Salvation			
		15. Self-respect			
		16. Social recognition			
		17. True friendship			
		18. Wisdom			

Table 12.2 Research on "emergent values" (Peterson 2006, pp. 178, 179) and values relationship with culture, ideology, and institutions

W. Scott (1965)	G. Hofstede (2001)	T. Kasser (2005)	P. Freire (1970), Braithwaite (2000)
Emerging values in fraternities and sororities in US campus during the 1960s	Common values in the same international corporation Cultural dimensions: feminine/masculine Proximity/distance to power; individualistic/collective	Time as "affluence" an affordance, a personal good to specific groups in society	"*Conscientization*" – becoming aware of own life social constraints (what about "blessings"?) *Empowerment* seen at micro, meso, and macro levels of life

self-confrontation was a strategy for inducing change in values. It involved presenting individuals with feedback and interpretations concerning the values, attitudes, and behaviors of themselves and their significant others. The theory is that for some, this information will induce a state of self-dissatisfaction by making them aware that they hold beliefs that violate their sense of themselves as moral and competent. As a mean of reducing this dissatisfaction, these individuals will change their values, attitudes, and behaviors to become more consistent with their self-conceptions.

Also worth noting by its consequential and transformational potential is the study done by Sandra Ball-Rokeach, Milton Rokeach, and Joel Grube – *The Great American Values Test: Influencing Behavior and Belief Through Television* (1984). In it the authors compared the influence of attitudes toward people of other races, genders, and the environment, using an educationally and research-designed TV show.

12.3.3   The Study of Values and Economy

One of the aims of this chapter consists in drawing attention for the need in integrating new ways to think of economy, especially in what concerns the issues related with the study of values. At this level it is also worth considering a historical perspective. For example, Jeffrey Skansky (2002) analyzed what concerns the fruitful relationship between Social Psychology and the US economy models after the Civil War. In fact, during the seventeenth century, the US economy was in a crisis situation since its models were failing to account for changes in manufacturing, labor relations, and property ownership. During that time, the notion of an independent "economic man" was no longer sufficient. The author adds, "the self governing individual, endowed with the natural faculties of rational will and productive labor, entitled to the natural rights of property and popular sovereignty." However, Social Psychology research and literature made available by the new emergent discipline, economists were enabled to respond and to "reconceive market society as a fast moving mainstream of culturally created desires, habits and mores, instead of an

unchanging arena of contract and competition among independent proprietors."
Additionally, accordingly to Sklansky (2002) "Social Psychology of that era represented a progressive challenge to reigning ethics of competition and accumulation
which had become loosely identified with the old science of wealth" (idem pp. 9,
10). This meant the at-the-time emergent Social Psychology helped economy to
overcome a stalemate and find appropriate ways of development.

Recent ways of thinking made available in the social sciences additionally provided new mentalities that could be applied to economy. Because of this, the New
Economic Foundation (among others) draws attention to the consideration of
unusual indicators of development beyond the GDP, such as the ecological footprint
left by progress. Table 12.3 sums up some of the contributions made to this issue.
See also Chap. 10 by G. Burns' in this volume.

Aligned with the need of considering new ways of thinking in economy are
investigations done by economists such as Richard Layard that used research done
in Positive Psychology and on happiness studies and integrated it in a new area of
empirical study (Layard 2005). This line of thought, which incorporates data from
well-being studies, became known as the Economy of Happiness. In the United
Kingdom, an official research branch was created in order to provide official public
policies with research originated in well-being and Positive Psychology studies.
Other economists assumed the "mandate" of integrating research on subjective
well-being and Positive Psychology with Economy. In France, an official committee was created including Nobel laureates Amartya Sen and Joseph Stiglitz, who
produced what was labeled as the "Sarkozy report" (Stiglitz et al. 2009). In a close
relationship between religious-societal values and the need to rethink the foundations of economy, relating it with other Human and Social Sciences, it's worth
mentioning the work undergone by Luigino Bruni of Italy, one of the promoters of
the so-called Civil and Communion Economy (Bruni 2012) and, in the United
States, Daniel Finn (2006), author of *The Moral Ecology of Markets: Assessing
Claims about Markets and Justice*. This integration between different domains of
the social and human sciences mirrors a famous observation made by Alex
Tocqueville, a French intellectual of the nineteenth century:

> Should I call it a blessing from God, or a last malediction of His anger, this disposition of
> the soul that makes men insensible to extreme misery? Plunged in this abyss of wretched-
> ness, the slave hardly notices his ill fortune: he was reduced to slavery by violence, and the
> habit of servitude has given him the thoughts and ambitions of a slave. (Tocqueville
> 1969/1839, cited in Menzel 1999)

Tocqueville's and Sen's thinking perspectives challenge mainstream economy
models but also some Positive Psychology assumptions, in particular when Positive
Psychology makes the *Reductio ad Unum* of sternly considering rigor in the collection of data coming from strict individual evaluations, with no consideration of
context and its values. This is particularly evident in Sen's work especially
concerning his idea of capabilities.

The ideas related with the capabilities model from Martha Nussbaum, one of the
most influential and eminent current social thinkers, are an enlargement and a recon-
sideration of Sen's work (Nussbaum 2003). Based on their approach, we developed
a set of "conscientization" (Freire 1970) questions made explicit on Table 12.4.

Table 12.3 Positive Psychology and Community Psychology milestones in the context of some Human and Social Science's discontinuities

Social psychology	Economy	Demography and ecology	Education	Community psychology	Positive psychology
Hadley Cantril (1965): *Patterns of Human Concern*		Rome Club Report			
Social Psychology crisis	Tibor Scitovsky (1976): *The Joyless Economy*	Richard Easterlin (1974): "Easterlin Paradox"		Rappaport (1977): *Community Psychology: Values, Research and Action*	
K. Gergen (1974) Social Psychology research as History	Amartya Sen (1977): *Rational Fouls*				
R. Harré and P. Secord (1972)			Michael Patton (1980): *Qualitative Evaluation Methods*		
Discursive Psychology (UK) Social Constructionism (USA)		Edward Wilson (2002): *The Future of Life*	H. Gardner (1983) Theory of Multiple Intelligences		American Psychologist January 2000
	Economy of Happiness and Communion	New Economics Foundation	*Good Work Project*		Akumal Manifesto; VIA (Peterson and Seligman 2004)

Table 12.4 Martha Nussbaum and Amartya Sen's capabilities, VIA virtues, and transformative-appreciative questioning

Capabilities (cfr. Nussbaum and Sen 1993)	VIA: Virtues (Seligman and Peterson 2004)	Transformative-appreciative *Conscientization* questioning
1. Living a normal life span	Wisdom and knowledge Humanity	"What's your main purpose in life? What do you want to accomplish?"
2. Bodily health, adequate nourishment and shelter	Humanity	"How does the health and the infrastructures of people around you invite you to take initiatives on their behalf?"
3. Bodily integrity (including freedom of movement and security against assault, as well as freedom of choice in reproduction and in matters of sexual satisfaction)	Humanity Temperance	"What's the smallest step for you to feel free, safe, and to make your own personal choices?"
4. Being able to use the senses, the imagination, and thought (including freedom of expression, religious exercise, and adequate education) and being able to have pleasurable experiences	Transcendence Temperance	"Please describe one situation that you were at your best. How was that possible? What did you offer to the situation and the people involved?"
5. Experiencing normal human emotions	Courage Humanity Temperance	"How would you describe your most common feelings and disposition? What does this say about your character?"
6. Development of capacities for practical reasons (liberties of consciousness and religious freedom)	Temperance	"When did you feel you should stand for your rights and the rights of other people?"
7. Capabilities for affiliation, caring, and commiserate with others	Humanity	"When did you feel more in touch with people in need? How did they respond to your helpful initiatives?"
8. Living with other species	Humanity	"What was the most important lesson that you learned from the relationship you have with your pet? From the animals of your farm?"
9. Play, including enjoying recreational activities	Wisdom and knowledge	"Please describe a situation when you and your significant others felt enthusiastic and alive while playing, enjoying nature, doing sports, and performing arts"
10. Control over one's environment (political participation, freedom of association, equal opportunities)	Temperance	"When did you most enjoy a collective expression of needs and wants? How did you help the situation to make it fruitful?"

Another of Sen's most cited quotations concerns the "happy slave," an apparent oxymoron referring to a very consequential paradox of consciousness. In a parenthetic note, we decided to "transform" this quotation into a poetic form (Richardson 1992) for reasons that will become explicit in the second part of this chapter, the "alternative research margin." Again, giving a new form to Sen's words while respecting profoundly its intended meaning:

The "happy slave" poetic quotation

If a starving wreck,
ravished by famine,
buffeted by disease,
is made happy by some mental conditioning,
the person will be seen as doing well
on this mental states perspective. (Sen 1985, p. 188)

The defeated and the downtrodden
come to lack the courage to desire things
that others,
more favorably treated by society,
desire with easy confidence. (Sen 1985, p. 15)

It's difficult to maintain a strict scientific standard when facing human flaws simultaneously at the individual and collective levels. This process of *interiorization* and *subjectification* of oppressive supra-individual structures is one of the major challenges for the Social and Human Sciences. Some historical processes and events like slavery (cfr. Edmond Morgan's *The Big American Crime*, 2003), the holocaust, or even recent examples of genocide, inequality, and abuse strike us as humans and scientists. However, the situation is not hopeless. In the recent history of Social and Human Sciences, examples are abundant. We will consider Paulo Freire's "*conscientization*" approach (1970) given its conceptual proximity with our own transformative-appreciative model. Some of these chapters inspired by Positive Psychology scientific literature also address dramatic and inhumane historical and social events in a more than promising way (see, for instance the chapters in this volume referring to South African and Brazilian solutions to historical and social circumstances). Besides, wasn't it seeing and doing things differently one of Positive Psychology's major aims and tenets?

Next we will continue to consider the importance of values from a Community Psychology theory and practice perspective.

12.3.4 Values in Community Psychology

Community Psychology is a well-defined field with a specific history and emergence (Rappaport 1977). Beyond the disciplinary links with Psychology and Psychiatry-Clinical, Social, Psychometrics, and testing practices, liaison Psychiatry – the disenchantment of some of its first-generation proponents was, and still is, obvious. This still-observable disenchantment with the mainstream was also related with the civil rights movement that brought a new kind of social conscience to the USA and to the western world. A new moral order emerged and its consequences were very clear to the first generation of Community Psychologists in the USA. However, other major influences originated in South and Central America. Two examples, among others, are the work of Paulo Freire, a Brazilian educator, with illiterate citizens in Brazil and Martin-Baró, a Jesuit priest, who gathered people from impoverished areas in San Salvador. They conceptualized the concepts of community empowerment through a social collective process of "gaining awareness," in Spanish *darse cuenta*. As mentioned before, Paulo Freire coined the word "conscientization," an English neologism, derived from the Portuguese *conscientização*.

In fact, some of the questions initially addressed by Community Psychology include community leadership, well-being at the level of local communities, social integration and cohesion, quality of life, empowerment, and social justice. All of this is linked directly with marginalized and oppressed populations.

In a vivid metaphor, a well-known community psychologist, Isaac Prilleltensky, once asked an audience in a Positive Nations Conference held in Lisbon in 2010 to consider the following situation: "Imagine you own a palace in Venice, right in the Grand Canal. As the years go by you started noticing that the median water level is rapidly climbing each year, putting your property at risk. Whatever you can think of doing in your palace does not solve the problem. What are you going to do?" Of course, the needed solutions require simultaneously global and local actions. This metaphor also applies to other areas of the world, like New Orleans, or other ocean and river shores, for instance, in Bangladesh. Another dramatic story when a community-driven solution was needed occurred during an epidemic of cholera that arose in London in the nineteenth century. John Snow, a physician, carried out one of the first epidemiological studies and interventions and was able to detect the origin of the problem: an infected water pump on Broad Street, used by locals as a water source. After the pump was closed, the epidemic started to recede. Remarkably, John Snow solved the problem without the scientific understating of what caused the epidemic, since a microbiological bacterial theory wasn't established at the time (Prentice 2000). However, beyond the dramatic consequences of climate change and biological hazards emergent in different areas of the world, other socially complex phenomena deserve, at least, the same level of complex solutions. Another well-known and remarkable example relates with the studies and interventions done in Ypsilanti, Michigan, with preschoolers. In fact, using a *quasi*-experimental design methodology, the head authors, Mary Hohmann and David Weikart (Hohmann and Weikart 1995), were able to compare the long-term results of the regular preschool curriculum and an approach in the USA based on the research done by Swiss developmental psychologist Jean Piaget. Twenty years later, the students involved with the new program had a higher rate of high school completion, lower number of arrests, and higher levels of economic achievement. Even though a causal link couldn't (and shouldn't) be established, those results were really remarkable, especially since the population of students involved belonged to an impoverished social community in the Chicago area.

However, following the scientific and value-based path described briefly before, we need to go well beyond a mere list of interventions and case studies, even when they show remarkable results. It is our conviction that values shouldn't be lost while accumulating data and results in the scientific literature. When considering the link between Positive Psychology and CP, several issues are raised, given the fact that the two domains have different histories and the scientific communities, researchers, and practitioners involved are only marginally connected. Even concepts have different meanings, methods of assessment, and application. It is worth considering that facing gaps and edges is a part of the growing pains and the expansion of every Human and Social Science.

If we aim to address issues related with the consequences of a possible merge between Positive Psychology and CP, it's important to consider events and situations from the recent history of the human and social sciences. In a remarkable historical example, Leon Festinger, a preeminent social psychologist, gave a speech to the Social Psychology researchers and raised one aspect of the issue: "Social Psychology is 99 % North American" (Festinger 1962, cit. in Kruglanski and Stroebe 2012, p. 8). Implicit was the need to expand and adapt to other cultures. Scientific domains, subdisciplines, and application fields need to build bridges but also need to learn from the past. A Positive Psychology that is almost exclusively North American and English-speaking and a CP that is mostly South American creates a tremendous waste of specific information for scientists, practitioners, and the populations they serve. We think that the cross-fertilization should be more than a mere metaphor for Positive Psychology and CP. The subdiscipline cross-fertilization should be simultaneously accompanied by some historical and cultural consciousness and sensitivity.

Within the CP frame of theory and practice, a clear conscience emerged leading to consider all its interventions rooted in diverse types of values. Some authors like Nelson and Prilleltensky (2005) emphasize and typify values according to their roots:

(a) Some are rooted in an ideal tradition deriving from moral, political, and spiritual thinking.
(b) Others are based on the studies of social sciences of communities, emphasizing the understanding of actual conditions, stressing the related needs.
(c) A third group is rooted in the psychological way of analyzing the experience and the needs of individuals belonging to certain communities.
(d) Finally, from a social activist point of view, some people base their social and community action derived from espoused theories of social change.

We will try to focus on the relationship between the use of values in the strategies of CP and some Positive Psychology ways of assessment, particularly the VIA, and others described in the empirical literature techniques. We will also point to the use of discursive strategies used by the authors in the transformative-appreciative, speech act land social episode level, conscience-raising frame. The foundations of this model have its roots in the coordinated management of meaning model (Pearce 1994). The practical features involved were derived from the appreciative inquiry model (Srivastva and Cooperrider 1999) and Mertens' (2009) transformative approach.

Table 12.5 From values for community praxis to relationship between values and behavior and to transformative-appreciative *conscientization's* inducing dialogues (cfr. Prilleltensky 2001; Peterson 2006; Marujo and Neto 2011)

Community praxis values (Prilleltensky 2001)	Criteria for enhancing relationship between value and behavior (Peterson 2006, p. 168)	Appreciative-transformative questions to induce "conscientization" (Freire 1970; Marujo and Neto 2011)
Self-determination	Circumstances: "Values stemming from direct experience are more consistent"	"What were the circumstances the last time you experienced any kind of self-determination in the community?"
Health	Identity: "The degree to which a value helps to define a person's self-image"	"Given your health status, how might the community help you? How do you see yourself possibly making a difference in the community?"
Personal growth	Self-consciousness: "Mindful enacting of social scripts makes behavior more consistent with values"	"Please describe a situation when you felt competent, acknowledged, and contributing to your community"
Social justice	Evaluation: "A person's evaluation of the particular behavior that supposedly reflects the values in question"	"When was it possible for your community to share resources and goods with the people in need? How did you accomplish that?"
Support for enabling community structures	Generality: More global and abstract values are less predictive of consistent behavior	"Please tell me the solutions your community found to solve housing and situations where infrastructure is needed."
Respect for diversity	Scope, relevance, frequency: "Behaviors are more likely to reflect values if we look at the total of what someone does"	"Can you please give examples of inclusion you remember from your community? How can that be amplified in the future?"
Collaboration and democratic participation	Circumstances	"When was the participation of community members to solve common issues in society more significant?"

We exemplify its use while pointing to the relationships between the use of values in CP's praxis (Prilleltensky 2001) and the criteria to enhance the association between behaviors and beliefs (Peterson 2006). We will present examples in Table 12.5 in its two parts. The first links Prilleltensky's praxis values (2001) and Peterson's (2006) empirical results of circumstances that strengthen the link between beliefs and behavior. The second part links that with some exemplars of transformative-appreciative questioning aimed to induce dialogues for "conscientization" and critical consciousness. Another table also points to the interventions at the speech act and communicational to empower level, crossing CP praxis-based values with VIA character strengths (Peterson and Seligman 2004). Finally, we crossed those with applied transformative-appreciative-conscientization questions, in order dialogues (cfr. Table 12.6).

Table 12.6 Values for community development praxis, self-others, mind-heart dimensions and relevant VIA strengths and proposal of appreciative-transformative questions

Community praxis values (Prilleltensky 2001)	Character strengths (Peterson and Seligman 2004) more relevant for community values	Empowerment-transformative-appreciative questions to induce dialogue (examples of possible questions) (Marujo and Neto 2011)
Self-determination	Creativity Learning Bravery Perspective Perseverance Self-regulation Open-mindness	1. "When were you at your top while experiencing creativity/perspective (etc.)?" 2. "What gave/brought life to that experience?" 3. "How do you think you can replicate that in the future?"
Health	Curiosity Creativity Zest Learning Teamwork Fairness Modesty Leadership	1. "Please tell me when your curiosity about the health situation of the community leads to an experience of teamwork in the community you were working with"
Personal growth	Curiosity Zest Hope Social intelligence Beauty Religiousness	1. "When were you at your top when experiencing curiosity/zest (etc.)?" 2. "What gave/brought life to that experience?" 3. "How do you think you can replicate that in the future?"
Social justice	Teamwork Leadership Forgiveness Kindness Gratitude Love Humor	1. "When were you at your top in a social justice context (teamwork, leadership, etc.)?" 2. "What gave/brought life to that experience?" 3. "How do you think you can replicate that in the future?"
Support for enabling community structures	Fairness Modesty Authenticity Prudence	1. "When were you at your top (experiencing fairness, modesty, etc.) in an enabling community situation?" 2. "What gave/brought life to that experience?" 3. "How do you think you can replicate that in the future?"
Respect for diversity	Teamwork Leadership Forgiveness Kindness Gratitude Love Humor	1. "When were you at your top in a context (teamwork, leadership, etc.) that respects diversity?" 2. "What gave/brought life to that experience?" 3. "How do you think you can replicate that in the future?"

(continued)

Table 12.6 (continued)

Community praxis values (Prilleltensky 2001)	Character strengths (Peterson and Seligman 2004) more relevant for community values	Empowerment-transformative-appreciative questions to induce dialogue (examples of possible questions) (Marujo and Neto 2011)
Collaboration and democratic participation	Fairness Modesty Authenticity Prudence	1. "When were you at your top (fairness, modesty, etc.) in a situation of collaboration and democratic participation?" 2. "What gave/brought life to that experience?" 3. "How do you think you can replicate that in the future?"

12.4 "Bridge Building from the Research Margin": Bringing in More Humane-Scientific Methods

> The gentleness of a methodological question remains as long as it stays fruitful
>
> (Bruni 2012).

> Science must begin with myths, and the criticism of myths; neither with the collection of observations, nor with the invention of experiments, but with the critical discussion of myths, and of magical techniques and practices.
>
> (Karl Popper 1963/1984, p. 50).

Research in Positive Psychology and Community Psychology is empirical and methodologically scientific in nature. However, it follows different purposes and modus operandi, according to the degree of historical evolution and context of each subdiscipline. Like in the above description of values, definition, assessment, and general usefulness, the status and goals of research share obvious features but also include significant differences in Positive Psychology and CP.

In order to identify the potential in the similarities and differences in research of the two subdisciplines, we are going to consider:

(a) Firstly, some specific methods, some of them unique, that defined the identity of the fields
(b) Secondly, to comment and infer about possible cross-fertilization of approaches, methods, and techniques
(c) Lastly, to give examples and make suggestions to a new generation of researchers-practitioners

12.4.1 Jacob's Ladder "Take II"

One symbol from the Bible is Jacob's ladder. In it, angels come up and down making communication possible between heaven and earth. The ladder is indeed a very vivid metaphor to describe the flux of life and communication between different realms. Given the importance of Hadley Cantril (1965), one is tempted to use "ladder methodology" as an upgrade of the Old Testament's symbol. However, there's a huge difference (to say the least): while angels could move in the old ladder, participants in social science research using Cantril's ladder stay frozen on the point of the scale they select. We give much importance to this "little-big" detail. This is because we have decades of experience in the scaling question, which is part of the solution-oriented psychotherapy tradition (Shazer et al. 2007). In this technique, instead of a fixed reality, like material steps in a ladder, the numbers of the 1–10 scale are used to identify objectives and promote change in the client's life. The individual research participant is without doubt in a different situation. She or he isn't a researcher's "client." However, especially in face of self-attributed low ratings in happiness, should the researcher leave the field and the research participant in that situation? The situation seems analogous if someone with a broken arm heading to the hospital was just given an X-ray and a diagnosis: "You have a broken arm!" and … that's all! As social and human researchers, we have a mandate that goes well beyond the mere extraction of qualities and numbers from social realities and humans involved in it. Serious community and social situations exemplify the evolving awareness of this issue, such as Grant Rich's quoted "Alaska case" (see his Chap. 2 in this volume).

The research situation in Positive Psychology should be an empowering moment for the participant and the researcher, as already is the case with most of the research done in Community Psychology, given its own transformative nature and critical consciousness raising consequences.

12.4.2   Pandora's "Take II": Opening the Paradox Box – Happiness in North and South America

One of the most fruitful and useful questions recently rose by the Social and Human Sciences appeared in the studies of the Economy of Happiness and is related with the so-called happiness paradox. Since the research done by Richard Easterlin (1974), the association between happiness and income was found to be nonlinear. In fact, in the same country, not all the rich people are happy, and when comparing between countries, the poor countries aren't necessarily less happy than the rich ones. This finding is called the "Easterlin paradox" and is still open to criticism and debate. This line of research exemplifies the use of objective methods being heavily based on statistical procedures and huge amounts of impersonal aggregates of data. This is very understandable given the background on Demography from Richard Easterlin. The "Easterlin paradox" attracted the consideration of other powerful paradoxes to the scientific literature of the Human and Social Sciences: David Myers (2001) called attention to *The* [North] *American Paradox*, while Ruut Veenhoven (2011) pointed out that the levels of happiness found in South America were lower than what would be expected, labeling the phenomenon the "South American paradox."

These kinds of polemics have a relevant social function in science since it helps scientists to popularize science findings. However, it simultaneously obscures social realities. Most of the time, people are able to withstand incredibly difficult situations. More than strictly discussing the quality of scientific representations of lived experience, it would be significant to know how people endure extreme life situations and survive well beyond the identified paradoxes such as the mentioned "Happy Slave." The ESM (Experience Sampling Method), the DRM (Daily Reconstruction Method), and the transformative-appreciative "conscientization" model are examples of methodologies in Positive and Community Psychology aimed to that endeavor.

12.4.3 The Use of "Systematic Phenomenology" in Research

Since their origin, the methods used in Positive Psychology are common to other areas and disciplines, especially Social Psychology. This is so due to a clear epistemological stance that requires an analogous position with mainstream empirical Psychology research methods. However, while some Positive Psychology researchers started to rebel against what was labeled as a "variable-centric world" by Kashdan and Steger (2011), others advocate an integration to mainstream Psychology (Sheldon 2011). This plurality of Epistemology frames and methods might be a sign of maturity within a phase of growth in the Positive Psychology field. It parallels other situations such as Herbert Blumer's presidential address to the American Sociology Association on the exclusive use of quantitative data and methods, titled *Sociological Analysis and the Variable* (Blumer 1956). More recently it also parallels the Social Psychology crisis during the 1970s. However, Positive Psychology's origin stood closely linked to "normal science": being empirically based and relying on an objective stance. Even so, there are remarkable methodological innovations in the set of scientific methods adopted in Positive Psychology. Some of them are clearly distinctive in the larger frame of the social and human sciences. Beyond the previously mentioned cases of M. Csikszentmihalyi's ESM (Experience Sampling Method) and Daniel Kahneman's DRM (Daily Reconstruction Method), we also should consider Christopher Peterson's interview based on the Values in Action, VIA assessment questionnaire. All of these methodologies have a distant but powerful root and a rigorous and, simultaneously, meaningful phenomenological stance. In one of Mihaly Csikszentmihalyi's concepts, they refer to "systematic phenomenology," meaning to be able to see through the research participant's eyes how he or she sees his or her life and experience – while using empirically and scientifically validated methods (Csikszentmihalyi 1997, p. 4). We claim that other methods besides the ones described above are simultaneously empirically sound, reproducible, and suitable to be trained, learned, and validated. Importantly, they are already available in the literature. However, they are not sufficiently acknowledged, especially by positive psychologists. Considering this, we would like to underline Christopher Petersons' attention to Scott's (1965, cited in Peterson 2006, pp. 170, 171) "interview strategy" to study emergent values with students in the USA:

> Think about the various people you admire, and try to reflect on what it is about them that is admirable. Now consider the general question: What is it about any person that makes him/her good? What personal traits would you say are particularly admirable? ... Please think about the traits you have mentioned ... which ones do you think are inherently good, and should properly be regarded as good by all people?

This is an outstanding example of a research question that is parallel, in our view, with the appreciative and transformational and with the "conscientization" at the speech act and social episode model herein advocated (see Tables 12.4, 12.5 and 12.6). This type of interview is frequently used in diverse qualitative studies done in various domains and settings. At this level, and aiming to enhance the amount of methods in use, we would like to call to attention the analytic work of Laurel Richardson (1992). She uses a poetic frame as an interview analysis strategy, which is very unique even for qualitative study methodologies. An empirical use of poetry has an ancient intellectual ancestry, going back to Aristotle's *poietike techne,* an empirical and useful means to reach and dive into the constant flux of the "river of life."

12.4.4   Research Suggestions and Some Final Words Concerning Big Historical Processes

Positive Psychology and Community Psychology opened up huge windows of possibility to enhance individual and collective lives. At the same time, we live in a historical moment full of challenges and perils. One of these, as Jurgen Habermas' reflections pointed, is to see the future as a repetition of the past, not including the "other" in our experience (Habermas 1971, 1982). As previously done in the aftermath of 9/11, it's time for a Positive Psychology and Positive Community Psychology to address historical challenging processes such as the Truth and Reconciliation Commission experience in South Africa, Collective Forgiveness episodes like the one reported in Brazil, and Spain's Historical Memory movement. Colleagues in this volume address some of these issues brilliantly.

References

Adorno, T. W., Frenkel-Brunswik, E., Levinson, D. J., & Sanford, R. N. (1950). *The authoritarian personality.* New York: Harper & Row.

Allport, G. W. (1937). *Personality: A psychological interpretation.* New York: Macmillan.

Allport, G., Vernon, P., & Lindzey, G. (1960). *A study of values* (3rd ed.). Boston: Houghton Mifflin.

Ball-Rokeach, S. J., Rokeach, M., & Grube, J. W. (1984). *The great American values test: Influencing behavior and belief through television.* New York: Free Press.

Blumer, H. (1956). Sociological analysis and the "variable". *American Sociological Review, 21*, 683–690.

Bok, S. (1995). *Common values*. Columbia: University of Missouri Press.

Braithwaite, R. L. (2000). Empowerment. In A. Kazdin (Ed.), *Encyclopedia of psychology* (Vol. 3, pp. 193–194). Washington, DC: APA /Oxford University Press.

Bruni, L. (2012). *The wound and the blessing: Economics, Relationships and happiness*. New York: New City Press. (Published originally in Italian in 2007)

Cantril, H. (1965). *The pattern of human concerns*. New Brunswick, NJ: Rutgers University Press.

Csikszentmihalyi, M. (1997). *Finding flow: The psychology of engagement with everyday life*. New York: Basic Books.

Easterlin, R. A. (1974). Does economic growth improve the human lot? In P. A. David & M. W. Reder (Eds.), *Nations and households in economic growth: Essays in honor of Moses Abramovitz*. New York: Academic Press, Inc.

El Diario. (2008, December). *Toni el Suizo y Walter Yánez construyeron 14 puentes*. http://www. eldiario.com.ec/noticias-manabi-ecuador/101388-toni-el-suizo-y-walter-yanez-construyeron-14-puentes/. Accessed Sept 2012.

Finn, D. (2006). *The moral ecology of markets: Assessing claims about markets and justice*. Cambridge, MA: Cambridge University Press.

Freire, P. (1970). *Pedagogy of the oppressed*. New York: Herder & Herder.

Gardner, H. (1983). *Frames of mind. The theory of multiple intelligences*. New York: BasicBooks.

Gergen, K. (1974). Social psychology as history. *Journal of Personality and Social Psychology, 1973, 26*, 309–320. Reprinted in *XIP readings in psychology*. Xerox College Publishing, 1974.

Giddens, A. (1994). *Beyond left and right: The future of radical politics*. Cambridge: Polity Press.

Habermas, J. (1971). *Knowledge and human interests*. Boston: Beacon.

Habermas, J. (1982). *Theory of communicative action*. Boston: Beacon.

Harré, R., & Secord, P. F. (1972). *The explanation of social behaviour*. Oxford: Blackwell.

Hofstede, G. (2001). *Culture's consequences: Comparing values, behaviors, institutions, and organizations across nations* (2nd ed.). Thousand Oaks: Sage Publications, Inc.

Hohmann, M., & Weikart, D. (1995). *Educating young children*. Ypsilanti: High Scope Educational Research Foundation.

Inglehart, R. (1990). *Culture shift in advanced industrial society*. Princeton: Princeton University Press.

Inglehart, R., & Klingemann, H. D. (2000). Genes, culture, democracy and happiness. In E. Diener & E. M. Suh (Eds.), *Culture and subjective well being* (pp. 165–183). Cambridge, MA: MIT Press.

Jayawickreme, E., & Pawelski, J. O. (2012). Positivity and the capabilities approach. *Philosophical Psychology, 2012*, 1–18. doi:10.1080/09515089.2012.660687.

Justice. *Feminist Economics, 9*(2–3), 33–59.

Kashdan, T., & Steger, M. (2011). Challenges, pitfalls and aspirations for positive psychology. In K. Sheldon, T. B. Kashdan, & M. F. Steger (Eds.), *Designing positive psychology: Taking stock and moving forward* (pp. 9–21). Oxford: Oxford University Press.

Kasser, T. (2005). Personal aspirations, the "good life", and the law. *Deakin Law Review, 10*, 33–47.

Kekes, J. (1993). *The morality of pluralism*. Princeton: Princeton University Press.

Kruglanski, A., & Stroebe, W. (2012). *Handbook of the history of social psychology*. New York: Psychology Press.

Kuhn, T. S. (1977). *The essential tension: Selected studies in scientific tradition and change*. Chicago: The University of Chicago Press.

Layard, R. (2005). *Happiness: Lessons from a new science*. London: Penguin.

Marujo, H., & Neto, L. (2011). Investigação Transformativa e Apreciativa: Um elogio da Subjetividade na Contemporaneidade. *Ecos, Revista de Investigação Contemporânea da Subjetividade, 1*(1), 1–14. http://www.uff.br/periodicoshumanas/index.php/ecos/article/view/714/546. Accessed May 2012.

Massicampo, E. J., & Baumeister, R. (2011). Finding positive value in human consciousness: Conscious thoughts serves participation in society and culture. In K. Sheldon, T. B. Kashdan, & M. F. Steger (Eds.), *Designing positive psychology: Taking stock and moving forward* (pp. 175–189). Oxford: Oxford University Press.

Menzel, P. (1999, April 1). *How should what economists call "social values" be measured?*. Society for Ethics meeting at the Pacific Division, American Philosophical Association, Berkeley, CA.

Mertens, D. M. (2009). *Transformative research and evaluation*. New York: Guilford Press.

Morgan, E. (2003, December 3). The Big American Crime, *New York Book Review, 45*, 19, 14–18.

Myers, G. D. (2001). *The American paradox: Spiritual hunger in an age of plenty*. Yale: Yale University Press.

Nelson, G., & Prilleltensky, I. (2005). *Community psychology: In pursuit of liberation and well-being*. London: Palgrave Macmillan.

North, M., & Fiske, S. (2012). A history of social cognition. In A. W. Kruglanski & W. Stroebe (Eds.), *Handbook of social psychology*. New York: Psychology Press.

Nussbaum, M. C. (2003, July/November). Capabilities as fundamental entitlements: Sen and social justice. *Feminist Economics, 9*(2 & 3), 33–60.

Nussbaum, M., & Sen, A. (1993). *The quality of life*. Oxford: Clarendon.

Patton, M. (1980). *Qualitative evaluation and research methods* (2nd ed.). Newbury Park: Sage.

Pearce, W. B. (1994). *Interpersonal communication: Making social worlds*. New York: Harper Collins College Publishers.

Peterson, C. (2006). *A primer in positive psychology*. Oxford: Oxford University Press.

Peterson, C., & Seligman, M. E. P. (2004). *Character strengths and virtues: A handbook and classification*. Oxford: Oxford University Press.

Popper, K. (1963). *Conjectures and refutations*. London: Routledge & Kegan Paul.

Prentice, D. (2000). Community psychology: Prevention and intervention. In A. Kazdin (Ed.), *Encyclopedia of psychology* (Vol. 2, pp. 219–224). Washington, DC: APA/Oxford University Press.

Prilleltensky, I. (2001). Value-based praxis in community psychology: Moving toward social justice and social action. *American Journal of Community Psychology, 29*(5), 747–778.

Rappaport, J. (1977). *Community psychology: Values, research & action*. New York: Holt, Rinehart & Winston.

Richardson, L. (1992). The consequences of poetic representation: Writing the other, rewriting the self. In C. Ellis & M. G. Flaherty (Eds.), *Investigating subjectivity: Research on lived experience*. Newbury Park: Sage.

Rokeach, M. (1968). *Beliefs, attitudes, and values*. San Francisco: Jossey-Bass.

Rokeach, M. (1973). *The nature of human values*. New York: Free Press.

Rokeach, M. (1979). *Understanding human values*. New York: Free Press.

Schwartz, S. H. (1992). Universals in the content and structure of values: Theoretical advances and empirical tests in 20 countries. *Advances in Experimental Social Psychology, 25*, 1–65.

Schwartz, S. H. (1994). Are there universal aspects in the structure and contents of human values? *Journal of Social Issues, 50*(4), 19–45.

Schwartz, S. H. (2001). Existem Aspectos Universales em la Estructura y Contendio de los Valores Humanos? In M. Ross & V. V. Gouveia (Eds.), *Psicologia Social de los Valores Humanos* (pp. 53–73). Madrid: Biblioteca Nueva.

Scitovsky, T. (1992 [1976]). *The joyless economy: The psychology of human satisfaction* (Rev. ed.). Oxford: Oxford University Press.

Scott, W. (1959). Empirical assessment of values and ideologies. *American Sociological Review, 24*, 299–310.

Scott, W. A. (1965). *Values and organizations: A study of Fraternities and Sororities*. Chicago: Rand McNally & Co.

Sen, A. K. (1977). Rational fools: A critique of the behavioral foundations of economic theory. *Philosophy and Public Affairs, 6*(4), 317–344. http://philpapers.org/rec/SENRFA

Sen, A. K. (1985). *Commodities and capabilities*. Amsterdam: North-Holland.

Sen, A. K. (1999). *Development as freedom*. Oxford: Oxford University Press.

Shazer, S., Dolan, Y., Korman, H., Trepper, T., McCollum, E., & Berg, I. K. (2007). *More than miracles: The state of the art of solution-focused brief therapy*. New York: Haworth Press.

Sheldon, K. (2011). What's positive about positive psychology? Reducing value-bias and enhancing integration within the field. In K. Sheldon, T. B. Kashdan, & M. F. Steger (Eds.), *Designing positive psychology: Taking stock and moving forward* (pp. 421–429). Oxford: Oxford University Press.

Sheldon, K., Kashdan, T. B., & Steger, M. F. (Eds.). (2011). *Designing positive psychology: Taking stock and moving forward*. Oxford: Oxford University Press.

Sklansky, J. (2002). *The soul's economy: Market society and selfhood in American thought, 1820–1920*. Chapel Hill: University of North Carolina Press.

Srivastva, S., & Cooperrider, D. (1999). *Appreciative management and leadership* (Rev. ed.). Euclid: Williams Custom Publishing.

Stiglitz, J. E., Sen, A., & Fitoussi, J. A. (2009). *Report by the commission on the measurement of economic performance and social progress*, OECD.

Tocqueville, A. de (1969). *Democracy in America*. New York: Anchor Books. (Originally published in 1839)

Veenhoven, R. (2011). *Life satisfaction in nations*. Published in French in Securité Sociale CHSS 6/2011, 9:298–302 ISSN 1420–2689

Wilson, E. O. (2002). *The future of life*. London: Abacus.

Chapter 13
From South-West Africa to Namibia: Subjective Well-Being Twenty-One Years After Independence

Martina Perstling and Sebastiaan Rothmann

13.1 Introduction

Formerly known as South-West Africa, Namibia, under the administration of South Africa, was governed according to a policy of apartheid. The apartheid regime, as early as 1945, gradually started segregating nonwhite from white people. The harshest was the homeland policy, put into practice by President Verwoerd of South Africa in 1962. Stratifications in terms of access to resources were determined by race and migrant labor contributed to the wealth of white-owned economic resources. In opposition, SWAPO (South-West African People's Organization) struggled for human rights and equality. A prolonged bush-war eventually led to the independence of Namibia in 1990. The United Nations was called in to secure a peaceful election during the 7th and 11th of November 1989. SWAPO consequently took the reign over Namibia from the South African Administration in 1990.

New legislations, assuring equality in terms of accessibility of resources, helped to create a sense of security in the culturally diverse nation. Churches did not get involved in the liberation struggle. They consistently supported the people of Namibia since 1971 by not condemning those who did partake and advocated love and peace as opposed to violence. The first president, Dr. Sam Nujoma declared his commitment to national reconciliation, including former detainees and military opponents. Former labor migration and the liberation struggle took its sacrifices in terms of disrupting family life and trust between people, especially in the northern

M. Perstling (✉)
Department of Psychology, Faculty of Humanities and Social Sciences,
University of Namibia, Windhoek, Namibia

Clinical Psychologist Private Practice, Windhoek, Namibia
e-mail: martinap@mtcmobile.com.na

S. Rothmann
Faculty of Humanities, North West University, Vanderbijlpark, South Africa
e-mail: ian@ianrothmann.com

H. Águeda Marujo and L.M. Neto (eds.), *Positive Nations and Communities*, Cross-Cultural
Advancements in Positive Psychology 6, DOI 10.1007/978-94-007-6869-7_13,
© Springer Science+Business Media Dordrecht 2014

regions of Namibia. Eight years after independence, the detainee question could not be resolved. This led to the National Society of Human Rights and the CCN to call for a truth and reconciliation commission to bring closure.

Namibia is susceptible to postwar consequences. Past educational disadvantages together with a limited self-sustaining industry, Namibia's economic development was hampered. Liveability in terms of happiness is influenced by economic affluence, political freedom and rule of law, state welfare, income inequality, and tolerance. Recently, researchers initiated the assessment of subjective well-being of Namibians. Initiatives to incorporating existing colonial monuments and historical artifacts in museums are continuously enriched by traditional artifacts and historical monuments – a visible indication of an ongoing effort to incorporate the past into the present aiming to build a constructive future.

13.2   Europeans Influence Over Southern Africa

In order to better conceptualize Namibia as a nation, one cannot avoid the historical background. Many cultures are united in one common geographical space, with many different languages, dialects, and traditions. Through events within the past centuries, African traditional life has been distorted and a new lifestyle has developed as a result of early European influences.

A term for the Afrikaans word apartheid is "separateness" (Goosen et al. 2007; O'Callaghan 2011). Before independence in 1990, Namibia was called South-West Africa, at first a German colony and finally under the political and economic administration of South Africa. To better understand Namibia's struggle for freedom, an epigrammatic venture into the intertwined history and sociology of South Africans and Namibians, former South-West Africans, is needed.

13.2.1   Demographical Overview

Before the existence of geographical borders in Africa, the people of southern Africa constituted a few main cultures with many subcultures. Namibia's Africans at large stem from the South African Bantu (Ovambo, Herero, Kavango), San, and Khoikhoi (Nama, Damara, San) communities. The Khoisan community stems from a mixture of tribes (O'Callaghan 2011; Hishongwa 1992). The Ovambo, also referred to as Oshiwambo, settled in the northern, most fertile regions. The Ovambo tribe has seven subcultures. It is estimated that at precolonial times, the Ovambo constituted half a million people (Hishongwa 1992). In 1886, the population within the borderlines of Namibia was approximately 200,000 indigenous people and 200 Europeans (Breyer 1979), while the census of 1991 showed a population of 1.4 million and in 2001 rose to 1.8 million (National Planning Commission 2001). In 2001 the Ovambo represents 48 % of Namibia's population, while non-African (white/European, Colored, and Baster) communities jointly accounted for 11 %

(National Planning Commission 2001), indicating a decline in white (European) societies since it was estimated that during 1977, 12 % alone constituted white (European) people (Hishongwa 1992).

13.2.2   Europe Conquers Africa

Prior to European settlers, African livelihood was determined by a self-sustaining lifestyle (O'Callaghan 2011). Rainfall determined fertility of land, which influenced survival, health, and population growth (Hishongwa 1992). Communities lived in tribes, called chiefdoms. Land usage was granted by the respective chiefs. Sometimes tribes would consolidate for the purpose of maintaining power over other communities. Land was not owned or fenced in. Usage of a specific area was granted for a particular period of time only. Tribes consisted of large family systems, mostly paternally related (Hishongwa 1992; O'Callaghan 2011). Communal ownership, equality, and family unity indicate that socialism is a preexisting condition to traditional African societies (Goosen et al. 2007).

Settling in southern Africa gradually started with the discovery of the sea route to India by Portuguese sailors during 1486. The first landing in Namibia was at Angra Pequena, today called Lüderitzbucht. Later a natural harbor, called Walvis Bay, in Namibia was used in addition. The desert and murky water discouraged sailors for many years to proceed to the inland (Hishongwa 1992). The Cape was inhabited by the Dutch in 1652, serving as a supply base. With the increase of the European community, later known as the Boers or Afrikaners, they started to move inland. Boers mixed with Khoikhoi tribes, creating semi-Westernized communities, living similar lifestyles as the Western settlers, including utilization of clothes, horses, ox wagons, and weapons. As the settler community increased, they continued to push inland and were fought off by African tribes. In 1806 the British Government took reign over the colony, of which the legal system commanded equal land for all and abolishment of slavery of African communities. This was not well received by the Boers, as Africans were used as cheap labor and frequently poorly treated. Boers, who had settled at the inland borderlines of the colony, were increasingly at risk to be raided by African tribes. Since the British Government did not support the Boers in their struggles at the borderlines, the Boers decided to move further inland. This mass migration in 1835 was called the Great Trek, and the participants were referred to as the Voortrekkers (O'Callaghan 2011). A new society with a new lifestyle formed. The danger, hardships, and death came with the Great Trek. With their victories over African communities in the venture to create their own colony, they developed a sense of superiority among Boers (Kros 2010; O'Callaghan 2011).

Boer families lived in a patriarchal family tradition, strictly in accordance with the Calvinist-Reformed doctrine. As a result of the hardships endured by women, during the Great Trek and Anglo-Boer war, women were seen as an icon within the family and society. Henceforth, they were referred to as the "Volksmoeder" (van der Watt 2009), creating a traditional role of women being the head of the house, while men were the head of the household.

The Great Trek laid firm foundations for the Boers to socially and politically dominate the European community in South Africa, which for the British meant weakened control over the colony (O'Callaghan 2011). However, after the Anglo-Boer war during 1899 and 1902, the Boers lost the two republics: Orange Free State and Transvaal (Goosen et al. 2007).

For Africans, the disaster started with the Great Trek. It meant loss of land, lives, and mostly independence. The Great Trek laid the foundations for over a century of oppression, regardless of which European power would dominate (O'Callaghan 2011).

13.2.3 Europe's Contribution Toward Exploitation

Europe's industrial revolution (1760–1830) contributed to Africa's colonization. People emigrated from Europe as a result of change in family system from the agricultural society to the nuclear society, which reduced the quality of life detrimentally. Industrialization decreased income from formerly handmade products, forcing people to seek work in factories. Child labor in factories was on daily order just as much as fatal accidents (May 1987; Parsons 1977). Workers were described as dark shadows, rushing to work, struggling for survival on meager wages and extensive labor-intense hours, alienated from families (Brown 1992). Capitalism was growing in Europe and extended its greedy arms to Africa, given that Africa harbored much sought after raw materials. The growing population as a result of improved health care in Europe, as well as decreased quality of life due to the transition from a community-based existence to nuclear existence, became a push factor for Europeans to emigrate. The new colonies had hope as a valuable pull factor, hope for a better life, especially in terms of capitalism (Brown 1992; May 1987). Raw materials were extracted from colonies such as cotton, tea, coffee, and unrefined mining material, creating countless opportunities. Ironically, once refined, the same raw products returned to the colonies as commodities, obviously at an increased price. France, for example, would import raw materials at the worth of 199 million pounds during 1815 and export-refined commodities worth 422 million pounds (Clough and Cole 1966).

Taking Europe's conditions pertaining to the labor force into consideration, it is clear that humane treatment regarding laborers was not a work industry's concern at that time. This, together with Europeans motivation to gain economic wealth, influenced human mistreatment in Africa.

13.2.4 Inhabitation of Namibia (Former South-West Africa)

Europeans which chose to emigrate from Europe to the arid, former, South-West Africa were described to the least, of being adventurous, while others described them as rather suicidal (Breyer 1979; May 1987).

Contradicting general perception, land acquisition in Namibia during the nineteenth century was a gradual process (Vedder 1985). European traders started to trade with indigenous tribes. In exchange for alcohol, weapons, and material, Europeans received ostrich feathers and eggs, cattle, as well as farms. The first sold farms in Namibia were the Farms Haruchas, for 215 lb, and Farms Tsawisis, Holoog, and Groedorn for 800 lb. Those farms were sold to white settlers by Chief Willem Cristian, of Warmbad, against the will of the Herero Chief Maharero. During 1880, 150 Europeans lived as missionaries, hunters, merchants, and farmers in Namibia. Lethal wars between tribes led to respective African Chiefs to seek support of Europeans in their struggles. As from 1870s Boers attempted to settle in Namibia. Typically, the permission of the tribal Chief, having jurisdiction over the respective region, was to be obtained before settlers were allowed. This did not always go smoothly. For example, the van Zyl clan sought such permission from Chief Maharero in the Okahandja region. First obtaining that permission but then losing it consequently van Zyl fled, was sheltered by missionaries however, still ended up murdered by his bushman servant (Vedder 1985).

Predominantly, settlers stemmed from Boer inhabitants in former South-West Africa, due to land scarcity in South African regions and the increasing interest of Portuguese and German Europeans (Vedder 1985). Eventually, Germany took control over former South-West Africa, during 1880, henceforth calling it "Deutsch Süd-West Afrika" (German South-West Africa).

A German businessman, named Lüderitz through his accountant of Jewish descent, one Vogelsang, obtained permission to purchase land from the Chief of Bethanie. Angra Pequena was renamed Lüderitzbucht: a small coastal desert town in the south, of which the surrounding area is still rich in diamonds (Breyer 1979). Before realizing the riches, Vogelsang, in the name of Lüderitz (Breyer 1979), bought Angra Pequena and surrounding land, in a 5 mile radius, from the Chief of Bethanie for 100 lb in Gold and 200 Westley-Richards rifles. He continued purchasing land for Lüderitz, forming the basis for the German colony. Consequentially, from 1884 Lüderitz' land was under the formal protection of the German Government. Between finding the first diamond and 1914, the surroundings of Lüderitzbucht gave off seven million carats of diamond for the German colony.

Germany did not interfere in the trading for land between the respective Chiefs and Europeans (Vedder 1985) nor did Germany buy land from the Chiefs. Germany did however enter agreements of protection with the Herero and Nama Chiefs, initiated by the delegates, Göring and Büttner. After having suffered over a decade of tribal warfare, the tribal Chiefs welcomed the protection offered by the German Government. As a result, the Chiefs Manasse (Hochachanas and Omaruru regions, respectively), Hermanus van Wyk (Rehoboth region), and Maharero (Okahandja region) signed peace treaties in 1885. During the time of negotiating the peace treaties, there was the unfortunate death of Lüderitz, by drowning, in 1886 (Breyer 1979). His land was transferred to the German Government, since there was no heir. Borderline agreements between Germany and Portugal as well as Britain were disrespected, and the land was taken by the Germans. This marked the founding of the German colony in 1884 (Breyer 1979; Mlambo 2011). German ruling focused on creating an infrastructure based on capitalism, not one of formal oppression (Mlambo 2011). Europeans, mainly Germans, as well as Boers continued to settle in former South-West Africa. Under the German Government the most fruitful areas, called the Police Zone, were restricted for use by the indigenous people according to the Native Regulation. Outside these areas, Africans had more freedom. Migrant laborers within the Police Zone were negotiated with the respective Chief (O'Callaghan 2011). Only half a century after German colonization, oppression was formalized by legislation under the administration of South Africa. Migrant labor was introduced during colonial times.

13.3   Oppressing Equal Social, Economic, and Educational Development Through Apartheid

After the start of World War I, South African military defeated the German forces in former South-West Africa. After Germany lost in World War I, among others, according to the treaty of Versailles, signed on the 28th of June in 1919, they had to give up all overseas colonies. Hence, German colonies were handed over to the newly formed League of Nations, which created mandate territories, to be governed, but not owned, by members of the League. Former South-West Africa was placed under the mandate of South Africa during 1919 (Anderson 2008; O'Callaghan 2011). The aim of mandates was to guide former colonies into an independent state, and ideally, international supervision should protect its people from oppression. During 1922 and 1923, the Bondelswarts and Rehoboth community of former South-West Africa fought South Africa's oppression – unsuccessfully. The League dissolved. South Africa saw its chance to request the incorporation of former South-West Africa into South Africa from the United Nations Organization (UNO), who replaced the dissolved League. However, the UNO declared all mandated territories of the League to be under their supervision (O'Callaghan 2011). All mandate holders adhered, apart from South Africa (Anderson 2008). The fact that power was never transferred to the UNO from the League of Nations before it dissolved suited the South African government well in their future refusals to accept the UNO as authority while holding on to former South-West Africa. Power plays continued with former South-West Africa as an ideal platform. South Africa maintained the mandate over former South-West Africa, aggressively supporting their action with the argument that the UNO was not the inherent descendant of the League of Nations (Irwin 2010). The reluctance of the UNO to allow incorporation into South Africa was a product of increasing requests from Namibia's Africans for their rights and prevention to incorporate Namibia into South Africa (O'Callaghan 2011). In 1968 the UNO recognized "Namibia" as the name for former South-West Africa (O'Callaghan 2011). It was however only until after 1990 that the name changed from South-West Africa to Namibia by the countries' inhabitants. For clarity purposes, former South-West Africa will henceforth be called Namibia.

Although the make-belief to the external world was that Namibia was a dry arid country being an economic burden to South Africa (Anderson 2008), during the twentieth century, commercial farming bloomed under the white settlers occupying 50 % of the farmland, while indigenous people were confined to 25 % of the land (Hunter 2004). Unequal land distribution (Horsthemke 2004), divided a multicultural society into two distinct groups, generating two separate developmental structures differentiating even more so through the initiation of the apartheid regime.

The worldwide propaganda advocating freedom and end of oppression encouraged black South Africans/Namibians to conceptualize and act in favor of racial equality. During World War II, only white militants were allowed to carry arms, assigning the role of noncombat support to African volunteers. This decision rooted in fear that adequate military training may result in war against the minority white-dominating population of South Africa. Still, the South African government, to which Namibia was subordinate, relaxed the racial bar, increasing job opportunity for Africans. Public talks by the Secretary of Native Affairs, Douglas Smit, encouraged the government in 1942 to abandon unjust segregation. This was however not to the taste of the opposing party, being the National Party (NP). By 1945 the NP theorized that "...every race has a unique destiny of its own and a unique cultural contribution to make to the world. Different races should therefore be kept separate, so that each can develop within their own cultures. In the case of South Africa this meant that each race should be allocated an area of the country as its 'homeland' where it could live in its own way" (O'Callaghan 2011, p. 280). Practically, however, the formal apartheid system was merely an extension of the racial segregation and exploitation which had taken place since 1910. Homelands would be 12 % of South Africa's soil to be assigned to black Africans. Homeland was land without mineral resources, industry, and ports. Therefore, all social and political powers were minimized (O'Callaghan 2011). Resulting from developments, such as South Africa withdrawing from the Commonwealth, international isolation grew from 1960 onward. Prime Minister Dr. Hendrik Frensch Verwoerd, a former psychology professor and driving implementer of the segregation system, survived an attempted of assassination by a white farmer in 1960 and deceased consequential to another attempt by a black parliamentary messenger in 1966. Although the requirements for a parliamentary messenger were to be a white South African, the assassin slipped through the bureaucratic system despite a gloomy past and being of Swazi-Portuguese descent, originating from Mozambique. It is not clear how this could have happened, as South Africa took social segregation, in terms of employment policy, serious at the time (Lauren and Swartz 2011).

According to the 1924 Native Reserves Regulation, Africans were confined to reserves in order to eradicate African "vagabonds" from the so-called white areas. Africans had no right to land ownership outside the reserves. The 1920 Vagrancy Proclamation secured the obligation of Africans, who seemingly could not sustain themselves, to work for the white-owned industry (Mlambo 2011). The dissatisfaction of the UNO grew at the rate that the apartheid policies tightened. During 1948 the UNO condemned the National Party (NP), led by a minister of the Dutch Reformed Church, Daniel F. Malan, for their "...nationalist paranoia and God-ordained white supremacy..." (Anderson 2008, p. 313), marking the official beginning of the apartheid system in 1948 under the leadership of the NP leading to the legalized apartheid system of South Africa in 1948 (O'Callaghan 2011).

Various Acts were developed in order to assure segregation between black, Asians, as well as colored people and the white community. For example, the marriage between white and nonwhites was not allowed (Prohibition of Mixed Marriages Act of 1949), prohibiting sexual contact between whites and nonwhites (Immorality Act of 1950), classification according to race (Population Registration Act of 1950), separation of residential areas according to race (Group Areas Act of 1950), to remove surplus natives to emergency camp (prevention of Illegal Squatters Act of 1951), every black person outside the native reserves was to carry a passbook (Native Abolition passes Act of 1952), and nonwhite students were not allowed to study the same syllabus as white students (Bantu Education Act of 1953). As in the Mines and Works Act of 1911, skilled work was reserved for whites and unskilled work for nonwhites (Mines and Works Act of 1911) (Goosen et al. 2007).

According to the late local sociologist Annelie Odendaal (Isaak and Lombard 2002), the only nonracial form of oppression transcending cultures and religion throughout pre-independent Namibia's societies was patriarchy. This was confirmed in that especially white women, who crossed the race barrier, were regarded as nymphomaniacs, consequentially institutionalized and declared as deviant and insane. In contradiction typically white men having sex with black women was of no concern. The case history of Bessie Head (Pucherova 2011), being an illicit child of an upper class white woman and black worker, stated that her mother committed suicide after having been in a mental hospital for 6 years as a result of illicit sex with a black man. Bessie was given up for adoption as newborn and raised by a colored family.

Although the resistance against oppression started as early as 1946, in which African leaders repeatedly sought support from the UNO, the Odendaal Commission was set up by South Africa in 1964. Implementation of the homeland policy became reality (O'Callaghan 2011). The Odendaal Report validated the homeland setup with the promise to grant indigenous people control over their local, tribal, and territorial interactions, supported by time-consuming and monetary investments in social modernization programs aimed to enable their self-government (Irwin 2010). Almost 30 % of Namibian Africans were relocated to the reserves, naturally with resistance (O'Callaghan 2011). Evidently, forthwith violations against human rights were inflicted upon (Irwin 2010).

13.4   Migrant Labor and Its Effect on the People

Initially, the migrant labor system was formally introduced by the Native Administration Proclamation No. 11 of 1922, and until 1972 only African men were allowed to migrate (Winterfeldt 2002). Labor migration was connected to land distribution based on the Odendaal Commission in 1963. In accordance with the Odendaal

Commission, roughly 40 % of land was divided into 11 African reserves, or native homeland areas, for 88.5 % of Namibia's population. The remaining 60 % were divided among the 11.5 % of the white population. The latter areas consisted of the most fertile land as well as the land with most mineral resources (Mlambo 2011). As early as during the German colonial times, the contract labor system was introduced but until 1940 was at large limited to the Africans within the Police Zone (Winterfeldt 2002). Tribal chiefs received remuneration from the German Government for each laborer that they would recommend to work in mines, build infrastructure, and cultivate farms (Goosen et al. 2007; Mlambo 2011; Winterfeldt 2002). Even though contract labor system had its origin during the German colonial time, the northern part of former South-West Africa, being Ovamboland, was not under direct German rule and therefore also not subject to colonial taxation or expropriation policies. These were only introduced under the South African regime. For the Ovambo people, to resort to migrant labor was at large attributed to socioeconomic factors mainly as a result from environmental challenges (Winterfeldt 2002).

Work contracts would vary between 9 and 18 months, after which the worker would be sent home. The contract labor system had advantages as wages for the employees could be kept rather low due to sufficient supply of laborers from the tribal areas (Goosen et al. 2007; Mlambo 2011). Africans would not be able to easily settle in the so-called white areas and so become a possible political threat (Winterfeldt 2002). One African, Reverend Michael Scott, investigated matters in the former South-West Africa for the UNO, as South Africa opposed any outside observers about African's living conditions. Scott immediately understood the relationship between land ownership, economic advantages, and labor migration (Anderson 2008).

13.4.1   Migrant Laborers and Basic Psychological Needs

It is documented that during 1975 a vast difference in terms of wages between white unskilled laborers and migrant laborers existed. Migrant laborers could hardly sustain themselves economically. During 1971 migrant workers accounted for 88 % of the total labor force of Namibia (Mlambo 2011). There were no fixed working hours for contract laborers, which resulted in exploitation (Hishongwa 1992). Workers were allocated according to physical strengths and had no choice in the work they were allocated for (Goosen et al. 2007; Mlambo 2011).

Working conditions for migrant laborers were rather disastrous. The rationale was that workers would return home to their families after the contract was fulfilled; therefore, there was no need to supply housing. Instead they were housed in compounds, or hostels, of which the conditions were often cramped and described by workers as "prison-like" sleeping arrangements and food supply (Goosen et al. 2007; Mlambo 2011). Compounds were segregated between black and mixed-race workers. Fifteen black African workers would share one room as mixed-race African workers would share a room among four workers. At Rössing Uranium Mine, for example, toilet facilities for black workers were in one long room, allowing no privacy (Goosen et al. 2007; Mlambo 2011). Interviews with migrant workers described their housing in general as dreadful, overcrowded, and lacking privacy, a stench of urine hanging over the compounds (Hishongwa 1992). Other mines were not less dreadful. Compounds were in general poorly maintained however sometimes less crowded. Mines like CDM, Uis Tin Mine, and TCL housed 4–12 workers in one room. White workers were accommodated in free-standing houses per family. In the compounds, food was often poor, served strictly at certain times which led to logistical problems preventing workers frequently from one or other meal intake due to shifts and distance between workplace and dining hall. No choice was provided. Food was of basic nature and extreme poor quality (Hishongwa 1992). Others angrily described the conditions in general as inhumane (Goosen et al. 2007; Mlambo 2011), forced to wear identification around the neck, similar to dog tags, creating a feeling of humiliation (Mlambo 2011). According to Maslow's self-actualizing theory (Meyer et al. 1997), consisting of five hierarchical needs, the most basic psychological need determining survival includes the need to satisfy hunger, thirst, sleep, activity, sensory stimulation, and sexual gratification. These needs have been reduced to the minimal by the migrant labor system.

There were little safety precautions and health care for workers (Mlambo 2011). Health-care services were minimal for black Africans, with small and poorly staffed clinics often lacking medical specialists. Especially in mines and fishery industry, the nature of work led to ill-health conditions among African workers, which were only randomly attended to. Unsanitary conditions of compounds also brought illnesses, as serious and contagious as tuberculosis (Hishongwa 1992). Farm workers were reported to have been vulnerable to physical assault, sometimes resulting in death (Mlambo 2011). Once the most basic psychological needs are satisfied (Meyer et al. 1997), other secondary needs such as safety, in terms of security, stability, protection, structure, law and order, and freedom of fear were also been jeopardized.

Women in the tribal areas, or homelands, were often left alone and needed to take the traditional roles of their husbands over. This meant plowing land, farming and taking care of the cattle, and building and maintaining their houses in addition to their own traditional chores: cultivating fields, milking cows, raising small stock, cooking, and taking care of children, the sick, and elders. Often being overworked reflected negatively on education, health, and production standards of food (Goosen et al. 2007). Social disruptions implicated that men would not live with their families, in average for one quarter of their lifetime (Hishongwa 1992; Winterfeldt 2002). Some never returned home and others ended supporting two families, one in the urban and the other in the rural area (Hishongwa 1992). Often adulterous affairs caused marital and economic distress, as frequently the man's much needed wages needed by his family at home were shared with a mistress (Goosen et al. 2007; Mlambo 2011). Traditionally, adultery within the Ovambo culture was deeply immoral, causing a psychological struggle between loneliness and deviance (Hishongwa 1992). Psychological effects were alienation from wives and children, resulting in emotions of sadness, bitterness (Hishongwa 1992), and longing for their loved ones

(Goosen et al. 2007; Hishongwa 1992; Mlambo 2011). Marriage often affected since couples as tradition forbid couples to live together before marriage and men were sent at an early age, often also to earn their dowry. Out of economic need, or fear of not being reemployed, men remained home only for short periods, often not long enough to know their new wives, witness the birth of their children, and take care of the traditional responsibilities and presence at birth. Women were equally helpless and had no influence over their husband's urban life. Whether a man chose to return from urban life, extend an existing contract, or abandon his rural family altogether was solely based upon the husband's morality and goodwill. During 1970 a migrant laborers' time with his family varied between a few weeks to 6 months per year (Hishongwa 1992). The third need for love and affiliation has also been jeopardized by this time-constraining situation impacting family life and (Meyer et al. 1997) disturbing intimacy and belongingness within families. One can safely argue that neglecting the three basic hierarchical needs automatically jeopardized the remaining two hierarchical needs, being the need for self-esteem and self-actualization.

13.4.2   The Effect of the Migrant Labor System on Traditional Life

One would assume that the decision of migrant laboring should improve the socioeconomic status of the family, a win and lose scenario, as generally the family as a system is disturbed, but would gain economically in exchange (Lu and Treiman 2011). A survey of 1970 revealed that women were sad, felt abandoned, and miserable for being without their husbands; however, they understood the necessity as otherwise they would be poverty struck (Hishongwa 1992). Apart from cumbersome wages earned by the men (Hishongwa 1992; Mlambo 2011), researchers found that mostly additional income was rather consumed instead of invested in terms of poverty reduction (Lu and Treiman 2011). As a result of the migrant labor system, Namibia's traditional and community life underwent drastic changes, especially Namibia's northern Ovambo culture.

Within the Ovambo culture, the traditional hierarchy in family life was most vulnerable. Traditionally, a man as head of the household, not being able to provide for those residing under his roof, was regarded as a "good for nothing." Furthermore, Namibian contract laborers lived with ongoing concerns about the well-being of wife and children. Subsistence farming contributed to their worry of how the family coped, as well as the sufficiency and quality of food production in their absence (Hishongwa 1992). Typically for migrant laborer families, women were faced with additional agricultural and household duties, exhausting themselves, while children too had to contribute in labor (Lu and Treiman 2011; Hishongwa 1992). Some women, especially those who had no children, out of the wedlock, that could help out were overwhelmed by work and responsibility. As a result from time to time, a woman was found to abandon the common household. In addition women failing to meet the production target and surplus for unproductive months were ridiculed by the entire community, perceived as lazy and hopeless, and potentially faced divorce (Hishongwa 1992).

Although life for women was marked with hardship in absence of their men, studies revealed that generally women in sub-Saharan Africa gained self-confidence from their new roles, even though the migrant labor system did not contribute to female independence or empowerment as decision-making power remained with the husbands. Still, women had to make decisions in the absence of their husbands on their behalf pertaining to agricultural activities and household matters. Poor decisions reflected badly on the husband, making her susceptible to punishment (Hishongwa 1992). Assistance from kinsmen was offered, however found not to be adequate (Hishongwa 1992; Lu and Treiman 2011). Women were also not allowed to consult kinsmen in private matters. Other forms of communication through letters and verbal messages were often time-consuming or jeopardized by illiteracy or distortions of verbal messages. Traditionally, women had no control over their part of the family income or property, in their husband's absence. The husband symbolized economic survival as women had no alternative to earn an income or any social welfare. This left women feeling inferior, despite their abilities and hardships, enhancing his position of power in the household. In the event of death of the husband, all property and means of income the woman worked for would automatically be inherited by the husband's maternal relatives (Hishongwa 1992).

Within migrant families emotional intimacy and social support are regarded to be crucial (Lu and Treiman 2011). The Ovambo culture demands a husband to take exceptional care of his pregnant wife, name the child, and organize a festivity in honor of the birth. Often men were only home long enough to father a child and returned a year or two later. Children often perceived their fathers as strangers (Hishongwa 1992). As a result, fatherhood was challenged to the maximum (Goosen et al. 2007). Older children going to secondary schools were home during holidays only, which did not necessarily fall into the same time slot the father would be home, resulting in children often not seeing their fathers for many years (Hishongwa 1992).

Contemporary researchers have found that 170 million people in developing nations resort to migrant labor. As a result, 30 % of children live in a single-parent household. Compared to children living with both parents, single household parenting influences the child's development negatively, and low income is also negatively related to school enrollment and attendance among South African migrant laborers (Lu and Treiman 2011). Confirmed by Hishongwa (1992), who described a typical case in which a family of ten children allowed children to take turns, thus, each child would miss one school day to work on the land or with the livestock and attend school for the remaining nine consecutive days. This family was regarded lucky to be blessed by many children. Furthermore, Hishongwa (1992) described the educational institutions as extremely unpleasant for African children. The South African educational system followed the rationale that the standards between European children and African children had such a degree of difference that the lower-level Bantustan education system would be sufficient for African children (Irwin 2010; Lu and Treiman 2011).

Overexploitation of women and child labor decreased quality and sufficiency in food production, frequently resulting in undernourished children, mostly lacking protein (Hishongwa 1992). Typically, a community would consist of women, children, and elder men as men within their productive years worked as migrant laborers (Hishongwa 1992; Lu and Treiman 2011). Consequently, decision-making was left to the elder men, who often feared change and appeared rigid in the drastically changing lifestyle of the Ovambo people. As a result of their obligations toward the South African government, the elder leaders were often regarded as disloyal toward their own people.

The absence of men directly influenced the decline of traditional thanksgiving for good harvest, called "oshipe." As a result of living close to the poverty line, women commercialized their self-made pottery and baskets, that which originally was a cultural artifact lost its traditional value through commercialization. Other joyful traditions such as youth assemblies to sing and dance deteriorated as a result of a shortage in adolescent boys and disapproval of the church. These events transformed into female gatherings in which women came together to express their feelings of sorrow in songs and dances. These songs were also sang in the field and while threshing corn (Hishongwa 1992).

13.4.3   Migrant Labor and the Consequences on Well-Being

The "Bantustan" system of 1977, under the South African Administration, among others, delegated the health-care responsibility, to the relevant tribal representatives, who functioned as the ethnic authorities. This caused fragmentation in the health-care systems, as not all communities were equally able to initiate and sustain such a system (United Nations Institute of Namibia 1988).

Furthermore, HIV/AIDS has been found in direct relation to war and migrant labor (Edwards 2006; United Nations Institute of Namibia 1988). Studies in other African countries have confirmed that migrant populations in countries, such as Sierra Leone, DRC, Rwanda, and western Sudan (Edwards 2006), are vast contributing factor to the spreading of HIV/AIDS and other venereal diseases (Edwards 2006; United Nations Institute of Namibia 1988). For black Namibians under the apartheid system, access to health care was scarce, resulting in medically related problems such as high rates in maternal, neonatal, and young children's morbidity and mortality. Many black people were undernourished due to unequal distribution of resources under the apartheid regime. In addition, poor education about gastroenteritis became the major contributor for infant mortality among black people (Namibia United Nations Institute of Namibia 1988). Alcoholism was another danger which detrimentally affected many migrant workers and remained uncared for by the system (Hishongwa 1992; United Nations Institute of Namibia 1988). Workplaces were often a health hazard for migrant laborers. For example, exposure to toxic materials in mines, accidents from unprotected machinery, and insanitary conditions caused illnesses and injuries. Poor accessibility to water and lack of education resulted in unhygienic water reservoirs as breeding places for snails and malaria mosquitoes (United Nations Institute of Namibia 1988). Education for black children was of lower level and often quality was compromised. School enrollment figures of black children decreased, as level of education increased toward secondary and tertiary education (Lu and Treiman 2011).

13.5 Ending the Apartheid Regime

The migrant labor system led to unity among Africans. White supremacy together with poor working conditions and inhumane treatment led to emotions of dissatisfaction, anger, and hatred among black Africans. A statement of a white Afrikaner recollected by John ya Otto during the apartheid regime verified that white people were aware of the toxic emotions created by supremacy and full of fear of retaliation (Hishongwa 1992). The latter was however not the initial intention (Klein 2011; Katjavivi and Shimming-Chase 2012).

13.5.1 Political Forces

World economy played a significant role in not being able to dismantle the power of a white minority in South Africa and Namibia. The Western world economically gained through South African mining resources and market-competitive products as a result of a cheap labor force (Hoyle 1981; Katjavivi and Shimming-Chase 2012). In spite of the Western world's repulse toward South Africa's apartheid regime, global economic affairs did not allow weakening South Africa's economy, until the involvement of the Soviet Union (Irwin 2010). The killing of African protestors during the Sharpeville massacre in South Africa, 1960 (Irwin 2010; Lauren and Swartz 2011), became a landmark for the UNO to act against racism in South Africa (Irwin 2010). This was not a matter of race any longer. The dynamics of the cold war were transformed by nationalist supporters, leading to the alienation of South Africa from their economic and political partners (Irwin 2010).

The UNO's increasing resistance to the mannerism of South Africa's ruling over Namibia strengthened Africans in their opposition. While South Africa reduced the former South-West Africa's value by describing it as wasteland, the UNO questioned the financial investments made as well as the continuous pleas to incorporate South-West Africa into South Africa (Anderson 2008). By 1960, approximately 120 petitions requested the UNO's assistance against oppression (O'Callaghan 2011), one of the very few rights within a mandate system (Anderson 2008). During 1957 it was named the Ovamboland People's Congress, later renamed to Ovamboland People's Organization (OPO) and finally renamed again to South-West Africa's People Organization (SWAPO). This organization was formed, aiming to eliminate the migrant labor system. The Windhoek massacre during December 1959 was one of the major landmarks increasing resistance against the South African oppressors. The Windhoek massacre resulted from a demonstration against relocation of Africans from Windhoek's Old Location to the new apartheid township named Katutura. Eleven Africans were killed and 54 wounded (O'Callaghan 2011).

During 1663 the South African regime activated against African opposition. Consequently, communism was forbidden. Solitary confinement without charge and detention was introduced. The African National Congress and Pan-Africanist Congress were outlawed (Lauren and Swartz 2011). The International Court of Justice failed to declare South Africa's ruling over former South-West Africa as illegal, since it was not perceived as a security threat. Furthermore, the ruling was substantiated by legally flawed motivations and evidence, therefore not of full legal usefulness. African movements lost trust in Western Courts. The Western societies speculated that the African bloc's only alternative for support would be the Communistic bloc (Irwin 2010), not an unwarranted notion. Already, as a direct reaction to the Sharpeville massacre during 1962, the British Anti-Apartheid Movement (AAM) called broad attention to opposing apartheid. They actively promoted the African National Congress (ANC) since 1959, enhancing ANC's international credibility. Both organizations shared their communist ideology and relations with communist organizations (Klein 2011).

After the ruling, the International Court of Justice, Prime Minister Verwoerd, declared self-righteously that no grudges would be held against the opponents, making the ruling at international level unmistakably impartial (Irwin 2010). This was an affront to Africans, especially since accumulated evidence set out to neglect well-being and social and human rights of the South-West African people; it included aspects such as economic growth, citizenship rights, freedom of movements, security, rights of residence, and educational opportunities for former South-West Africans (Irwin 2010). Almost simultaneously, Nelson Mandela won ground on international level with the assistance of the AAM. After a representation of the ANC at the Pan-African Freedom Movement, ANC obtained recognition by the Organization of African Unity (OAU), which in turn paved the way for the UNO to grant the ANC observer status in 1973. This resulted in the South African regime being banned to represent South Africans (Klein 2011). The OAU was a result of Pan-Africanism based on experiences during slavery and Civil Rights Movement aimed to join all people of African descent and made it their business to assist all Africans to break the chains of colonial oppression and exploitation (Riruako 2006).

For Africans, losing the trail meant to forsake the attempted reinforcement of universal human rights as justification for the liberation struggle against racial oppression. For the NP the aim was not only to put off sanctions and armed struggle but to maintain the power of segregation. The African bloc at the time consistently continued to oppose South Africa maintaining the mandate over former South-West Africa (Irwin 2010). Yet, the National Party remained rather uncontested. During the Rivonia Trial in 1964, the NP had reached a state of certainty that the African National Congress (ANC) and Pan-Africanist Congress (PAC) could not threaten their position (Irwin 2010), unacquainted with the international magnitude that the anti-apartheid movement was about to reach, in years to come. With the support of

AAM and their operational office in London, the ANC's endless quest to obtain international solidarity to become South Africa's legitimate representative paved the way to future victory over apartheid (Klein 2011).

The relationship between ANC and SWAPO, together will all other parties of southern African regions, was intertwined (Katjavivi and Shimming-Chase 2012). Africans did not lose sight of their goal to end the apartheid regime. Objectives serving this purpose were to, firstly, cooperate with and support African campaign against apartheid; secondly, to raise global awareness; and thirdly, to end it (Klein 2011). Undoubtedly, these objectives explain the high degree of unity among leaders of various organizations aimed at liberation in favor of a nonracial and nonsexist society (Katjavivi and Shimming-Chase 2012). Furthermore, the AAM, with endless effort, supported the awareness campaign against apartheid across European countries leading to the formation of world bodies concerned with racism, such as the United National Special Committee Against Apartheid (Klein 2011).

The beginning of the end of nonviolent opposition against the Apartheid regime started with the Rivonia Trial, 1963. South African police found a hideout at a Rivonia of anti-apartheid activists, kept them in solitary confinement until they were trialed in Pretoria. Among eight suspects were Athur Goldreich, a former member of the Israeli underground movement (Linder 2010), as well as ANC leaders during the 1950s and 1960s Govan Mbeki, Walter Sisulu, and Nelson Mandela (Klein 2011; Linder 2010). Mandela was perceived to play a leading role among the conspirators (Linder 2010). In particular Nelson Mandela would serve a prison sentence of 30 years, of which 18 was served at Robin Island, partially under solitary confinement (Linder 2010).

For Namibia to gain independence, the engagement of the UNO has been hindered throughout the armed struggle, with increasing urgency, by South Africa through a sequence of strategies. For example, 1980 South Africa changed their constitution to a pyramid structure of institutions. Henceforth, the Administrator-General of Namibia was under direct control of Pretoria. A three-tier system was put in place. The first tier constituted a Council of Ministers, equivalent to a cabinet over which the Administrator-General had the power to veto any decision. The second tier represented the "homelands." The third tier constituted the municipalities and village boards. Furthermore, the establishment of a political party, namely, the DTA (Democratic Turnhalle Alliance), was aimed at redirecting workers and peasants from SWAPO, creating a false impression of widespread support and so international credibility, unsuccessfully. Furthermore, attempts like bantustanization as well as the homeland consolidation delayed progression toward Namibia's independence (United Nations Institute for Namibia 1988).

13.5.2   Military Engagement

Clearly, the years of nonviolence were over (Linder 2010). The first major incident for Namibia was the fight at Ongulumbashe in Ovamboland on the 26th of August 1966, between SWAPO guerrilla fighters and SADF (South African Defense Force)

(Klein 2011). Although SWAPO was defeated, the attack served as a psychological enhancer since South Africa was unprepared and caught off guard (Saunders 2002). The disbelief of the South African leaders for guerrilla war to actually take place was uncovered by the hasty enactment of the Terrorism Act in 1966 which was made retroactive to 1962 (Goosen et al. 2007). Furthermore, South Africa did not take the might of the global anti-apartheid movements into consideration (Klein 2011).

In 1966 SWAPO officially assumed armed struggle against South African rule, forming a military wing, called People's Liberation Army of Namibia (PLAN) (O'Callaghan 2011); hence, the joint intention for a violence-free transition in accordance with Mahatma Gandhi's example failed (Katjavivi and Shimming-Chase 2012). Over 100 African men were arrested in Namibia under the Terrorism Act. February 1968, Toivo ya Toivo, the founder and leader of SWAPO, was sentenced by the Pretoria court to 20 years of imprisonment at Robin Island (Goosen et al. 2007). Consequently, Sam Nujoma was destined to become Toivo ya Toivo's descendant (Nortje 2003).

By April 1974 the 30-year war started in Angola, north of Namibia (Nortje 2003), once again emphasizing the racial issue being less significant than the cold war. The African party MPLA (Movimento Popular de Libertação de Angola), supported by OAU, Zambia, and Tanzania, was supplied with weapons by the Soviet Union, while FNLA (Frente Nacional de Libertação de Angola) and UNITA (União Nacional para a Independéncia Total de Angola) were funded by the USA. Furthermore, in exchange for weapons from Pretoria, FNLA joined forces with SADF against SWAPO, and therefore against communism, as from 1975 onward (Nortje 2003). Although the involvement of the communistic Soviet Union was no secret, their involvement on platoon level only became evident in 1981, about 100 km north of Namibia when soviet soldiers were captured and killed as part of a SWAPO convoy (Hoyle 1981).

SWAPO used the southern Angolan territory as catalyst to invade Namibian borders. The operation included setting up various training bases in Angola. SWAPO militants were trained in Zambia and Cuba. Middle 1980 PLAN (the military wing of SWAPO) fighters mutated into efficient military units under the military leadership of Domo Hamambo (Nortje 2003). During 1981 it was estimated that 400–2,500 East Germans and 20,000 Cubans and 1,000 military and economic advisors from the Soviet Union actively supported SWAPO in Angola. Being aware of the seriousness of the matter and the danger of siding with either party, as this was not merely a racial struggle any longer but had become an East–west matter, the United Nations managed to pave the way to a cease-fire and supervised free election in Namibia (Hoyle 1981).

With the political heat increasing for South Africa, during 1975, the Turnhalle Conference was launched in order to enable South Africa to grant Namibia's independence. This move was primarily investigated as a result of the increasing global pressure against apartheid (Klein 2011; Mlambo 2011) as well as the bush-war in southern Angola and northern Namibia (Nortje 2003; Mlambo 2011). According to historian, Peter Katjavivi (Mlambo 2011), this merely served as deception, based on two argumentations: firstly, participants were nominated by the South African government and, secondly, presented by members of different ethnic groups. However, not any of the genuine and banned political parties included SWAPO. Nevertheless, temporarily the Turnhalle Conference served its purpose and granted minor changes but, however, failed later. Reason for failure was that the Turnhalle Conference and consequential elections, in 1978, were not recognized by SWAPO and the UNO, as it was not concise with Resolution 435 of the UNO, namely, to honor free and fair elections (O'Callaghan 2011).

During 1970–1972 SWAPO, as a political party, was actively involved in establishing the National Union of Namibian Workers (NUNW), supported by workers and peasants for protection against violence and harassment. NUNW engaged workers in strikes, demobilizing economic activities, until the South African system compromised. Increased oppression merely intensified resistance over the coming years. The resilience of Africans gave voice to grievances and led to positive modifications (Hishongwa 1992).

Bush-war was an environmental challenge for all parties. The average length of service among SWAPO and NDF soldiers was between 7.5 and 26 years (LeBeau 2005). At the border of Namibia and Angola, the northern border of Namibia and the southern border of Angola are bestowed with rather dense grass, bush, and tree landscape. Fundamentally, this physically impaired sight and control over immediate geographical surroundings. An environment which communist activists described as ideal, dubbing bush war as the "war of fleas" connected to the analogy that one flea cannot hurt a dog; however, if the dog (referring to the noncommunist alliances) is manifested with fleas (communist alliances), the dog dies (Breyer 1979). Foot patrols were the norm due to the density of the bush, among all parties. Underground bunkers served as storage facilities and protection. 1978 SADF trained special units in reconnaissance, young adults who were recruited after graduating from the School of Infantry. Training was extremely harsh which only the fittest survived to be called henceforth "reccies." Reccies were frequently assigned in very small groups with minimal military support from their base, to locate the enemy and report back for the battalion to launch an attack. Physical contact and shootings were frequent (Nortje 2003). It may be debatable whether civilians truly were ever a target and not accidental casualties based upon the environment and platoon activities, resembling a labyrinth of environmental and military challenges, paired with immediate combat reaction. Fact however remained, as per Nortje (2003), that occasional civilian casualties, including women and children, were a reality.

The war zone was overburdened with war refugees. Including those from Angola, Zambia, and Namibia, 100 and 1,000 refugees were documented. Hence, refugee camps were established providing educational and health services as good as possible (Mlambo 2011). The autobiography of Lucia Engombe (2004) described her early years around 1976 in a refugee camp, called Nyango. This camp housed about 2,000 refugees, before she was transported to East Germany during 1978 as an exile child to be educated. She reported having been chronically hungry, resorting to insects as food supply, and later mice and birds, bothered by dirt and lice. As a pre-scholar in her venture to search for food, she reckoned to be adequately fed at the day care center of Nyango which supplied food three times a day to children. Yet, in her experience only the bigger and stronger children gained forceful access to this valuable and scarce resource. Engombe further described how children believed it was a game, initiated by mothers and other supervising mother figures, to hide under trees for hours until an occasional plane flew over the area, in reality a threat to their lives. She described transparent tents, in which the refugees hid at night and did not understand the haste, silence, and fear of the adults at the time.

One of the most hurtful massacres of Namibia's Africans was the Cassinga event in 1978, which delayed, at the time speedily progressive, negotiations over Namibia's independence with the UNO for over 10 years (Goosen et al. 2007). How the Cassinga massacre developed is not certain. Later in East Germany, Engombe (2004) met a woman, named Erika, who survived the massacre at Cassinga. She described how early one morning many warplanes dropped bombs over Cassinga, immediately transforming the camp into a bloodbath, followed by parachute soldiers dropping from the sky to kill the survivors. Erika could rescue her two boys, her husband died. Her sister in law died in the bullet hail protecting her two surviving sons with her body. At the time of the attack (Goosen et al. 2007), approximately three to four thousand men, women, and children lived in Cassinga, a SWAPO refugee camp. Casualties accounted 700 civilians of which 300 were children, 600 were wounded, and 200 taken prisoner by SADF. Attacking civilian camps was against the international agreement to protect refugees and resulted in accusing SWAPO of having been warned but failed to remove the civilians from the camp. A report from the Times (Anon 1978) stated that the attack on Cassinga occurred one day after SWAPO attacked a hydroelectric station at Ruacana Falls. Reports from South Africa were alleged to claim having raided Cassinga as a military headquarter, destroying large supplies of ammunition during 12 h, while the Angolan government insisted that Cassinga was only a refugee camp.

Case histories of NDF and SWAPO ex-soldiers (LeBeau 2005) reported that witnessing injury of civilians had a more lasting negative effect than witnessing the injury or killing of a soldier. Negative emotions were also associated with threats of being killed, accidentally killing a fellow soldier or being seriously injured, killed children, and injured people by bombs and landmines.

Throughout the guerrilla war, SWAPO's national and international supporters increased and strengthened, respectively. In return, South Africa's international credibility weakened over time, and their economic resources were exploited through maintaining their military force. In addition, the economy of South Africa declined as a result of a shortage of young men within the employment sector. Furthermore, the prolonged and increasingly strengthening guerrilla war demoralized soldiers and induced insecurity in the white society of Namibia. Consequently, numerous white farmers sold their property and emigrated (United Nations Institute for Namibia 1988).

The consequence of war on soldiers has been investigated by the PEACE center in Namibia, from a sample population, equally distributed Namibian SADF and SWAPO ex-soldiers. It has been found that ex-soldiers (SWAPO and SADF) had a high degree of social dysfunction symptoms but a low degree of depression.

Only 7 % suffered from posttraumatic stress disorder (LeBeau 2005). Even though this figure may appear very low, it indicates pathology and low levels of well-being. Studies have shown that soldiers engage in ad hoc sexual activities due to loneliness and use rape as a weapon of war. Seventeen percent of rape war victims have been tested positive for HIV/AIDS in Rwanda (Edwards 2006). Merely 14 % reported psychological or physical impairment as a result of war and 20 % reported to have received counseling, through churches, relatives, and foreign governments. The most prominent needs for improving their living conditions in 2005 were the most basic needs: money for survival, employment (employment opportunity for SWAPO ex-soldiers is 43 % and for SADF ex-soldiers only 18 %), and housing (LeBeau 2005).

13.6 Independence

The UNO has been involved in protecting Namibia from South Africa's incorporation since 1947. After the decision in the International Court of Justice 1966, the UNO Security Council was engaged. Although the UNO Security Council could not apply for mandatory economic sanctions against South Africa, they requested that the South African government's authority was not to be recognized over Namibia. Only in 1972 the South African government agreed to Namibia obtaining separate international status and offered to lead Namibia to independence. Yet, actions were cumbersome in this regard, implying a strategy of delay. Hence, Resolution 385 (1976) of the UNO Security Council stipulated that "…free elections under the supervision and control of the United Nations be held for the whole of Namibia as one political entity…" and that "…the United Nations should establish necessary machinery within Namibia to supervise and control such elections…" as well as "… to enable the people of Namibia to organize practically for the purpose of such election…" (United Nations Institute for Namibia 1988, p. 49). Unfortunately, the resolution remained unimplemented. South Africa set various conditions, for example, to insist on the withdrawal of Cuban troops out of Angola. SWAPO as well as South Africa were determined to not lose sight of their objectives, and both adopted various strategies to achieve them. As SWAPO's supporters increased, South Africa's supporters decreased. After years of negotiations the UNO independence plan according to Resolution 385 (1976) was approved and independence of Namibia could finally be realized (United Nations Institute for Namibia 1988).

Elections took place in November 1989 supervised by the United Nations Transition Group (UNTAG) involving teams of 8,000 UNO officials and soldiers, monitoring elections and witnessing the victory of SWAPO (O'Callaghan 2011). On 21st of March, 1990, Namibia's official date of independence (Saunders 2002), Sam Nujoma was sworn in as the first President of Namibia. Sam Nujoma grew up in the northern regions of Namibia. Based upon his political engagement and increasing power among Namibians in his capacity as SWAPO leader, Sam Nujoma had to flee into exile in 1960 (Saunders 2002). After SWAPO won the elections by 41 seats, the

72 members strong Constituent Assembly formulated the Namibian Constitution (O'Callaghan 2011). African leaders maintained their personal styles and so influenced dynamic processes (Katjavivi and Shimming-Chase 2012). Although decisions about how to attain their target were not necessarily in accord, the leaders remained united in the objectives, vision, and goal in terms of working toward a race- and gender-free society.

Independence for Namibia meant much more than the freedom of Namibian citizens. According to Katjavivi and Shimming-Chase (2012), Namibian independence as a fifth province of South Africa served as testing grounds for South Africa's independence. South Africa's new leaders were able to learn through the Namibian model. Katjavivi pointed out that Namibia managed and paved a way for a peaceful transition in government, including abolishment of the apartheid system and thereby positively influenced South African independence. While leaders shared in their experiences of the independence of Angola, Zambia, Zimbabwe, and Mozambique, Namibia served South Africa as a role model, which was never appropriately accredited.

13.7   The Role of Churches

Churches have played a large role in Namibia since 200 years ago. The first German and Finnish missionary introduced Christianity. Currently 90 % of Namibians are Christians (Mlambo 2011; Goosen et al. 2007). An African branch of churches has developed, distancing themselves from discriminatory white-led churches (Mlambo 2011). During the apartheid years, church leaders contributed by responding to the needs of their black members by developing their sense of worth, advocating for better education under the Bantustan system, creating a global network of churches, and confronting South African political practices of oppression (Goosen et al. 2007).

One of the earliest examples within the history of Namibia, Reverend Michael Scott, an Anglican priest, freedom fighter and idealist, as well as dubbed communist, played a significant role in Namibia's history. After convincing himself physically about the devastating living conditions of Namibians under the South African mandate during 1947, he managed to present a petition from the Hereros, Damaras, and Namas to the international world, through UNO. On grounds of this petition, the International Court of Justice was involved. He was stripped of funds and his parish and church as a consequence (Anderson 2008).

The ELOC (Evangelical Lutheran Ovambo-Kavango Church) referendum led, in 1971, to the revision of the 1966 decision of the International Court of Justice, declaring that South Africa's mandate over Namibia was illegal. ELOC and ELC (Evangelical Lutheran Church) managed to give a voice to 48 % of the total population opposing South African rule (Goosen et al. 2007). South African resistance brought about an open letter by Bishop Auala and Pastor Paulus Gowaseb to South Africa's Prime Minister, John Vorster, on the 30th of June 1971. The letter identified the position of the church as an authority within the community, pointed out aspects of oppression and acts of inhumanities toward black people, being against the UNO declarations in 1948. As a result, the open letter joined all nonwhite political and tribal forces of Namibia. Furthermore, a pastoral letter was disseminated to all congregations as well as the South African Prime Minister. Ignorance of the Prime Minister resulted in the churches mobilizing a strike among workers during 1971 and 1972 demanding the abolishment of the migrant labor system and freedom of movement. Consequently, a state of emergency was called. During 1973, conditions for migrant laborers improved somewhat. However, churches in Namibia were repressed by the South African rule.

While church leaders supported their members and voiced their disapproval in the Christian toward oppression, many leaders remained pacifists during the armed struggle. In spite of that they did not condemn those who part-took in the armed struggle (Goosen et al. 2007).

In terms of reconciliation religion played a significant role for Namibians (Isaak and Lombard 2002). SWAPO liberation fighters made use of Western contact groups throughout their political struggle, therefore signaling willingness to abstinence from racial retaliation. In addition, the concept to involve opposing forces, retaliation versus forgiveness, acts as a motivator toward social change.

13.8   Truth and Reconciliation for Namibians: The Ex-detainee Question

Truth and reconciliation is not based upon "forgetting" and forgiving the past (Dobell 1997), it is about "Ubuntu." Ubuntu is an African term that can be described as an indigenous sense for community; interconnectedness among individuals; "I am you"; an honorable term for a kind, generous, compassionate, hospitable, and caring person; an affirmative and non-threatening approach toward others; transcending religion; and the knowledge of holistic existence (Krog 2008; Murithi 2009). In the Namibian Oshiwambo (Ovambo) culture, three words describe reconciliation: "ediminafanepo (you forgive someone and he/she in turn forgives you), ehanganifo (someone takes the hand of one person and then takes the hand of another person, thus bringing them together), and etambulafano (two people accept one another following a quarrel; acceptance takes place on an equal footing)" (Isaak and Lombard 2002, p. 93). Other languages, such as Otjiherero (okuhangana means peace and okuisirisana means to forgive another) as well as Khoekhoegowab and Tswana, each have terms or verbs indicating togetherness above quarrel.

The truth and reconciliation concept originated in post-independent South Africa. Its aim was, at first, to give victims a platform to share past injustice and hurt inflicted by inhumane treatment. Secondly, the perpetrator is allowed to express his remorse and share own suffering. Thirdly, instead of revenge by the victim, the way toward forgiveness is paved. Finally, reconciliation is sought (Dobell 1997; van Zyl 1999).

This resembles the psychological trauma treatment approach. In brief, trauma treatment is based on sharing and acknowledging the traumatic events and feelings associated with it, under psychologically controlled conditions. This serves the purpose to put an end to unresolved and pathological emotions (Riggs and Foa 2004). Taking this one step further toward traumatic growth would be to consciously transform the traumatic experience into a new, positive activity (Linley et al. 2004). However, during trauma treatment, the perpetrator is not present in person and therefore no realistic threat at the given moment.

Fundamentally, truth and reconciliation within the southern African context and on societal level focuses on restoring the dignity of the victim and not on judging the perpetrator. It is not about forgetting the past, but to create a platform to openly share injustice endured by victims and remorse felt by perpetrators, working toward reconciliation (Dobell 1997).

Dr. G. Straker (van Zyl 1999) explains truth and reconciliation as a chain of therapeutic processes, functioning on personal and social level. Through the victim creating a narrative of trauma, the traumatic event is not only contained but also given meaning, on social as well as personal level. The rationale is that feelings of aggression start to resolve in the victim, through witnessing that also the perpetrator suffers as a result of having inflicted pain in the past. Therefore, the perpetrator's presence and voicing an admission of guilt is important to the victim. Once feelings of aggression within the victim are resolved, psychological repair can begin. Truth and reconciliation is underpinned by the Christian belief in forgiveness.

Furthermore, Nelson Mandela, as a role model, has refrained from any vengeful feelings toward his oppressors, which set an exceptional national and international example of forgiveness. However, Krog (2008) argues that although forgiveness rises above the deed, it can only proceed to reconciliation if the perpetrator is acting upon through (1) wanting to change and (2) takes action toward change through his or her contribution to society. Completion of this cycle also coincides with the fundamental processes of traumatic growth by transcending traumatic healing (Linley et al. 2004).

The Namibian approach toward truth and reconciliation differs somewhat. Namibian leadership has embraced all races and forfeited retaliation against former oppressors, but it seems that rather a veil of silence is drawn over the past. Leaders are cautious to fulfill the full spectrum of the truth and reconciliation concept. They feel that to take precautions in not endangering the racial, social, and economic reconciliation better serves the purpose. This is based on the assumption that reviving the past would be counterproductive as successful transition is based upon cooperation of former enemies (Dobell 1997) and not to blame them. Feelings of regret are clear approximately 15 years after independence and the end of war. Research confirmed (LeBeau 2005) that 60 % of SADF ex-soldiers felt if they had full disclosure at the time, they would not have participated, while the majority of SWAPO ex-soldiers found the struggle for freedom worth its while. Possibly, the Namibian government reluctance to revive the past is not as unfounded as it may appear, since residual negative feelings are related to blame with 30 % of both

SADF as well as SWAPO soldiers, despite over 80 % of the soldiers reported to accept their former enemy (LeBeau 2005).

The Namibian situation pertaining to the exile and former detainee situation seems blurred, and it is claimed that the Namibian government never officially acknowledged violations against human rights. It is reported that suspected nonconformists to SWAPO have been subjected to mistreatment, torture, and vanished in dungeons during the apartheid years (Dobell 1997). A counteraccusation that these individuals have been spies and traitors jeopardizes the true essence of truth and reconciliation.

Namibia's SWAPO government is criticized for not admitting atrocities against alleged nonconformists of SWAPO, while ANC has acknowledged violations against human rights in their camps (Dobell 1997). Even during in-depth interviews with SADF and SWAPO ex-soldiers, the questions about committing atrocities or inducing inhumane acts toward others, including rape and killing of fellow soldiers, remained unanswered (LeBeau 2005). War has a direct relation to rape as a weapon of war. African studies have confirmed that predominantly refugee women were at risk, since they needed to leave the camp to collect wood for survival (Edwards 2006). Only 12 % of ex-fighters, half of each force, have reported to have been imprisoned themselves, at average longer than 6 months and mostly in Namibia and Angola. More than 30 % experienced torture, with increased risk for women (LeBeau 2005). During 1994 a former detainee demanded name lists of 2,100 unaccounted individuals and the issue of formal death certificates of these persons, so that guardianship over their children can be legitimized, and new marriages can take place by remaining spouses (Dobell 1997).

Critics appose to include the "wall of silence" in Namibia's reconciliation. They claim that it only works well for Namibia's economic elite and excludes the proportion of the society with low living standards and who are unemployed. When addressed, responsibility herein is delegated to corruption by urban government officials (Dobell 1997).

Another aspect of criticism is the unresolved detainee questions. Whether the detainee question is a matter of Namibia's government not being able to accept criticism and admit fault, or whether the matter is blown out of proportion in order to create a new dividing climate, is not certain. Fact is however that a petition was presented to the Council of Churches (CNN) by former detainees; consequently, a committee called Breaking the Wall of Silence (BWS) has been formed. The members constitute former detainees and supporters and CNN employees. Gatherings have developed in disclosure of emotions and grievances to channel emotions of anger into forums for political activity. Forceful encounters of former detainees to evoke admission of guilt by SWAPO resulted in SWAPO accusing this minority population to threaten Namibia's peace and stability. One may argue that the formation of the BWS is positive toward a democratic society or whether it is a potential danger to the still fragile new Namibia (Dobell 1997). Churches in Namibia maintained their autonomy yet still managed to functionally interact with Government and its political forces. Ninety percent of Namibians are Christians (Isaak and Lombard 2002). Churches in general create platforms to act toward reconciliation and share the pain. Religion may not be able to change the past; however, it changes the meaning of events for people. Instead of being isolated in pain, churches actively encourage the start of emotional healing and that people should integrate themselves within society.

13.9   Legislation Changes to the Benefit of Well-Being and Equality

Change in legislation at large protected Namibia's previously disadvantaged society from further exploitation and inequality as the first step toward social change. Social change is not an overnight process. The Namibian Constitution has been drafted with regard to democratic rights, humanitarian treatment, and freedom for each resident of Namibia. The Racial Discrimination Prohibition Amendment Act of 1991 (26) (Government Gazette 152, 1991) made it punishable to practice any form of racial discrimination or apartheid. This included the provision to render good health, educational, and religious service to all members of the society. All acts resulting in racial disharmony or victimization are to be punished by law henceforth. Many other Acts have been promulgated, the most prominent ones concerning the livelihood of Namibians through land ownership, condition of employment and dismissal, as well as gender equality are addressed herein seeing that these are fundamentally relevant to this chapter.

13.9.1   Land Ownership

As the United Nations has sharply noted, the main emphasis of colonies was to maintain control over land and increase economic wealth from its resources. Based on the weight of self-sustained farming, women of the north had to bear as a result of migrant labor, while all economic power remained with their husbands. Already during 1977, SWAPO managed to change this as per legislation Act 5 of 1977. Article 48 explicitly states that "property acquired by spouses through work in the course of marriage shall be their joint property" (Hishongwa 1992, p. 101).

Rhodesia, renamed after its independence in 1980 to Zimbabwe, served as a good role model for the new Namibian government of how not to redistribute land to attain equality. Zimbabwe was counterproductive in their haste to implement a fundamentally acceptable the Act and jeopardized a peaceful transition, based on ideological plans and overambitious decisions. Agriculture dominated by the white population was the economic backbone of Zimbabwe (Stiff 2000).

The question of land ownership has also proven central after Namibia's independence in order to reinstate equal land distribution across race. Namibian leaders learned to avoid two pitfalls as a result of the Zimbabwe model. For one, Namibia kept by the willing seller/willing buyer principle and secondly broke this pathway down into achievable proportions over a long period of time. The Land Reform Act 6 of 1995 stipulates among others that market-related compensation is to be offered as well as an advisory committee consisting of stakeholders and land tribunal to solve possible disputes between private seller and government. According to Article 14(1) of the Act, beneficiaries should not possess any additional or adequate agricultural land. The Act should serve socially, economically, or educationally disadvantaged population resulting from past discriminations (Werner 2002).

This also includes in compensating for gender inequality in terms of women of all races now also having the equal right to purchase, own, and sell land on their own. The objective of the Resettlement policy 2001 was to increase opportunity for self-sustained farming, increase employment opportunity, to introduce small holdings to the economic farming industry, and to alleviate agricultural pressure in communal areas (Werner 2002).

In practice however the land reform proved to be a social, economic, and political challenge. The prerequisite to much desired wealth through farming is based upon responsible farming within the environmental context. Furthermore, production must be compatible with international markets. In addition, poor land management can result in desertification (Seely and Zeidler 2002).

13.9.2 Labor Law

Labor laws have been drafted for the protection against exploitation of workers in Namibia. For example, the Labor Act 1992 (6) (Office of the Prime Minister, 1992) regulates labor aspects such as working hours on a weekly basis, employees working on a daily basis, and shift work. Regulations pertaining to overtime, Sunday or Public Holidays, night work, and meal intervals are regulated, as well as conditions are stipulated in the event that the employee resides on property of the employer. Calculation and payment of remuneration, annual leave, sick leave, maternity leave, as well as child labor is regulated Protection from victimization and freedom of association is offered. Under the Labor Act 1992 (6), labor court rules were established in order to regulate labor disputes in terms of fair hearings for all parties involved as well as possible arbitration or settlements.

The Affirmative Action Act 1998 (29) (Government Gazette 1962, 1998) assured equal opportunity based on Article 23 of the Namibian Constitution. The aim of this act was to eliminate past discriminatory practices based on conditions of disadvantage in the employment sector. Prospective employees, sufficiently trained and educated, must be given preference if they stem from the "previous disadvantaged" population group.

13.9.3 Gender Equality

Before-mentioned acts had been implemented allowing women to purchase, own, and sell property, as well as equal remuneration for women and men based upon experience and qualification. In the family and workplace however, the Namibian society remains a male-dominated society, and in practice it is not only men's obligation to take a step backward but also women should overcome their culturally indoctrinated submissiveness (Isaak and Lombard 2002).

Namibia's legislation compensating for gender inequality is regarded as revolutionary and progressive on an international level with particular reference to the Namibian Combating of Rape Act 4 of 2003 and the Domestic Violence Bill. In practice however the male supremacy is culturally deeply rooted to the degree that many Namibian men regard it as their cultural duty to beat their wives as a disciplinary measure, according to Odendaal (Isaak and Lombard 2002). That change is in progress, proven by a survey, during 2006, on 327 university students, where 166 were male and 161 female. Only 30 % males and 22 % females reported negative experiences related to violent behavior in relationship. Increased figures on male subjects may possibly be an indicator of increased assertiveness in females. Further, 77 % males and 83 % females were willing to attend a workshop dealing with abusive behavior in relationships (Haidula et al. 2007).

13.10   Namibia Today in Practice: Change Is a Challenge

Fundamentally change is subordinate to commitment. Within the context of the Namibian liberation struggle, certainly a strong commitment toward change was the foundation. The youth of Namibia (Katjavivi and Shimming-Chase 2012) tends to criticize Namibia's progress yet omit to see the different stages of development which went hand in hand with the decade-long struggle to change the life of Africans in a concrete and above all consistent manner. According to Shimming-Chase (Katjavivi and Shimming-Chase 2012) the only explanation for impatience and critical analysis of the youth is that they have not been part of the struggle and do not understand the patience and endurance going with it. The contemporary problems which Namibia's youth faces pertaining to unemployment, corruption, and poverty are another developmental stage in the holistic picture.

Impatient demands toward the government to resolve these problems are supported by numerous newspaper reports. Similar reports to the latest articles are surfacing regularly causing debates. For example, defending (Kotsebi 2011), and condemning (Absalom 2011), women offering their babies for sale as a result of poverty instead of giving them up for adoption. The link between poverty and crime is heavily criticized. One of the latest reports voices heavy disapproved of Namibia's distribution in wealth (Heita 2011), claiming that an economic worth of N$82 billions is distributed at large among 22 % of the population with 700,000 households being unable to meet their livelihood. Economic and political commentator Uhuru Dempers counters that this is due to a poor education system which should serve as equalizer. In support, Gonzo and Plattner (2003) has found that

38 % of unemployed population have attained 10th grade and 17 % even 12th grade (the highest secondary school grade). At a minimum, these individuals should have school education and received some job training, for example, mechanic, electrician, and gardener. Not being able to find work decreases self-esteem, nurtures help-lessness, induces stress, and depression (Gonzo and Plattner 2003). In opposition to unemployed, some of the employed population resorts to greed. Reports on corruption, for example, one former government employee accused of having embezzled N$2.8 million, is no isolated case (Menges 2011), and it is questioned whether Namibia is breeding "fat cats" in their economic elite society. One explana-tion could be that a new elite is emerging (Fumanti 2002), similar to the bourgeois classes of Europe. In African traditions, in this particular case, the Kavango's of the northern regions of Namibia, a man's prestige is measured in accordance with his ability to accumulate wealth, which was mostly measured in terms of cattle. Based upon the traditional, redistributive community-oriented culture, this not only determines the degree of power in the community but also sets the parameter for expectations from the community. In contemporary times however, cattle are exchanged for cash and Western commodities have achieved local value exceeding the basic needs of food and shelter by far. The predicament is a typical elite dilemma, as often extended family members rely on this one source of income and are dis-appointed when the man cannot deliver.

The newly developing challenge for Namibia's next 100 years of existence will be to grow and resolve arising problems (Katjavivi and Shimming-Chase 2012). The very traditional African way to deal with conflict is to allow the elder to guide the younger to attain a newly formulated goal to iron out economic inequality within the society. An unwelcome companion of poverty is criminality which Namibia needs to control, especially among youths. A particular newspaper report titled "Gangsterism on the rise" stands currently out. Members are mostly younger than 18 years of age and dropped out of school. Considering their tender age, they show admirable skill in terms of their operation modus and respecting each other's turf (Ekongo 2012). There is no lack of energy for Namibia's youth to fight for their livelihood, even if not in the most constructive manner for their social environment. In this particular case, according to Wilfried Immanuel, the Director of the Kuisebmond Community Against Crime (KCAC) has identified the expertise of the youngsters. To change in terms of betterment, a rehabilitation program is planned. The aim is to utilize this knowledge, by involving the juvenile gangsters in the solution of crime. Possibly programs like this can overcome the lack of education, particularly in the occupational niche of crime investigators. The unemployment rate, among youths between 15 and 19 years of age, has been a concern since 1997 (Mufune 2002). Rural areas accounted for 72 % and urban areas 57 % of youth crime, opposed to 30 % non-youths. Only 1 % of the unemployed have post-secondary education. Scarcity in terms of job availability forces people to seek alternative income in the form of crime, often petty crime such as stealing and hustling or street work. All of these activities are illegal. Education plays a significant role as it has been found that 48 % of street workers are school drop outs, of which 88 % failed to go beyond grade 7 and 52 % dropped out at the second grade, making them functionally illiterate.

Who better to solve crime than one who has firsthand experience from such a young age? Only time will prove success.

Very typical to the pathway of the liberation struggle, once again Namibian's find themselves on the road of trial and error, adjusting to situations and circumstances, disagreeing about how to deal with each and every challenge, yet not losing sight of the goal and applying a great deal of flexibility in counteracting problems on hand.

13.11 Post-independent Well-Being of Namibians

Very little research has been done particularly within the parameters of positive psychology. No research could be found in particular to psychological well-being during the apartheid and pre-apartheid years. It is however not difficult to understand that psychological well-being must have been impaired based on the evident hardships of the formerly oppressed Namibian society. Supporting documentation in the form of petitions as well as case histories clearly indicates many negative emotions pertaining to satisfaction with life. Subjective well-being is a term originated within the positive psychology paradigm indicating individual's well-being as a matter of degree in terms of self-assessment of their overall life domains (Diener et al. 2008). Subjective well-being is not a constant state although it remains relatively stable over time and is used to assess general happiness (Diener and Ryan 2009). Even though Namibia is a postwar society, it is questionable whether this is in fact a pathological state.

Investigation, within recent years into the well-being of Namibians, revealed the following results: social workers show surprisingly average scores in well-being, despite daily surviving efforts in a postwar society with related trauma issues: poverty, HIV/AIDS, orphans, disabled population, and violence-related cases. Compared to many other countries, social workers of Namibia are exposed to the full scope and do not only operate in one particular niche for some time (Perstling and Rothmann 2012). It has been found that students as well as public service employees of Namibia, deriving from a sample population of 147 university students and 116 social workers, do experience equal levels of life satisfaction. This implies that the majority of Namibians experience an average level of life satisfaction (Diener 2006). However, improvement in some domains is desired with the aim to move to higher levels through some life changes.

Studies from South Africa have found that the quality of life is related to living standard, having an inverse relationship with the fear of crime (Davids and Gaibie 2011). Given that within Namibia, newspaper reports indicate that crime and poverty are related, more specific studies would be needed to study how crime influences well-being on various living standard levels, including the unemployed population. Data collectors have been instructed to record their participant's reactions to the Positive Nations Questionnaire in an unstructured interview. The unemployed population reacted similar to the Positive Nations Questionnaire in the following manners: It was recorded that the unemployed population, who were exposed to the Positive

Nations Questionnaires, in general responded with ease. Of the 81 documented cases, noncompliance was mostly traced back to poor understanding of questions and impatience of the respondents as a result. Only isolated cases shared grievances. Most participants welcomed the data collectors and shared some personal information. Prominently, the difficulty of finding employment and their method of survival was shared. Many tried to work as street vendors or handyman to survive. In general, apart from economic distress, the data collectors perceived the respondents relatively content with their lives. Isolated cases indicated that there are no grudges against the previous oppressors and that they look forward to opportunity.

Signs of reconciliation can be seen in the Museums of Namibia housing numerous artifacts throughout the history on Namibia from all cultures. Effort is made to promote Namibia's heritage and not lose historical value as a result of political change. One of the many visible signs of reconciliation on national level is the Olukonda National Monument (Museums and Libraries in Windhoek 2012), in the northern region of Namibia. Olukonda was a finish mission station during the German colonial time and has been declared as a National Monument in 1992. The Nakambele Museum, on the premises of the National Monument, is a symbol of the Church missions and local cultures of the region, showing consideration for both cultures in the past and present.

References

Absalom, J. (2011, December 16). Ministry condemns selling of children. *Economist*, 21.

Anderson, C. (2008). International conscience, the cold war and apartheid: The NAACP's alliance with the Reverend Michael Scott for South West Africa's liberation, 1946–1851. *Journal of World History, 19*(3), 297–325.

Anon. (1978). Hitting SWAPO where it lives to win its way to South West Africa, Pretoria gambles. *Times*, 111, 20. Retrieved on July, 7, 2011, from Academic Search Premier Database.

Breyer, K. (1979). *Moskaus Faust in Afrika*. Stuttgart: Seewald Verlag.

Brown, R. (1992). *Economic revolutions in Britain 1750–1850*. London: Cambridge University Press.

Clough, S. B., & Cole, C. W. (1966). *Economic history of Europe* (3rd ed.). Boston: Heath & Co.

Davids, Y. D., & Gaibie, F. (2011). Quality of life in post-apartheid South Africa. *Politikon, 38*(2), 231–256.

Diener, E. (2006). *Understanding scores on the satisfaction with life*. Copyright Ed Diener, 13th February 2006. Retrieved on December 23, 2010, from the World Wide Web: http://internal. psychology.illinois.edu/~ediener/SWLS.html

Diener, E., & Ryan, K. (2009). Subjective well-being: A general overview. *South African Journal of Psychology, 39*, 391–406.

Diener, E., Kesebir, P., & Lucas, R. (2008). Benefits of accounts of well-being: For societies and for psychological science. *Applied Psychology: An International Journal, 57*, 37–53.

Dobell, L. (1997). Silence in context: Truth and/or reconciliation in Namibia. *Journal of Southern African Studies, 23*(2), 371–387.

Edwards, L. (2006). HIV/AIDS and gender in Africa: Confronting our sexuality and inequalities. In B. F. Bankie & K. Mchombu (Eds.), *Pan-Africanism: Strengthening the unity of Africa and its diaspora* (pp. 105–118). Windhoek: University of Namibia.

Ekongo, J. (2012, January 10). Gangsterism on the rise. *New Era*, 1–2.

Engombe, L. (2004). *Kind Nr.95*. Berlin: Ullstein Buchverlag GmbH.

Fumanti, M. (2002). Small town élites in northern Namibia: The complexity of class formation in practice. In V. Winterfeldt, T. Fox, & P. Mufune (Eds.), *Namibia society sociology* (pp. 169–177). Windhoek: University of Namibia.

Gonzo, W., & Plattner, I. E. (2003). *Unemployment in an African country: A psychological perspective*. Windhoek: University of Namibia Press.

Goosen, D., van Wietersheim, E., Katzao, J. J., Mbumba, N., O'Callaghan, B., Patemann, H., van Staden, E. I., & Tait, D. H. A. (2007). *Understanding history in context*. Windhoek: Longman Namibia (Pty) Ltd.

Haidula, L., Perstling, M., Riekert, C. A., Naweya, M., Manuel, T. L., Sibanda, T., Langfellner, J., Theron, S., & Hamibili, H. I. (2007). Student perceptions of abusive behaviours in male–female relationships. *New Voices in Psychology, 3*(2), 92–102.

Heita, D. (2011, October 14). Poverty in a sea of riches. *New Era*, 1–2.

Hishongwa, N. (1992). *The contract labor system and its effects on family and social life in Namibia. A historical perspective*. Windhoek: Gamsberg Macmillan.

Horsthemke, O. (2004). Land reform in Namibia: Opportunity or opportunism. In J. Hunter (Ed.), *Who should own the land?* Windhoek: Konrad Adenauer Stiftung, Namibia Institute for Democracy.

Hoyle, R. (1981, September 14). Marching to Pretoria's beat. *Time*, 0040781X, *118*(11).

Hunter, J. (2004). *Who should own the land?* Windhoek: Konrad Adenauer Stiftung/Namibia Institute for Democracy.

Hitting SWAPO where it lives to win its way in South West Africa. (1978, May 5). *Times 0040781X, 111*(20).

Irwin, R. M. (2010). Apartheid on trial: South West Africa and the International Court of Justice 1960–66. *The International History Review, 32*(4), 619–642.

Isaak, P., & Lombard, C. (2002). Religion and its impact on Namibian Society. In V. Winterfeldt, T. Fox, & P. Mufune (Eds.), *Namibia society sociology* (pp. 87–123). Windhoek: University of Namibia.

Katjavivi, P., & Shimming-Chase, E. (2012, January 9). *In honour of ANC's 100th birthday*. Discussion forum on the Namibian Broadcasting Channel.

Klein, G. L. (2011). Publicising the African National Congress: The anti-apartheid news. *South African Historical Journal, 63*(3), 394–413.

Kotsebi, L. (2011, December 16). Women not the only ones at fault. *Economist*, 5.

Krog, A. (2008). This thing called reconciliation: Forgiveness as part of an interconnectedness-towards-wholeness. *South African Journal of Philosophy, 27*(4), 353–366.

Kros, C. (2010). Public history/heritage: Translation, transgression or more of the same? *African Studies, 69*, 63–77.

Lauren, H., & Swartz, S. (2011). The professionalization of psychology within the apartheid state 1948–1978. *History of Psychology, 14*(3), 249–263.

LeBeau, D. (2005). *An investigation into the lives of Namibian ex-fighters, fifteen years after independence*. Windhoek: PEACE Centre.

Linder, D. O. (2010). *The Nelson Mandela (Rivonia) Trial: An account*. Retrieved on January, 25, 2012, from the World Wide Web: www.law2.umkc.edu/faculty/projects/ftrials/mandela/mandelaaccount.html

Linley, P. A., Joseph, S., & Seligman, M. E. P. (2004). *Positive psychology in practice*. Hoboken: Wiley.

Lu, Y., & Treiman, D. J. (2011). Migration, remittances and educational stratification among blacks in apartheid and post-apartheid South Africa. *Social Forces, 88*(4), 1119–1144.

May, T. (1987). *An economic and social history of Britain 1760–1970*. London: Longman Group.

Menges, W. (2011, October 14). Shalli's bank account frozen. *The Namibian*, 1–2.

Meyer, W. F., Moore, C., & Viljoen, H. G. (1997). *Personology: From individual to ecosystem*. Sandton/Johannesburg: Heinemann.

Mlambo, A. (2011). *Discover history*. Sandton: Heinemann.

Mufune, P. (2002). Youth in Namibia: Social exclusion and poverty. In V. Winterfeldt, T. Fox, & P. Mufune (Eds.), *Namibia society sociology* (pp. 179–195). Windhoek: University of Namibia.

Murithi, T. (2009). An African perspective on peace education: Ubuntu lessons in reconciliation. *International Review of Education, 55*, 221–233.

Museums and Libraries in Windhoek. (2012). *Olukonda National Monument.* Retrieved on April 4, 2012, from the World Wide Web: www.namibweb.com/olukonda/html

National Planning Commission. (2001). *Namibia 2001 population and housing census.* Retrieved on January 13, 2012, from the World Wide Web: www.npc.gov.na/census/index/html

Nortje, P. (2003). *32 Battalion: The inside story of South Africa's elite fighting unit.* Cape Town: Zebra Press.

O'Callaghan, B. (2011). *Understanding history: The world and Africa.* Windhoek: Longman Namibia (Pty) Ltd.

Parsons, T. (1977). *The evolution of societies.* Englewood Cliffs: Prentice Hall.

Perstling, M., & Rothmann, S. (2012). Well-being and secondary traumatic stress of social workers in Namibia. *Journal of Psychology in Africa, 22*, 1–9.

Pucherova, D. (2011). A romance that failed: Bessie Head and black nationalism in 1960s South Africa. *Research in African Literature, 42*(2), 105–124.

Riggs, D. S., & Foa, E. B. (2004). Posttraumatic stress disorder. In C. D. Spielberger (Ed.), *Encyclopaedia of applied psychology* (Vol. 2, pp. 83–90). Maryland Heights: Academic Press/ Elsevier.

Riruako, H. (2006). Which way Africa: A multifaceted/dimensional discourse shaped by paradoxes that characterize both Africans and Africans in the diaspora. In B. F. Bankie & K. Mchombu (Eds.), *Pan-Africanism: Strengthening the unity of Africa and its diaspora* (pp. 27–30). Windhoek: University of Namibia.

Saunders, C. (2002). Namibia's freedom struggle: The Nujoma version. *South African Historical Journal, 47*(1), 203–212.

Seely, M., & Zeidler, J. (2002). Land distribution and sustainable development. In V. Winterfeldt, T. Fox, & P. Mufune (Eds.), *Namibia society sociology* (pp. 75–84). Windhoek: University of Namibia.

Stiff, P. (2000). *Cry Zimbabwe: Independence, twenty years on.* Alberton: Galago Publishing.

United Nations Institute for Namibia. (1988). *Namibia: Perspectives for national reconstruction and development.* Lusaka: United Nations Institute for Namibia.

Van der Watt, L. (2009). *The comradely ideal and the Volksmoeder ideal: Uncovering gender ideology in the Voortrekker tapestry.* Retrieved January 5, 2012, from the World Wide Web: http://www.tandfonline.com/loi/rshj20

Van Zyl, S. (1999). An interview with Gillian Straker on the Truth and Reconciliation Commission in South Africa. *Psychoanalytic Dialogue, 9*(2), 245–274.

Vedder, H. (1985). *Das alte Südwestafrika – Südwestafrikas Geschichte bis zi, Tode Mahareros 1890.* Berlin: Martin Warneck Verlag.

Werner, W. (2002). *The current state of land reform in Namibia – Some facts and figures.* Unpublished master's dissertation, University of Namibia, Windhoek.

Winterfeldt, V. (2002). Labor migration in Namibia – Gender aspects. In V. Winterfeldt, T. Fox, & P. Mufune (Eds.), *Namibia sociology* (pp. 39–74). Windhoek: University of Namibia.

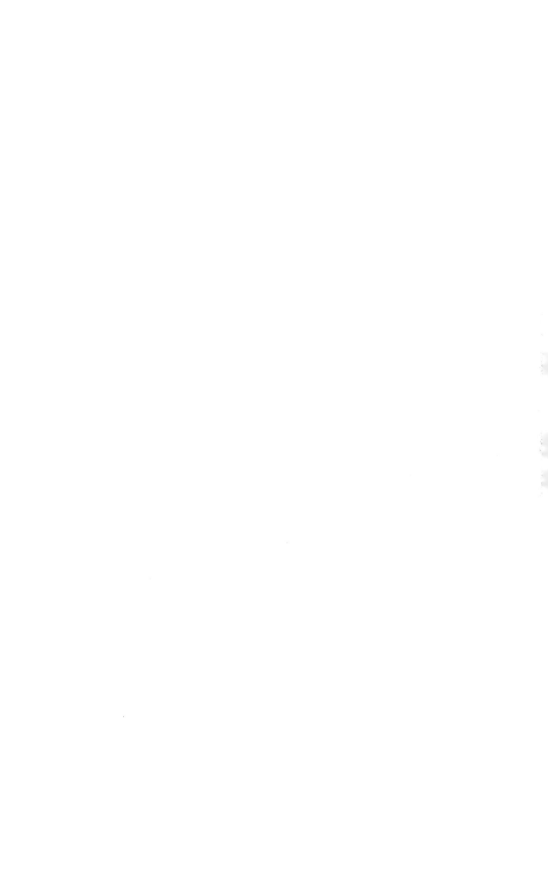

Printed by Publishers' Graphics LLC